PRIMUM
NON NOCERE

THE ULTIMATE GUIDEBOOK TO MEDICAL SCHOOL ADMISSIONS

FROM A 2.96 GPA TO YALE SCHOOL OF MEDICINE
CAROLINE ECHEANDIA-FRANCIS

TABLE OF CONTENTS

INTRODUCTION 7
PREMED VOCAB 11
THE MEDICAL SCHOOL "IT" LIST. 13

01. MAKING THE MOST OF YOUR UNDERGRADUATE EXPERIENCE 16
    ATTENDING A TOP 20 UNDERGRADUATE SCHOOL
    VERSUS ALL OTHER SCHOOLS 17
    ATTENDING A RESEARCH UNIVERSITY VERSUS A
    LIBERAL ARTS COLLEGE. 21
    FINANCIALLY PREPARING FOR YOUR FUTURE 23

02. GRANNY'S ADVICE FOR ALL PREMEDS 28
    CRAFTING YOUR NARRATIVE. 29
    BUILDING STRONG FRIENDSHIPS AND AVOIDING TOXICITY 33
    DATING AND SOCIAL LIFE 35
    PREMED ADVISORS AND APPLICATION CONSULTANTS 38

03. ACADEMICS 41
    TESTING ANXIETY. 42
    ACADEMIC ACCOMMODATIONS 42
    TO WHAT EXTENT DOES GPA MATTER.. 42
    DOMINATING SCIENCE CLASSES 47
    ACING NON-SCIENCE CLASSES 53
    CHOOSING A MAJOR. 53
    RECOVERING FROM A GPA BLUNDER 54
    POST-BACCALAUREATE PROGRAMS VERSUS EXTRA CLASSES. . . . 56

04. ACTIVITIES AND HONORS 58
    RESEARCH 59
    CLINICAL EXPERIENCES.. 77
    RESEARCH, CLINICAL, AND PUBLIC HEALTH FELLOWSHIPS.. 82
    SHADOWING.. 93
    VARSITY SPORTS 94
    GREEK LIFE.. 95
    LEADERSHIP 97
    HONORS AND AWARDS.. 105

05. RESUME OF FAILURES — 118

06. PLANNING YOUR SUMMERS — 124
- FRESHMAN SUMMER 125
- SOPHOMORE SUMMER 128
- JUNIOR SUMMER 130
- SENIOR SUMMER 132
- GAP YEAR(S) 132

07. LETTERS OF RECOMMENDATION — 135
- HOW IMPORTANT ARE THEY? 136
- WHO TO ASK 137
- HOW TO ASK 143
- POLITE FOLLOW-UP FOR YOUR LETTER WRITERS 146

08. MCAT — 149
- TESTING ANXIETY 150
- MCAT ACCOMMODATIONS 150
- CHOOSING WHEN TO TAKE THE EXAM 159
- HOW TO STUDY 162
- POST-MCAT BLUES 190
- MCAT RETAKES 192

09. TO GAP YEAR OR NOT TO GAP YEAR — 199
- GAP YEAR: THE PROS AND THE CONS 200
- HOW MANY GAPS 202
- WHAT TO DO DURING YOUR GAP YEAR 206

10. MAKING YOUR SCHOOL LIST — 208
- HOW DO GPA AND MCAT AFFECT YOUR SCHOOL LIST? ... 209
- STATE SCHOOLS VERSUS PRIVATE SCHOOLS 210
- INTERNATIONAL APPLICANTS 212
- URM AND ORM APPLICANTS 216
- SAFETY SCHOOLS? FACT OR MYTH 218
- HOW MANY SCHOOLS? 221
- WHICH SCHOOLS? 222

11. EARLY DECISION — 226

12. ESSAYS — 230
- HOW IMPORTANT ARE MY ESSAYS? — 231
- WHEN TO WRITE — 232
- HOW TO WRITE — 246

13. CASPER — 249
- HOW IMPORTANT IS CASPER? — 251
- HOW TO PREPARE — 253

14. INTERVIEWS — 255
- HOW IMPORTANT ARE INTERVIEWS? — 256
- WHAT TO EXPECT FROM INTERVIEW DAY — 259
- HOW TO PREPARE FOR ONE-ON-ONES — 260
- HOW TO PREPARE FOR THE MMI — 263
- ANSWERING THE MOST COMMON AND IMPORTANT QUESTIONS — 265
- PRESENTING YOURSELF: VIRTUAL AND IN-PERSON — 274
- NAVIGATING VIRTUAL INTERVIEW BLUNDERS — 277
- WHAT TO DO IF AN INTERVIEW BOMBS — 278
- THANK YOU NOTES — 285
- LETTERS OF INTEREST AND LETTERS OF INTENT — 286

15. POST-INTERVIEW BLUES — 292
- COPING WITH THE BLUES — 293
- SENDING UPDATES — 294

16. PAYING FOR MEDICAL SCHOOL — 300
- SCHOLARSHIPS — 301
- FINANCIAL AID — 305

17. REAPPLYING — 306
- WHAT WENT WRONG? — 307
- APPLICATION REHAB — 308

18. RESULTS — 311
- ACCEPTANCES — 312
- WAITLISTS — 317
- REJECTIONS — 319

19. DECIDING WHERE TO MATRICULATE   321
     GETTING TO KNOW YOUR MEDICAL SCHOOL OPTIONS............ 330
     NEGOTIATING SCHOLARSHIPS................................. 333
     SECOND LOOK 334
     SELECTING YOUR SCHOOL AND WITHDRAWALS 335

ACKNOWLEDGEMENTS 337

APPENDICES.. 339
     APPENDIX A
     2014-2018 Aggregate Medical School
     Matriculant Statistics for WashU Undergraduates................... 340
     APPENDIX B
     List of Academic Term and Post-Baccalaureate
     Research and Clinical Fellowships 344
     APPENDIX C
     List of Summer Research and Clinical Fellowships................. 345
     APPENDIX D
     Out-of-State Applicant vs. In-State Applicant
     Friendliness Table (Accepted, 2022).............................. 375

ABOUT THE AUTHOR 383

INTRODUCTION

Hello everyone! My name is Caroline, and I began my first year at Yale School of Medicine in Summer 2021. After a successful medical school application cycle, I wrote this guidebook to use the knowledge I've gathered to assist other premed students.

As an undergraduate at Washington University in St. Louis (WashU), ***I recovered from a 2.96 freshman science GPA and ended up earning nineteen medical school interview invites – ten of which were to the top 20 research medical schools*** (*U.S. News & World Report*) during the 2020-2021 application cycle. This guidebook is for premeds anywhere along their path to medicine, but reading it sooner rather than later can hopefully help you avoid some of the many pitfalls that I found myself floundering in as a student. It covers everything from recovering from a prolonged GPA blunder, receiving stellar recommendation letters, and finding your "it factor," to writing winning application essays, plus much more (see Table of Contents).

To introduce myself and my background: I am the daughter of Mark Robertson Francis and Lauren Echeandia-Francis. My dad works in the technology side of healthcare, while my mom is the founder and president of a staffing agency. I am a sister to Claire, a University of Oregon graduate with a major in sociology. I am also a cat and dog mama to Hazel, Holly, and Max. While my sister and I were born in the San Francisco Bay Area, our family moved frequently during our childhood, living in Jacksonville, Florida, and Cincinnati, Ohio. In 2008, my family settled in Portland, Oregon. From an early age, despite limited exposure to the field, I somehow knew that I wanted to become a physician. There was a brief moment after watching *Legally Blonde* for the first time that I longed to become a lawyer clad in pink, but I quickly snapped back to dreams of a medical career.

WashU was my home for four years of undergraduate education. I chose the school because of its top-notch premedical curriculum, stunning campus, and kind, collaborative community. Although my time at WashU was incredibly dear to me, I can't deny the significant challenges that I faced, especially during the underclassman years. Difficult science classes that I was unprepared for, an ill-formed study strategy, and poor personal priorities were all obstacles I grappled with. But, despite this, WashU education taught me a crucially valuable lesson: *the power of dedication and hard work.*

My freshman and sophomore years were academically very difficult for me. Following two years of blaming my subpar academic performance on externalities, I decided to devote myself to my education fully and strive to get into the best medical school possible. If you had told me at the end of my sophomore year that I would attend Yale School of Medicine, I simply would not have believed you. Back then, I did not fit the mold of a competitive, top-tier medical school applicant, which was made clear by one of WashU's best premedical advisors when I met with her two years into college.

There was something about feeling as though I had nothing to lose at the end of sophomore year that finally pushed me to take my education into my own hands. I began to devote myself to my schoolwork, eliminate distractions, and pursue nearly every opportunity available - even those I considered to be out of reach (e.g., leadership positions, research fellowships, volunteer work, scholarships). Instead of looking at my circumstances and whining and moaning about the unfairness of it all (some of my favorite past excuses: my high school education didn't prepare me for college; scholarships and fellowships are rigged; I am not competitive enough for leadership positions), **I began to look in the mirror and ask myself what I could have done to change an outcome. It was this shift in mindset that transformed me.**

This transition molded me into the type of person I used to look at and wonder, *"how?"* How did they get into that school? How did they earn that fellowship? I learned that the answers to such "how" questions lie in realizing and embracing responsibility for your life. While this may sound harsh, knowing that you are in control of your outcomes is truly a relief. This autonomy is a tremendous privilege that is given especially to those who grow up in the United States. Personal responsibility and individual choice can transform who you are and where you are headed. No two people will ever have equal opportunity from the start. Some face significant hurdles that their peers do not. Rather than hyper-focusing on such disparities, imagine if we focused on leveraging every available opportunity.

How would we change? How would the people around us change? Where would we end up?

Among my peers at Yale School of Medicine, we all came from very different places. One of my classmates grew up in poverty, not knowing if he would eat on a given day. Some attended lesser known state schools. Others attended the best universities in the world. Though most are from the United States, three of my new friends are from Mexico, Ghana, and Ukraine. Our diverse paths converged in New Haven, Connecticut, working side-by-side as newly minted medical students. What choices will you make? Where will you go? I urge you to dare to answer these questions.

My objective of the guidebook is to allow you to learn from both my gaffes and achievements, enabling you to become a highly competitive and sought-after medical school applicant. The guidebook follows a chronological structure, beginning with the undergraduate years, progressing through the medical school application process, and ending in the selection of a medical school. I wrote the guidebook with all students in mind who aspire to attend medical school in the United States. Yet, there is also an emphasis on – and specific guidelines – for those who aim to attend a top 20 allopathic medical school. No matter your aspirations, I have no doubt that the following pages can bolster your chances of acceptance into any medical program – both allopathic and osteopathic.

My hope is, through reading this guidebook, that you find comfort in seeing that even a highly successful applicant makes many notable missteps along this long, demanding expedition. You and I will move arm-in-arm as we wade through the process of fashioning the stellar medical school applicant that you are certainly capable of becoming. I will be your mentor and cheerleader each step of the way, and by the end of our time together, perhaps a new friend – too sappy? Too flowery? Too bad. Let's get cracking!

DISCLAIMERS

This guidebook touches upon Caribbean medical schools. I fully acknowledge that many skilled and competent physicians have graduated from Caribbean medical schools and have gone on to become tremendous physicians who have serve thousands of patients in their communities. Such contributions are invaluable and deserve immense recognition. However, it is important to acknowledge that Caribbean medical schools are often not the first choice among applicants. Many of these programs have been known to have high attrition rates (Ideal Medical Care; *Forbes*). Students often lack time to sufficiently prepare for the USLME Step exams and their graduates often face more difficulty matching into U.S. residency programs (Ideal Medical Care; *Forbes*). Thus, Caribbean medical schools are the butt of some of my jokes and are used to exemplify less-than-optimal outcomes for applicants. You have been warned.

You will also notice that real people are referenced or used as examples throughout the guidebook. The names and personal details of these individuals have been changed to protect their privacy. However, the names of my recommendation letter writers have not been changed, as they are publicly known professors, researchers, and professionals.

Okay, now let's get after it!

PREMED VOCAB

Most of you will be familiar with at least some of these terms that are common in the premed and medical school worlds. I will use these terms throughout the book out of pure convenience, so here is a list of terminology in case any of this vocabulary is unfamiliar.

AAMC: The Association of American Medical Colleges

AMCAS: The American Medical College Application Service

cGPA: cumulative GPA

sGPA: science GPA

BCPM: biology, chemistry, physics, mathematics (GPA)

AO: all other (GPA)

URM: underrepresented in medicine – according to the AAMC, URMs include blacks, Mexican Americans, Native Americans (American Indians, Alaskan Natives, and Native Hawaiians), and mainland Puerto Ricans

ORM: overrepresented in medicine – all those racial and ethnic groups not defined as URM (AAMC)

IS: in-state

OOS: out-of-state

IMG: international medical graduate (students graduating from a medical school outside of the United States)

MCAT: medical college admission test

MCAT sections:

    C/P = chemical and physical foundations of biological systems

    CARS = critical analysis and reasoning skills

    B/B = biological and biochemical foundations of living systems

    P/S = psychological, social, and biological foundations of behavior

High-yield information: information that is very likely to show up on an exam

Low-yield information: information that is unlikely to show up on an exam but is still fair game to show up on test day (low-yield questions are often used to create bell curve distributions for standardized exams in which those knowing the most low-yield information score within the right tail of the distribution)

USMLE Step 1: the first part of the United States Medical Licensing Exam, typically taken during the second or third year of medical school

USMLE Step 2: the second part of the United States Medical Licensing Exam, typically taken during the third or fourth year of medical school

PI: principal investigator (head of a lab)

Impact factor: a measure of the frequency with which the average article in a journal has been cited in a particular year. It is used to measure the importance or rank of a journal by calculating the times its articles are cited (University of Illinois Chicago)

EMT: emergency medical technician

CNA: certified nursing assistant

Traditional applicant: an applicant taking a maximum of two gap years between college graduation and medical school matriculation

Non-traditional applicant: applicant taking three or more years between college graduation and medical school matriculation

Yield protection: the act of schools turning away top-tier applicants with the expectation that these individuals will not enroll in their program. These top applicants are not invited for interviews to protect their matriculation yield (the number of people who commit to enroll compared to the number of people offered an acceptance). Yield protection works to protect a school's ranking and keeps them from wasting their resources (the most notable being the number of interview spots) on people who will not attend their university. Mid-ranked and well-known schools such as Tufts, Tulane, and Boston University are well-known yield-protectors. Everyone from low-stat to high-stat applicants apply to these schools, forcing them to focus on the best students who, they believe, will matriculate to their program. Yield protection is fondly referred to as Tufts Syndrome (The Admissions Strategist)

THE MEDICAL SCHOOL "IT" LIST

This guidebook is chockablock full of information designed to shape you into a sought-after, capable, and confident medical school applicant. While reading through each section will provide crucial insights for navigating your undergraduate and post-baccalaureate years and then through the application process, I wanted to start by condensing the guidebook's key takeaways into a medical school "it" list. ***The medical school "it" list underscores the top items on your to-do list when striving to become a first-rate medical school applicant.***

You don't need to tick off every item on this list to earn a medical school acceptance. Heck, not all need to be hit to earn a top 20 medical school acceptance. However, the more achievements you can add to your resume, the more robust your application will be. While the "it" list may seem initially daunting, know that none of these "it" list items were a slam dunk for me. It took years to bolster my candidacy to a level where I became a successful medical school applicant. My journey was fraught with numerous trials and tribulations - all of which I am eager to share with you in the upcoming pages. Together, we'll work to make the "it" list a reality for you.

<u>**Let's start by seeing what I consider the medical school "it" list -**</u>

- **Plan your application timeline early**
    - Figure out if you are taking zero, one, two, or three+ gap years early on to ensure that you are building your application in a timely manner
- **Develop a compelling personal narrative that will anchor your application**
- **Invest your time in volunteer work and research or community projects that deepen and develop your personal narrative**

- **Showcase your research and/or community projects through publications and conference presentations**
- **Pursue leadership**
  - Serving as a Teaching Assistant demonstrates that you give back to other students, are trusted by professors, and have mastery over an academic concept
  - Working as a Resident Advisor or Peer Counselor shows that you, again, give back to other students and are trusted by the school administration
  - Club, sport, community service, and all other leadership are also excellent
- **Apply for fellowships, scholarships, and honors when appropriate - medical schools go gaga for these**
- **Build meaningful relationships with mentors and professors to prime the pump for outstanding letters of recommendation**
- **Earn a 3.5+ sGPA**
- **Smash the MCAT**
  - For top 20 schools, aim to score in the top 5%
  - For all other schools, aim to score in the top 20%
- **Maintain an upward GPA trend**
- **Don't sacrifice academic performance or meaningful extracurricular involvement for demanding relationships or friendships, athletics, Greek life, etc.**
- **Spend time writing engaging, thought-provoking application essays**
- **Practice and practice for your interviews**

MEDICAL SCHOOL "IT" LIST

- [ ] Plan your application timeline early
- [ ] Develop a compelling personal narrative
- [ ] Invest your time in volunteer, research, or community projects
- [ ] Showcase your work through publications and presentations
- [ ] Pursue leadership
- [ ] Apply for fellowships, scholarships, and honors
- [ ] Build meaningful relationships with mentors and professors
- [ ] Earn a 3.5+ sGPA
- [ ] Smash the MCAT
- [ ] Maintain an upward GPA trend
- [ ] Don't sacrifice academic performance or extracurricular involvement
- [ ] Write engaging, thought-provoking application essays
- [ ] Practice and practice for your interviews

CHAPTER

01

MAKING THE MOST OF YOUR UNDERGRADUATE EXPERIENCE

ATTENDING A TOP 20 UNDERGRADUATE SCHOOL VERSUS ALL OTHER SCHOOLS

If you look at the entering classes of most top 20 research medical schools, you will notice that many of the incoming students attended a top 20 undergraduate institution. This observation naturally raises several questions: How influential is a top university's reputation in medical school applications? How good of a shot do I have at getting into a medical school, including top medical schools, if I did not attend a top college? Let's discuss these questions.

Q: How influential is a top university's reputation in medical school applications?

A: Being a student at a top 20 college certainly offers an edge in the medical school admissions process. Yet, this advantage has much more to do with the unique opportunities that your university will afford you rather than the prestige of its name alone. Take my undergraduate institution, Washington University in St. Louis (WashU), for example – tied at #16 in *U.S. News and World Report's* "2021 Best National University Rankings." Both WashU and Johns Hopkins are recognized by medical school admissions officers for having the most rigorous premedical curriculums among U.S. colleges. Furthermore, these two universities are highly respected for their academic standards. Given this, how do WashU premed applicants fare in the admissions cycle, having both a stellar curriculum and name as their backdrop?

While numerous WashU alums I know are current students at the best medical schools in the country – Harvard, Mount Sinai, Yale, UCSD, UCLA (David Geffen), NYU (Grossman), Stanford, Columbia (Vagelos), Washington University, University of Pennsylvania (Perelman), University of Washington, University of Michigan, Vanderbilt, Northwestern (Feinberg), and Baylor – there are also those who had to reapply after not receiving a single interview offer, as well as those currently pursuing an M.D. students in Caribbean medical schools. How can there be such disparity in outcomes among equally motivated, intelligent students who attended the same undergraduate institution?

For my peers attending the highest-ranked medical schools, I have no doubt that WashU's reputation gave their applications a boost. However, be careful not to overestimate the impact of the name alone – it is a marginal bonus. My peers attending medical school at Harvard, Stanford, Baylor, etc., earned their seats by taking advantage of the abundant opportunities WashU offered. As our former chancellor, Mark Wrighton, stated at the Class of 2019's convocation ceremony: **"Take advantage of your advantages."** And this is precisely what my peers, who were admitted to the top medical schools, did. From working in leading research laboratories that pump out publications to earning one of WashU's distinguished undergraduate fellowships, the resumes that my peers built for themselves as college students were outstanding. In the upcoming chapters, we will go into comprehensive detail on how to build this bangin' resume.

Among my peers who either ended up at Caribbean medical schools or had to reapply to medical schools, the WashU name was not enough to guarantee them an interview at any of the U.S. M.D. and D.O. schools to which they applied – not even close. You may be wondering if they only applied to a few of the most competitive medical schools. They did not. Many of these students had extensive, well-balanced lists of institutions but still received no interviews. What could have possibly gone wrong?

Take "Malcom" for example. Malcom graduated from WashU with a 3.9 cGPA and sGPA and earned a 514 on his MCAT. Yet, despite having lab experience and a leadership role in a club, Malcom's involvement as a student was limited. He did not engage in significant volunteer work, fully immerse himself in his undergraduate research projects, or contribute significantly to his school or local communities. Simply put, he failed to take advantage of his advantages. This reflected in his application – Malcom struggled to find enthusiastic letter writers and wrote his essays last minute. Consequently, his application fell flat. It became lost among the thousands of other applications that, too, lacked a standout narrative and meaningful, prolonged extracurricular involvement. Malcom is now sunning his buns in the Caribbean – let's hope he packed sunscreen.

Now, let's look at reapplicant "Nyra." Nyra was an impressively involved student at WashU. She performed with competitive dance teams – one of which placed in national competitions. She headed WashU's largest annual cultural performance, was an executive of a prominent campus organization, and worked in a research laboratory for several years that studied women's reproductive health. Nyra continued her strong narrative of reproductive health immersion by leading first-year students through WashU's sexual assault prevention program and working as a sexual assault and rape hotline counselor. Nyra clearly has a stellar resume. How did she end up as a reapplicant? Nyra's grades slipped during her first year (which is not uncommon and completely rectifiable), and she did not recover her academic performance. Nyra chose a robust social life over academics – naughty girl. She graduated with a 3.5 cGPA and a 3.3 sGPA. Nyra also rushed her MCAT exam without properly studying. Such hastiness earned her a 508 when she was capable of a much better score. Her essays, also done without much care and attention, did not make a compelling case for her admission. As a result, despite her extracurricular excellence, Nyra received no interviews (even to her many in-state options as a New York resident). If only sweet Nyra had put away the buff, hairless frat boys in exchange for study time at the library. Better luck next time, Nyra. . .

Although the evidence laid out here is anecdotal, from my experience applying to medical school and watching dozens of my peers apply, I am confident that the value of a top college is in the rich opportunities afforded to students. A name cannot save your application.

Q: How good of a shot do I have at getting into a medical school, including top medical schools, if I did not attend a top college?
A: You can absolutely gain admission to any medical school, including top medical schools, without attending a top undergraduate institution. Part of the reason why top medical schools are filled with students from top colleges is because of selection bias. Those students who aim for and achieve academic excellence at the undergraduate level are naturally inclined to continue this trajectory. Hence, it's not just about the name of the undergraduate institution but the consistent effort and achievement of the individual.

Students at Yale School of Medicine (YSM) hail from a wide range of undergraduate institutions. In a class of 104, nearly 40 students graduated from schools not considered "top-tier" colleges. My peers attended the University of Oregon, University of Miami, Temple University, University of Central Florida, University of California - Riverside, University of California - Davis, University of Colorado at Denver, Lewis and Clark College, University of Texas at Austin, University of Illinois at Urbana-Champaign, Texas A&M University, Florida State University, Missouri State University, and University of Connecticut.

The key takeaway is clear: gaining admission to prestigious medical schools like YSM doesn't necessarily hinge on attending a top-tier undergraduate institution. More important is being someone who takes advantage of all the opportunities your university offers.

However, it's worth noting that applicants from less traditionally rigorous undergraduate institutions might face different expectations in that they will be given less leeway in their GPAs. For example, among WashU students who matriculated to Duke University School of Medicine from 2014-2018, their average cGPA was 3.75 (range: 3.31-4.00), while Duke's average GPA for matriculants is 3.88. Here is data on several other top schools (Washington University in St. Louis Undergraduate 2014-2018 Aggregate Matriculation Data):

	WashU average matriculant GPA and range	Average matriculant GPA
Columbia (Vagelos)	3.81 (3.21-4.00)	3.90
NYU (Grossman)	3.82 (3.42-4.00)	3.89
University of Michigan	3.68 (2.95-4.00)	3.80
University of Pittsburgh	3.70 (2.59-4.00)	3.78
Cornell (Weill)	3.79 (3.42-4.00)	3.90
Yale	3.68 (3.43-3.96)	3.83

WashU's rigorous premedical curriculum affords students some GPA breathing room, a leniency similarly seen in institutions like Hopkins with demanding premedical college programs.

For students at colleges with less rigorous curricula, a strong GPA becomes more pivotal. To put this idea into numbers, I would try to keep my GPA at 3.8 or above. That said, a 3.7 will likely not blacklist you from top medical schools. However, if your GPA hovers around 3.6 or 3.7, and you're from a less rigorous college, it's vital to focus time and effort on crushing the MCAT. *From what I have seen, many schools seem to gravitate toward the 3.6 GPA and 518 MCAT applicant over the 3.9 GPA and 513 MCAT applicant.* Admissions officers often have more confidence in academic abilities based on MCAT performance (due to it being a standardized exam) because, comparatively, curriculum difficulty, and thus GPA, varies widely from school to school.

ATTENDING A RESEARCH UNIVERSITY VERSUS A LIBERAL ARTS COLLEGE

Examining the incoming classes of top 20 research medical schools, there is a heavy skew toward students who attended large research powerhouse colleges. Why do we see this? Can students attending liberal arts colleges still gain admittance to the top research medical schools, and if so, do they have to prepare differently?

Q: Why do we see top research medical schools packed with students from large research universities?
A: The answer to this question is probably quite self-evident. Similar to why top medical schools are full of students who attended top colleges, there is a selection bias surrounding research-focused undergraduate institutions and medical schools. Students passionate about science and scientific research and who knew they wanted to pursue a medical career when choosing a college are more likely to select a large research powerhouse for their undergraduate education. Liberal arts colleges, while offering outstanding education, typically have a less pronounced research focus and fewer resources in this area. This is where the selection bias comes in – I suspect that this bias largely contributes to why we see the research medical schools' classes skewed toward students who attended research-heavy colleges.

Q: Can liberal arts college students still gain admittance to the top research med schools, and if so, must they prepare differently?
A: Liberal arts students are entirely capable of securing a spot at a top research-oriented medical school. In fact, a liberal arts education may help these applicants stand out among their slew of peers who attended large research institutions for college. However, given that top research medical schools value applicants with research-heavy resumes, there are some <u>strategies that I recommend liberal arts students take in order to increase their chances of admission:</u>

1. **Engage in Meaningful Research:** You do not have to attend a research powerhouse college to partake in gripping research. Find

a faculty member at your school or team up with hospital-based physicians involved in research that interests you. The key is genuine commitment and enthusiasm for the research process.

2. **Utilize Summers for Research Fellowships:** Consider applying for undergraduate research fellowships during your summers at other institutions. The Amgen Scholars Program is one of the most well-known and distinguished among these fellowships. A comprehensive list of summer research fellowships (encompassing basic science, clinical, and public health research) can be found in the section titled *List of Research, Clinical, and Public Health Fellowships*.

3. **Aim for Publications:** While a heavy emphasis is placed on publishing at the undergraduate level, this can often be difficult to do. We will dive into tips for getting published as an undergraduate in the Research section. Research powerhouses are known for pumping out publications, so where does that leave you if you attend a liberal arts college? Great work is being published at liberal arts schools across the country, even if research isn't the college's focal point. Looking at a faculty member's publication record and asking if they include undergraduates on the publications' list of authors can determine which mentors will help you become published.

4. **Don't Underestimate Conferences:** One of the most overlooked ways to help your research stand out is by presenting at conferences. The vast majority of the conferences I attended as a WashU undergraduate weren't university-sponsored but were local, regional, and national symposia to which I independently applied. In my experience, a student with an extensive presentation record with no publications can be easily favored over a published applicant. A common oversight is students getting credited as contributing authors but not sharing their team's findings with the broader scientific community. Demonstrating that you have actively participated in research conferences is a foolproof way to show that you are excited about your research, committed to your project, and knowledgeable in your field.

To add, conferences often have funding available to help students pay for lodging and travel to and from the symposium. Colleges will also sometimes set funds aside to cover these expenses for students attending symposia. As a liberal arts student, presenting a poster or giving a talk at conferences can be your secret weapon into the ice-cold hearts of admissions officers who guard the gates of top research med schools. Just kidding, my sweet honeys! Love ya!

FINANCIALLY PREPARING FOR YOUR FUTURE

Brace yourself. Here comes the debt!

It's no secret that the path to medicine is inordinately expensive. As of 2019, the average student loan debt for college graduates in the U.S. stood at $32,731 (ValuePenguin by LendingTree). By 2021, the average medical school debt escalated to $232,300 (Credible). Send help! Sugar daddies needed URGENTLY!

If you don't want to cozy up to an older man to help pay off mounting loan debt (or an older woman – no hate on you sugar mamas out there!), here are some tips on reducing debt during your college years:

1. Undergraduate Scholarships and Fellowships

One of the best ways to reduce your personal student debt is through applying to scholarships and fellowships – both for college and medical school. In the *List of Research, Clinical, and Public Health Fellowships* section, you will find a comprehensive list of the available medical school scholarships and summer undergraduate fellowships, respectively, that you can apply to. In these chapters, we will go into detail on writing winning essays for medical school scholarships and undergraduate fellowships.

When it comes to undergraduate scholarships, there are a ton that you can apply to both before and during college. Universities typically offer scholarships for both incoming and existing students. There are also numerous external scholarships available for college attendees. While it's impossible to document every such opportunity here, here are a few tips:

Finding ideal undergraduate scholarships can be made easier by understanding how these opportunities are organized. Funding is often set aside for certain racial and ethnic groups. Chinese, Polish, Hispanic, Black, Italian, Welsh, Scottish, Korean, etc. students can find awards specifically set aside for them (e.g., Hispanic Scholarship Fund). Women in STEM and minorities in STEM have plenty of scholarships available. Awards are also divided by location – see if your county, state, or region has specific aid. Like STEM awards, scholarships are open to those pursuing a particular profession (for you, this is medicine and healthcare!). Collegescholarships.org and scholarships.com are two of the most popular websites for finding college funding. My personal favorite scholarship search engine is cappex.com because, from what I have seen, they have the most comprehensive scholarship list. Cappex also has helpful scholarship sorting tools like the "competition level" (rated on a 1-5 scale). Check these out, and be sure to do your own thorough research to find many opportunities available to you! Even though applying for scholarships and grants is a tedious process, it will pay off (no pun intended) – especially when that compound interest starts accumulating on your loans!

2. Working During College

A breadwinner so soon? Working during college can be a great way to pay off debt and begin saving for grad school, future homes, and retirement. However, for us premeds, if it comes at the cost of our grades or meaningful extracurricular involvement, **working during college may hinder our medical school applications.**

Some of the best work for premeds is that which contributes to extracurricular activities. Positions such as a research assistant, teaching assistant, peer mentor, EMT, or CNA, among others, can enrich your skillset in research, clinical experience, or leadership. Other effective roles include working as a resident assistant (though this can be quite demanding), in the school library (which, at WashU, was basically a paid study hall), or as a tutor (which can help keep your own academic skills sharp). Lastly, summer fellowships offer compensation to conduct research, which will look great on your resume.

Depending on your financial needs and personal interests, see which options appeal to you and what is available at your university. At WashU, I worked as a teaching assistant, research assistant, and peer mentor during the school year (although I took course credit instead of cash in the research lab, and the peer mentor position was unpaid). I also undertook two research fellowships and an internship over three summers – all of which were paid. I will go into more detail on my personal activities in future chapters.

3. Gap Year Work

Working during your gap year can help you pay off college loans, save for your future, and help you take out fewer loans for medical school. Either part-time or full-time work can assist in achieving these goals. Throughout my two gap years, I have worked both full-time and part-time positions, some of which were completely unrelated to healthcare.

Remember that studying for the MCAT is a full-time job itself. If possible, I would encourage you to dedicate three months to focus solely on acing the exam. Pre-writing your AMCAS application and secondary applications is also incredibly time-consuming because of the sheer volume of writing that needs to be done at the highest possible standard. I experienced this firsthand; while working full-time at a clinic, I realized that I would not be able to prewrite my essays while sticking to my current work routine. I left that job for several reasons – we will get into that later – and spent the following month preparing and polishing all of my written application content. Thus, working part-time or taking a month or two off is recommended when writing essays if your situation allows for it.

Another vital point: the summer you submit your AMCAS application is your last chance to update your activities section with new experiences. I bring this up because I don't think people realize what a great time it is to squeeze in a fellowship or other distinguished opportunity that will stand out on your application. For me, the Summer of 2020 was spent completing a biostatistics and computational biology fellowship with the Harvard T.H. Chan School of Public Health. This activity had not yet begun when my AMCAS was submitted, but it served as an impressive final anchor for my candidacy. Consider pursuing similar positions. For those interested, comprehensive guidance is provided in the List of Research, Clinical, and Public Health Fellowships.

The big question when it comes to gap year work is whether to choose a research- or healthcare-related job that adds to a resume but usually pays poorly or, rather, choose a non-medical position with better pay. The answer hinges on your existing experiences. If your application is lacking in research, volunteer work, or clinical involvement, it is critical to use your gap year(s) to build up these pillars meaningfully. Common positions for recent graduates wanting research experience include research technicians and clinical research coordinators. EMT, medical scribe, or CNA roles are popular roles for those seeking solid clinical experience. A trick is that volunteering can often double as your clinical exposure if you engage with a patient population. This doubling trick is what I took advantage of.

Upon graduating from WashU, I initially felt pressured to pursue a medically-related job even though clinical involvement was the only area lacking on my resume. My first post-graduate job was working full-time as a research technician at the same lab I worked as an undergraduate. However, the full-time schedule left little room for the clinical work or volunteering experiences I desired. Several months into this position, I had to leave due to health issues and ended up returning to my hometown. It was here where I began the clinical job that I mentioned three paragraphs prior. However, I was soon unable to continue this role primarily due to a resurgence of health complications. This clinical job was not included in my activities due to the brevity of my involvement.

Unable to work full-time while overcoming my health obstacles, my focus shifted to volunteering with older adults to gain clinical exposure while pre-writing my application essays. I started up work once more (excluding the Harvard Chan School fellowship) at the beginning of my second gap year (Fall 2020) and continued this position until medical school began (Summer 2021). This final role has nothing to do with medicine. It was not mentioned in update letters to medical schools or during interviews. This job also paid double compared to what I earned as a research technician and at the clinic.

In short, if you have a strong resume, it seems safe to work a non-medical job, so long as you dedicate some free time to a healthcare-related activity such as volunteering. If your resume is lacking in necessary experience, prioritizing relevant professional experiences is recommended.

4. Investing your money: Motley Fool and *How Money Works*

Despite acing Calculus III and subsequently being offered the CFO position at McKinsey – thus becoming the company's youngest executive in its 100-year tenure (all at the tender age of nine), I must humbly admit that I'm not a financial expert.

The constant battle between my shopping habits and my love of financial security has caused me to think critically about how I save and spend money. Like many young people curious about finances, this led me to investing. Tragically, though, I knew nothing of finance, economics, or investing because our education system does not teach such integral life-learnings. Thankfully, a family friend gifted my sister and me *How Money Works: Stop Being a Sucker* by Tom Mathews and Steve Siebold. This book serves as an excellent introduction to basic savings and investing. After reading, I began conversations with my parents about how I would invest my savings (small as they may be) to profit from compound interest. If you are like me and have limited knowledge of finance, I highly recommend *How Money Works* as a first step toward financial literacy. This is not a paid advertisement for those who are wondering. Once you're armed with this knowledge, consider diving into the world of investing with the guidance of a family member, mentor, trusted friend, or financial advisor. This is where The Motley Fool comes in.

The Motley Fool is a favorite investing platform of my father's. Since its inception, The Motley Fool's average return on all stock recommendations has been 580%, while S&P's return has been 117% (HowTheMarketWorks). Not only are the people at The Motley Fool talented at investing, but they equip their users with frequent updates on investment strategies spanning over a couple dozen companies. My family and many others have reaped substantial benefits through The Motley Fool, prompting me to entrust my personal savings with their expertise. That way, my money will hopefully have strong growth over the four years I am in medical school. Again, this is not a paid advertisement.

Whether you choose to invest with The Motley Fool or another platform, learning how to invest money wisely and responsibly, in addition to increasing your financial literacy, are worthwhile endeavors. Efforts expended during your undergraduate or gap years to cultivate these goals will help you in the present and lay the groundwork for a financially secure and confident future.

… CHAPTER

02

GRANNY'S ADVICE FOR ALL PREMEDS

CRAFTING YOUR NARRATIVE

This is the most important piece of advice in the guidebook, so listen up, peaches! ***A well-crafted narrative can make your application***. An application lacking a narrative can freefall. If there's one reason I secured 19 interviews (10 being from the top 20 medical schools), it is my compelling personal narrative. If there is such a thing as the "secret sauce" to medical school admissions, your narrative is it. It's all about how you tell your story.

I have seen narratives lift those with ~508 MCATs to the top 5 medical schools – both URM and ORM applicants. I have also seen the absence of a narrative cause silence to echo through the cycle of a seemingly perfect applicant, ultimately leaving them scrambling to reapply.

The art of crafting your narrative should begin as soon as possible – I mean literally the moment you attend undergraduate orientation. If you missed this early start, no need to worry; we can work with what you have. But the earlier you start shaping your story, the better.

The biggest lie of the compelling personal narrative is that only *some* people have one. The lie is that these gripping stories are reserved for those who have lost a parent, lived through financial turmoil, experienced devastating discrimination, and a host of other examples. While such challenges undeniably shape an individual, many other ordinary circumstances and life events can be transformative. It is far less about *what* you have lived through and much more about analyzing the personal impact of your experiences and then conveying this narrative effectively through your writing.

Take me for an example. Besides moving quite a bit as a child, I have lived an exceedingly ordinary life. Two parents and a sister. A jolly, relaxed family. Both of my parents have been successful in their careers, involved in our upbringing, and have provided generously for my sister and I. Although my family is Hispanic, it is not obvious from appearance. There has only been one instance of a classmate making an insensitive ethnic remark. The illness that struck our family was my grandfather's decline from Alzheimer's disease. While devastating, forms of dementia are incredibly common among the elderly. Overall, an unexciting life, right?

As it came time to take stock of my narrative and how I wanted to share who I was through the big application essays (personal statement, diversity essay, overcoming challenge story), I chose to reflect on moments that had a profound impact, even though many of them, on the surface, were rather typical. For my personal statement, I focused on my grandfather's Alzheimer's, detailing its influence on my undergraduate activities and my envisioned role as a physician. For my diversity essay, I recounted my own experience with religious discrimination at the hands of a close friend. For my overcoming challenge story, I discussed overcoming my public speaking phobia. While none of these experiences at hand were particularly out of the ordinary, their power lies in the telling – *how* I told the stories and how they shaped my life choices. To see this brought to life through writing, my essays are located in the Essays chapter. We will go into more detail on how to achieve this type of storytelling in the *How to Write* section.

Back to crafting your own narrative! Early in college, spurred by my grandfather's diagnosis and my family's quest for answers, I decided to research Alzheimer's as one of my extracurricular activities. This drove my clinical involvement, leading me to volunteer with older adults with memory disorders, which not only complemented my research but strengthened my narrative. For my gap year activities, I contemplated working in a clinic serving the elderly or creating an online service answering the pressing questions that older adults and their caregivers are faced with when making eldercare decisions. Both choices, again, would enrich my narrative. I chose the latter activity for reasons I touched on in the Activities and Honors chapter.

Here are examples of other personal narratives that you could consider based on your passions and how to tailor your activities to match these passions:

- Liver cancer: basic or clinical liver cancer research; joining public health campaign connecting individuals with liver cancer to resources or focused on helping to spread awareness; hospice center volunteering where you will help care for and comfort those dying from the illness

- Single motherhood: public health research looking at differences in health outcomes among single mothers and their children compared to adults and children in two-parent households; involvement in public health efforts granting single mothers and their children greater access to healthcare; volunteer at a shelter for women and children

- Sexual assault and rape survivors: basic or clinical research on PTSD experienced by sexual assault and rape survivors; advocacy on behalf of fixing the backlog of untested rape kits; public health initiative to increase long-term access to mental health professionals for those who have experienced sexual violence; volunteer at a sexual assault and rape hotline
- Rural communities: basic or clinical research on long-term effects of toxin exposure in rural areas; public health campaign to increase the use of remote health monitoring and virtual health appointments among those living in rural areas; volunteer with mobile clinic team providing care for rural communities (volunteer work can be through advertising, patient check-in, scribing, etc.)
- Mental health: basic or clinical research on how mental illness can present as physical pain in individuals living in communities where mental illness is stigmatized; advocacy that spreads awareness of mental health and resources in Asian communities where mental illness can be heavily stigmatized; volunteer at suicide prevention hotline; join college organization where you are trained to provide counseling to your peers (at WashU this organization was called Uncle Joes)
- Black and Hispanic health: basic or clinical research on greater occurrence of polycystic ovarian syndrome (PCOS) in black and Hispanic women; public health awareness as to how hair products marketed to black and Hispanic women lead to reproductive issues, such as PCOS; teach medical Spanish at your university; volunteer in a clinic serving minority communities or serve as a Spanish translator
- International health: public health research on malnutrition and starvation crisis in North Korea; advocacy for wide-spread starvation and malnutrition affecting citizens of North Korea; mission trip delivering health supplies and food to North Korea

These examples illustrate how to expand a medical interest into sustained, multidimensional involvement before entering medical school. What I like about this focused approach is that it shows notable dedication to your passion.

Have you heard the saying, *"are you pointy or round?"*

Being pointy means you are an expert in one area, while being round means you are immersed in an array of interests. For medical school applications, being pointy can be dangerous. Too much research and the committee may wonder if you are committed to treating patients. Too much clinical care and the committee (at least at research powerhouses) may question your desire to advance scientific discovery (usually part of a research-heavy medical school's mission statement). However, being too round can hurt too. Simply checking off all boxes can lead to an unmemorable, unremarkable application. So what do I be? Be both. Think of a ball with a spike jutting out of one end. I will explain.

Centering your research (whether basic, clinical, or public health), clinical engagements, and volunteering around a core theme make you an "expert" in that domain. This ticks essential boxes (making you plump and bouncy), and your continued concentration in one area of medicine will differentiate you from other applicants (making your sturdy point a pillar of diversity to admissions committees). Taking one of the examples above, performing continued research and volunteering related to single motherhood could establish you as a leading voice on the topic among your cohort.

When addressing your future goals as a physician in essays and interviews, be sure to speak devotedly to the community or disease you've focused your activities on. Highlight your personal journey, detailing how it influenced your undergraduate pursuits and will subsequently shape your medical career. An important note: even if you do not actually want to continue with that patient population or disease in your career, say that you do. The truth is that nobody really knows what they want to do before beginning medical school. Some swear allegiance to OBGYN and end up in radiology. Others declare their love of working with inner city populations to end up serving a rural town. Nobody is going to say: "Hold on! You said you loved children in your primary application and now you want to work with older adults?" or, "You said you were going to become a urologist and now you're going into psychiatry?"

You are not lying when you express a long-demonstrated devotion to working with a disease or group of people, even if you think that you may change your mind. The point is to not waffle around during your interview and say, "Well, I know that I've spent the last three years investing in women's care, but now I'm feeling the vibes of pathology." Again, it's totally fine to make the change from women's health to pathology (or any other change) - just don't state this during the interview because it may come off a bit flip-floppy. I'll illustrate with a personal example of how my specialty preference evolved during the application process and how I navigated this change in feelings.

Are you pointy or round? Pointiness came to me in my research on dementia. I focused on Alzheimer's disease, I volunteered with older adults living with memory disorders, one of my gap year courses surrounded caring for dementia patients, and I founded and ran CaregiverZone - a platform bridging the gap between elders, caregivers, and leading aging research. This narrative helped me make a strong case as to why I was committed to working with older adults and improving care for our aging population. My experiences painted a picture of a future geriatrician poised to revolutionize geriatric care – a vision shared by admissions officers.

Yet, throughout undergrad, as I wrote my essays and during interviews, I wasn't entirely convinced about a geriatric specialty. I am still unsure. Currently, I am drawn to dermatology, but this may change over the course of medical school. While I love working with older adults and their families, most patients in our healthcare system (apart from pediatrics and obstetrics patients) are older adults. Almost every specialty will allow me to work with elders. Thus, in essays and interviews, I could keep my mind open while still being honest about my future in geriatric medicine. In fact, several of my interviewers encouraged me to explore each field of medicine before committing to geriatrics. They told me of their own stories of thinking they would become surgeons and ending up as psychiatrists. **College isn't the time to figure out your specialty. College is the time for you to figure out how to get into medical school.** Crafting your personal narrative around a focal point will help you achieve just that.

BUILDING STRONG FRIENDSHIPS AND AVOIDING TOXICITY

<u>When you arrive on campus, here are your first two objectives</u>: building a strong group of friends and getting into your academic groove. Once these two are nailed down, immerse yourself in other activities. Choose friends who are kind, loyal, supportive – and diversify beyond just premeds. People on other life paths provide a refresh-

ing array of perspectives. Assess if you have similar morals and values. As you will see below, some of the people whom I grew close to did not check these boxes. If given a chance to revisit my college years, I would be more discerning about the friendships I nurtured. I would have asked into people's values and surrounded myself with those with values that were closer to my own.

Premed culture is known to be toxic. Even if the people around you aren't schemers, it's easy to fall into the trap of comparison. As the saying goes, "Comparison is the thief of joy."

WashU was ideal for premeds because we were not pitted against each other in classes. With effort, anyone could excel. My peers were generous and collaborative, sharing resources and helping one another complete assignments, understand complex topics, and prepare for exams.

However, there were instances of toxicity among WashU premeds. One of my classmates would frequently brag about her near 4.0 GPA and make a scene if she earned an A- in a course. Years later, I learned that she had cheated throughout her four years of college. She wrote equations on her arms. She and another student would swap exams when the proctor was distracted to fill in blank questions for one another and correct the other person's mistakes. Ultimately, this young woman decided against becoming a physician. Thank the good Lord.

Another piece of hot WashU goss! Senior year, my classmate (whom I partnered with on a project) took credit for a scientific discovery that I made. This work ended up being the major finding in the first-author paper that we co-published. I was stunned by her dishonesty and had to clumsily explain to our professor that I had, in fact, done the work, not my classmate.

Despite WashU's collaborative culture, there were snakes in the grass. Slithering slippery reptiles waiting to bite. My advice to you is to cast your net wide in terms of friendships. Choose friends who are not all aspiring physicians. If someone takes advantage of you or is crossing the line, take steps back from the relationship. Tough conversations are never fun, but they are necessary. If you feel comfortable, politely tell people when they overstep the line. State the facts and how you feel. It will be up to them to correct their behavior, and if they fail to do so, it's time to re-evaluate your connection. I fully admit that I struggle with these conversations. They are awkward and unpleasant. But I have learned the hard way that it is much better to stand up for yourself than to continue being taken advantage of.

Other toxic pools are the premed community on Reddit and the Student Doctor Network (SDN). Even as someone who knows this, I still checked them occasionally during my application cycle. Rarely is there an occasion when I don't see online personas on Reddit and SDN spewing condescension and ridicule. Steer clear!

Now, if you can't find any non-toxic premeds who share helpful advice, consider watching Kaur Beauty and MedBros on YouTube. There is a fair amount of controversy surrounding whether medical school influencers and physician influencers are good for the field of medicine, but I personally enjoy these two channels. Kaur Beauty and MedBros are run by three siblings – two of whom are currently in medical school and one who is in his intern year of residency. They're hilarious and give helpful advice on effective studying, applying to med school, and plenty of other relevant topics.

DATING AND SOCIAL LIFE

One of the first pieces of advice I gave to my college mentees was "DON'T DATE!" (in college). Of course, this advice comes with caveats. You may meet the love of your life while they're sinking their teeth into a half-cooked cafeteria cheeseburger. Or perhaps you will gaze on as she elegantly performs a titration across from the lab table in chemistry. Mmm, college romance! But seriously, if you're fortunate enough to find "your person" in college, go for it! However, for the rest of us sad sacks, I would warn against haphazard dating and staying in relationships that suck the life and joy out of you. And yes, I speak from experience. I'll explain to you through a few anecdotes why I advise against certain relationships during undergraduate years for premeds. The ultimate takeaway is to avoid dating that makes you sacrifice your goals: good grades, meaningful extracurricular involvement, strong friendships, etc.

First, I want to acknowledge the allure of dating during college. Often, it's the first time away from home, where you are exposed to ambitious young adults pursuing their careers. Dating can be fun. But, like all things, dating comes with both costs and benefits. And for premeds, these costs can be particularly high.

Benefits of dating:

Reliable company: This wasn't the case for me, but if you're dating someone caring, then you have a reliable support system. Someone to bring you tea when you're sick or spend a Friday night watching Netflix.

Good vibes: Who doesn't feel like a naughty hotty with little totty on Lotty's snotty arm? Dating helps define our graduation from awkward, braces-ridden teenagers to sultry young adults – good vibes, good feels.

Learn what to look for in a partner: To me, this is the most important benefit of dating during college. You learn what to look for – or, in my case, what not to look for – in a partner. If you sidestep dating throughout college, you might graduate without experiencing a relationship. One of the best motivations to date during undergrad is to determine the qualities you like and dislike in your other half so you can date more efficiently in medical school and beyond.

Costs of dating:

Time suck: Dating consumes a significant chunk of time. You may think, "I only see my honey pot on Friday nights!" Wrong, you are! When it comes to time, it is not just the Friday night smooch fest. Days can be filled with daydreams of his popping biceps or anxiously awaiting her next text. And yes, maybe a touch of cyberstalking. Maybe you'll tell me that you two are productive because you study together. Big whoop. Your studying is much less efficient with the stolen glances and footplay under the table. Also, the downside of the "reliable company" benefit (see point one above): when your snug bug gets sick or needs a date to a party, you're on the hook.

Less time with friends: From my own experience in unhealthy relationships to friends experiences in healthy relationships, a sizable downside of college dating is having less time for lifelong friends. My early college "relationship" (actually a nightmare) took precious time away from making enduring, cherished friendships. When I finally reemerged (over one year later), I realized I never invested the time that I needed to in my friendships. While I had a bunch of casual acquaintances, none were close friends. I had to play catchup in the friend arena, and in truth, I ended college realizing that most of these friends and I didn't have similar values. Alternatively, my suitemate, who was in a happy relationship for 3.5 years (from the beginning of freshman year to the middle of senior year), was devastated when her husband-to-be ended things. She spent her final semester crushed that she, too, had few close, lasting friendships. Ultimately, my advice? If you want to date, make sure you identify loving friends and nail down your study strategies first.

Unlikely to end in marriage: Statistics show that approximately 72-80% of college relationships don't end in marriage (LoveToKnow). Still, not an insignificant portion does end in marriage. Focusing on your relationship is great if you are one of the lucky few who end up living happily ever after. However, if you don't find yourself bouncing to the palace in a pumpkin carriage, perhaps it is best to rethink your pursuit of the prince. He really may just be a swamp frog.

Less extracurricular involvement: Pouring time into your romance means less time for extracurricular activities, which means a less robust personal narrative. Simple as that.

Lower grades: This goes hand-in-hand with my "time suck" point. As explained earlier, more time spent in your relationship means less time studying. Below is a professional, in-depth analysis of how my relationship status correlated with my academic performance.

My grades perfectly correlated with the status of my relationship. Coincidence? Perhaps. . . perhaps not!

- Semester 1: beginning dating = 3.58
- Semester 2: relationship becomes more serious, but also more miserable = 3.19
- Semester 3: relationship ends = 3.58
- Semester 4: less damaging but still unhealthy, unhappy new relationship begins and then ends = 3.71
- Semester 5: no relationship = 3.90
- Semester 6: no relationship = 4.00
- Semester 7: no relationship = 4.00
- Semester 8: no relationship = 3.94

See! I just proved a scientific theorem. Dating = bad grades; no dating = good grades. It is infallible. Where is my Nobel?

While it's true that part of why my grades improved over time was because I learned how to study effectively in college, achieving those 3.90s and 4.00s in the last two years would have been unlikely had I been dating. Relationships simply sucked too much time out of my day for studying, extracurriculars, and friends. And those last three – grades, activities, and friends – are what defined my college experience. Enduring a few lonely Valentine's days was a small price to pay for medical school acceptance and gal pals for life.

PREMED ADVISORS AND APPLICATION CONSULTANTS

It is beneficial to seek outside input on one's medical school application. Given the multitude of moving application components, managing the ordeal can be daunting. Others can review your writing, provide insight on which activities need strengthening, and assist in finalizing a school list. The best advisors and consultants will have had experience in successfully guiding past students to medical school. If you are aiming for a top medical school, choose someone with a strong track record of helping advisees achieve this goal. While consultants should be proficient in editing essays, they will also know the value of preserving your own voice in your writing. Do not choose someone who will manufacture cookie-cutter personal statements, stripped of personality, sitting blandly, indistinct amid competing applications.

Be warned: While there are some gems in the advising industry, I have found the profession ripe with fraud. Specifically, frauds who prey on desperate students, offering minimal, ill-advised consulting work in trade for a large payday. How did I come to this conclusion? In high school, our school's college admissions consultant was utterly incompetent. He specifically advised against me attending Cornell after I had been admitted because "I should choose a school where I could succeed." How charming. Meanwhile, his daughter was failing out of a college that no one would consider particularly rigorous. Perhaps he should have tested his own advice on his own kids before doling it out to students whose capabilities and ambitions he did not care to know. Although I chose WashU over Cornell, I was able to succeed at an equally challenging institution – a feat that my high school consultant did not want me to attempt. Getting back to my point, this man's incompetence forced me and many of my peers to look outward for guidance throughout the college application process. Through this hunt for a mentor, I met many slimeballs in the consulting industry who gave just as ignorant guidance as our school counselor.

When searching for advice about my medical school applications, my previous experiences gave me forewarning that medical school consultants may also be trouble. While I liked my premed advisor at WashU, she told me to scrap my personal statement after she read it. My words and writing style were completely out-of-the-box, and she prompted me to take a more mainstream approach. Despite her guidance, I believed my personal statement truly reflected why I wanted a career in medicine. I would feel uneasy submitting a statement that was unauthentic, so I went against counsel and submitted my personal statement as it stood. While some may have seen this as a risky move, I believe you should strive to reveal the "self" through your writing. Throughout the interview cycle, my personal statement was highly praised by my interviewers at Northwestern (Feinberg), Mayo, Case Western, Tufts, Yale, WashU, etc. It's why I think I earned interviews and acceptances at numerous programs. Had I conformed to conventional advice, my application cycle would have turned out quite differently. **Don't feel pressured to follow the crowd in your writing.** Following the crowd and my advisor's advice would have likely cost me.

Several months before submitting my application in May 2020, I consulted an outside advisor (in other words, not my WashU premed advisor) to discern if my application was competitive for M.D. programs. Previously, I planned to apply to MD-Ph.D. programs, so I knew my application was research-heavy. Given this advisor's experience as a medical school admissions committee member and her reputation for successfully guiding students into the country's most competitive M.D. and MD-Ph.D. programs, I felt confident she could accurately assess my candidacy.

However, as we began our conversation, I was stunned to the point of being amused when she told me I had *no chance* of getting into an M.D. program. No chance! No chance of admission despite my extensive leadership experience, four research publications, graduating with honors from WashU, a top 5% MCAT score, etc. I was aghast! She told me she could get me accepted to medical school, but her rate was a $6,800 flat fee. That's when I knew things were really off. I was confident that I had a strong application to medical school. As soon as I got off our call, I knew I would not be working with her. Frankly, I came to this conclusion when we were on the phone.

Post-call, I immediately discussed this ordeal with my dad. We found ourselves bursting into harmonious laughter about my apparent dismal chances of medical school admission. It was clear that I would not be taking this woman's counsel. My application results vindicated my confidence: 19 interviews with M.D. programs, 10 acceptances, 7 waitlists, and finally, matriculation into Yale School of Medicine — all without her "essential" guidance.

The reason why I am sharing this story is to show that, unfortunately, there are people in this industry who prey on the anxieties, doubts, and fears of those who dream of becoming physicians. They undermine your significant achievements and crown themselves the gatekeepers between you and medical school. There is nothing wrong with working with a mentor, advisor, or counselor who is honest and has your best interests at heart. But please, do not be sucked into the traps of people who will exploit your angst and apprehensions in order to line their pockets. Buyer beware. If someone tells you that your hard work has amounted to a zero percent chance of your admission, proceed with skepticism. Have confidence in yourself. Consult the people you trust, and don't allow yourself to be devastated by erroneous and ill-founded advice. If people control your emotions, they control you. Keep calm and Vulcan on.

The best way to navigate the minefield of balancing your own voice in your application with advice from others is by truly knowing yourself and the personal narrative you wish to present. Advisors are there to strengthen and shape your application, not to entirely redo it. After each advisory meeting ack, be sure not to continuously feel that you are tearing down your application and then rebuilding it based on their feedback. Instead, consider their input and decide which parts align with your personal narrative. Remember, no one knows you better than you know yourself, and it is this *self* that medical schools yearn to see in the application.

CHAPTER

03

ACADEMICS

TESTING ANXIETY

Addressing testing anxiety is vital before discussing academics. Why? Because crippling testing anxiety can be detrimental to academic performance. Personally, I had never experienced extreme testing anxiety until my senior year of college. The prospect of tackling calculus for the first time since high school, combined with the pressure to secure a solid A to graduate with Latin honors in my biology major, turned me into a stress ball. Bibbidi-bobbidi-boo!

Frozen. That was my state when I took the first Calculus III exam. I made stupid mistakes on two questions and ended up with a B+ on the test. A B+ may not sound terrible, but for a girl desperate to graduate with honors, I was totally buggin'! That's when I turned to beta-blockers.

Those little gems (specifically a medication that lowers blood pressure and is shown to help with performance anxiety) granted me the calmness needed during calculus exams. With a clear mind, I was able to focus on the questions. I ended the semester with an A in the class. I graduated college with cum laude honors in biology! Without beta-blockers, I am truly unsure if I would have been able to overcome the dread that consumed me during exams. I highly recommend beta-blockers or any similar medication to help with test anxiety. Talk to your doctor or perhaps a therapist to get the deets!

ACADEMIC ACCOMMODATIONS

Surprisingly, I did not realize that academic accommodations were available in college until one of my professors set me straight during my first semester. Securing these academic accommodations during college can be instrumental in obtaining similar support like the MCAT and USMLE. If critical to your academic performance, get those testing accommodations during college!

TO WHAT EXTENT DOES GPA MATTER

1. Attending a Top 20 College

In the chapter on *Making the Most of Your Undergraduate Experience*, we dove deep into how attending a top 20 undergraduate institution can offer more leniency in terms of grades. Total matriculants to Yale School of Medicine, for example, had an average 3.83 GPA spanning 2014-2018, while WashU matriculants to Yale School of Medicine had an average GPA of 3.68 over these same years (Washington University in St. Louis Undergraduate 2014-2018 Aggregate Matriculation Data). This information on several medical schools can be found in the section *Attending a Top 20 Undergraduate School Versus All Other Schools*. Here's the skinny on what we know about college reputation leading to GPA leniency.

Prestigious undergraduate institutions are often more rigorous. Tougher classes equate to more GPA leeway. Therefore, if you attend a prestigious college, you are more likely to have greater leniency in your grades when applying to medical school.

Do not be mistaken – this GPA leniency is not overly generous. In fact, I believe most of this leeway applies to your first year or two of college. One of the hardest parts of attending a tough undergraduate program is adjusting to the classes during the first year. These first few semesters are when students become acquainted with rigorous academic demands and figure out how to succeed in this challenging environment. Thus, it seems that the GPA wiggle room comes from a rougher transition into the classroom. Successful medical school applicants from these top 20 or so colleges should work to overcome any GPA drop from their first few semesters. Such an upward GPA trend during the final semesters demonstrates to medical schools that you can triumph in difficult courses and master scientific material.

A 3.7+ cGPA or 3.6+ sGPA from a top 20 undergrad is excellent. These numbers can be used as a loose benchmark for academic accomplishment, with **an upward GPA trend being the primary marker for success.** Do not be discouraged if you don't match these exact figures. There are plenty of students below these marks who gain admittance to medical school, including top programs. Take me for example. I graduated with a 3.70 cGPA and 3.56 sGPA. My sGPA was below the 3.6 mark, but this didn't stop me from receiving 19 medical school interviews and 10 acceptances.

Only one medical school asked about my grades during interviews. The culprit? Vanderbilt! My interviewer (who is, in all seriousness, a very kind person) mentioned that the committee noted my science GPA was lower than that of most accepted students. She said that the committee did notice that my science GPA had a strong upward trend, as I only earned As (A-, A, or A+) in my science classes during the last two years of college. My interviewer then relayed that the committee was wondering if there was a particular reason for my struggles in science courses during my first two years. I went on to explain my high school's difficulty in finding competent science teachers, many of whom were fired after finishing the year with our class. More importantly, I took responsibility for not actively holding myself accountable for information that I should have learned in high school. Rather than using our textbook to teach myself, I took the easy A from teachers who designed oversimplified courses. I elaborated on how this poor foundation caused me to flounder in college-level science classes and how I took responsibility for my education by making up the information I had missed in high school.

The key aspect of my response was accepting responsibility for my own mistakes and how these actions led to lackluster grades. If you are questioned about your academic performance or need to address it in an essay, don't avoid accountability.

2. ORM vs. URM

Ah. . . the old ORM versus URM debate! No medical school applicant guidebook would be complete without dragging this chicken from the barn!

Applicants who are underrepresented in medicine include blacks, Mexican Americans, Native Americans (American Indians, Alaskan Natives, and Native Hawaiians), and mainland Puerto Ricans (AAMC, Underrepresented in Medicine Definition). Those overrepresented in medicine comprise all other racial and ethnic groups. This definition given by the AAMC can be found in the *~Trendy, Cool, Hip~ Premed Vocab* chapter.

Let's keep it short and sweet. URM applicants have more GPA latitude compared to ORM applicants (AAMC, Table A-18). Some informal consensus points to a 0.2 GPA difference in wiggle room between URMs and ORMs. To illustrate, if an ORM needs a 3.8 cGPA and 3.7 sGPA to be competitive for top 20 research schools, a URM needs a 3.6 cGPA and 3.5 sGPA to be competitive for the same schools. I want to stress again that these numbers are approximate. If you are below these ranges, you **can** still be admitted to top medical schools. But you will have to compensate with other strong aspects of your application. This was certainly the case for me.

One last thing – there seems to be slightly more grade forgiveness for URMs from black or Native American backgrounds compared to Mexican Americans and mainland Puerto Ricans (AAMC, Table A-18). Something to keep in mind if you fall into these respective groups.

3. Struggle story

Overcoming adversity isn't just a personal achievement; it's an essential quality that defines and shapes our ability to empathize and care for our patients. If the adjustment to college was particularly challenging for you, or you tanked a semester because of personal challenges, do not fret! Poor grades that stem from personal challenges can be explained in your personal statement or disadvantaged explanation essay (both being parts of the AMCAS primary application) or in the "anything else" essays, which are part of each school's secondary application.

What constitutes disadvantaged circumstances? Examples include growing up without financial security, in an unstable home, in a dangerous neighborhood, or attending a poorly funded school. I would recommend passing your disadvantaged explanation essay by a pre-health advisor. Approach this essay with caution: If it seems like you're claiming a disadvantaged circumstance when you are not actually disadvantaged, the admissions officers will get a good laugh out of it. And through their laughter, your chance of interviewing dwindles.

Experiences like the death of a family member or a loved one experiencing hardship (e.g., drug addiction, illness, unemployment, interpersonal violence, etc.) or your own journey overcoming major adversity (e.g., disability, assault, etc.) can be valid reasons for a dip in grades. Depending on the particulars, you can discuss these experiences in your personal statement, diversity explanation essay, or the "anything else" essay. Ask your advisor which essay prompt is most appropriate for your specific experience.

When you hear about an applicant with a 3.4 GPA and 508 MCAT getting into NYU Grossman, for example – a school with a 3.96 median GPA and 522 median MCAT score (NYU Langone Health: MD Admissions Requirements, 2020 matriculate statistics) – disadvantaged circumstances are often involved. These individuals have surmounted significant hurdles in order to become physicians and show devotion to caring for those in need. Their unique perspectives will grant them uncommon lenses through which to view medicine and the medical system, thus allowing them to understand patients in ways that many of their colleagues cannot. This is what allows for academic latitude.

4. "It" factor

Sorry hotties! Just because you're an "it" girl doesn't automatically grant you the medical school "it" factor. That is unless you used your "it" girl status to score you a sugar daddy on the medical school admissions board. You sneaky minx!

Let's define the "it" factor before explaining how it relates to GPA. The term "it" factor refers to the "hard-to-define quality that makes someone special or outstanding" (Lifestyle Dictionary). For our purposes, the "it" factor is an activity, accomplishment, or personal circumstance that makes you an exceptionally compelling applicant. While this list is not an exhaustive run-through of every medical school "it" factor, <u>these examples are some of the most common "it" factor candidates</u>:

- First-author research publication in a prestigious journal
- Multiple first-author research publications in lesser-known journals
- Recipient of esteemed scholarship/fellowship for post-graduate study and research: Rhodes Scholarship, Gates Cambridge Award, Mitchell Scholarship, Fulbright U.S. Student Program, Harry S. Truman Scholarship, Carnegie Junior Fellows, Churchill Scholarship, Marshall Scholarship, and more
- Recipient of esteemed scholarship/fellowship for undergraduate study and research: Barry Goldwater Scholarship, Udall Undergraduate Scholarship, DAAD Undergraduate Scholarship, Amgen Scholars Program, and more
- Surmounting significant and unusual personal hurdles that you choose to share with the admissions committee: escaping starvation in North Korea to come to the United States and become a doctor; surviving human trafficking and now pursuing a career in medicine; etc.
- Founding notably impactful volunteer efforts or organizations (e.g., delivering large quantities of fresh vegetables to the community without access to grocery stores and, as a result, helping the community lose an average of seven pounds per person)
- Leading notably impactful and well-known public health efforts (e.g., educating the community about the importance of regular breast exams and, as a result, watching breast cancer mortality fall 20% over the course of several years)

Remarkable achievements outside of medicine: Olympic athlete, United States Poet Laureate, *NYT* best-selling author, etc. (If this is you, what the hell!?)

Feeling bad about your application? Please don't! Each WashU student whom I know who has attended a top 20 medical school (including myself) does not have ANY of these "it" factors. Not a single one of them. You are totally fine if your resume is void of an Olympic gold medal or a first-author *Cell* publication.

Now, for those few applicants who have achieved one or more of these "it" factor distinctions, you may have significant leeway in your GPA. For example, if you are a Rhodes Scholar, a 3.2 GPA will likely not keep you out of the most illustrious medical schools. The same goes for Olympic athletes, first-author publishers in prestigious journals, those who escaped horrific circumstances to pursue medicine, and qualities or achievements of a similar caliber. DAAD Scholars, Amgen Scholars, first-authors in lesser-known journals, etc., may have slightly less GPA leniency. It's hard to put exact numbers as to what GPA range an applicant can still be competitive when in possession of an "it" factor. Regardless of the numbers, if you have an "it" factor, feel confident in applying to top medical schools. There's no guarantee of an interview or acceptance, but I would wager that your application will be a standout.

As I touched on above, there are tiers to the "it" factor. Accomplishments such as the Rhodes Scholarship, Olympic participation, first-author publications in a prestigious journal, and those of a similar caliber are at the highest tier. A notch below (yet still extraordinary) are accomplishments such as the DAAD Undergraduate Scholarship, Amgen Scholars Program, first-author publications in lesser-known journals, and those of comparable metric are still outstanding, yet of a slightly lower tier. These tiers are somewhat subjective; do your best.

DOMINATING SCIENCE CLASSES

Learning for Success

Not to fluff up my own feathers, but . . . WashU is known to have the hardest premed curriculum along with Johns Hopkins. The science classes were difficult but, most importantly, doable if you put in the work. As a survivor and eventual crusher of the WashU science classes, these guidelines should help any student and any university earn As in these courses.

First things first: Don't overload your schedule with science classes when beginning undergrad. Start slow and build your way up. Begin with just chemistry and chem lab in a semester. See how that goes before leaping into physics and biology concurrently. From my experience, science classes at WashU (and at most colleges) were far harder than anything I had encountered in high school – even in A.P. classes. Of course, some of you will be in majors requiring intense science courses from the get-go (I'm looking at you, biomedical engineering). If that is the case, let the Lord be with you and use your time productively. A few of you may even fall into the category of ~super genius~ – those who can wrangle the sciences like an Arizona cowboy after his heifer. Super geniuses: "*congratulations, do whatever you want, and f*ck you*" (Reddit user). Now, back to the normies.

The gradual foray into sciences grants you the luxury of time, which you can use to figure out how to study successfully and efficiently. I will share my studying tips and how they changed as I moved from a B student to an A student in the toughest courses. Yet, even with my advice and the advice of others, each person must identify their own best habits for acing exams.

Tip one for crushing your sciences is to attend class every day (either in person or through watching the recorded lectures). Personally, I prefer to go to class in person and sit near the front – this way, even in large classes, you can potentially form a bond with the professor. These bonds can often turn into research opportunities, mentorship relationships, teaching assistant positions, or strong recommendation letters. Small classes are optimal for earning glowing recommendations, so definitely attend small classes. The argument for watching recorded lectures is that you can play them at a faster speed and thus zoom through them more efficiently. This strategy may be best if you are in many large, time-consuming classes (e.g., taking both biology and chemistry at the same time) because you can have more time for studying and your activities by speeding up lectures. Be warned that there will be days when the recordings fail or when the videographer misses content written on the board. Of further note – if you choose to watch lectures instead of attending class, do not let the recordings pile up. Stay on top of them *every single day*. I can't tell you how many students I know who were twelve general chemistry lectures behind come test day freshman year. They did not do well on those exams, to say the least.

Hand-in-hand with regular class attendance is taking impeccably detailed notes. Your fingers should be flying during lectures. Classroom time for me was predominantly spent transcribing as much of what came out of our professors' mouths as possible. This high speech-to-transcription ratio was necessary because many professors heavily tested the spoken details that weren't included in the daily slides. The PowerPoint slides themselves were shells of the lecture, and the meat came from what our professors said. Taking detailed notes meant class was tiring because I listened actively and typed constantly. My hands would often cramp up. However, these efforts were worth it, as I could convert these notes into study flashcards. Insert Anki plug here.

Each day after class, take your notes and turn them into flashcards. Staying on top of your flashcard-making is critical to avoid a mounting backlog to get through in one sitting. Making flashcards helps to pinpoint challenging content; jot down your questions and present them during office hours. Now, since this is college, you can choose to go through a few cards each day to learn the material progressively or you can wait until there is an exam or quiz. I was, admittedly, in the latter group. If you are shooting for a 4.0 GPA or have multiple hard classes at once, the former approach is your best bet.

Do your homework. Do it on time. Tragically, homework assignments remain an integral part of the college experience. They count for part of your grade, so make sure to complete them. In most classes, I like to get my homework done as soon as possible so that I can turn my attention to other things like studying and extracurriculars for the rest of the week. Furthermore, don't just do your homework – ensure you understand it as well. Note down any confusing areas and clarify these during office hours. Understanding your homework as you complete it will make studying for exams much easier and allow you to focus on the very important practice exams. I can't tell you how many people at WashU were sloppy about homework assignments (submitted them late or made silly errors). These lost points became the difference between a B+ and A-, an A- and A, etc.

Seize every opportunity for extra credit. At WashU, an additional one percent credit was awarded to those who attended large lectures, serving as an incentive over simply watching the recordings. This number seemed small at the beginning of the semester. Yet, when I was scraping the barrel of the final exam to get over the hump to earn an A- rather than a B+, I wish I had earned the extra credit points.

Last piece of advice: Don't just memorize the material but aim to truly understand what you're learning. Obtaining a deep comprehension of material will make recalling and retaining facts much easier, especially when information begins building on top of itself. What do I mean by learning for understanding? I will explain with the following example.

You may know that the bases found in DNA are cytosine (C), guanine (G), thymine (T), and adenine (A). It might be tempting to memorize that cytosine pairs with guanine and thymine pairs with adenine. That's not too difficult, is it? Yet, a more effective way to remember the base pairings is to understand *why* cytosine pairs with guanine and thymine with adenine. To do this, know that cytosine and thymine are smaller in size compared to adenine and guanine. Cytosine and thymine have one carbon ring, while adenine and guanine have two carbon rings. Therefore, to have our DNA enjoy an even width throughout the strand, a small base needs to pair with a large base. Cytosine and guanine end up being a small-large pair because they both form three hydrogen bonds (they form these bonds with each other to make up the DNA backbone). A helpful way to remember is: "*C and G rhyme with 3!*" Meanwhile, adenine and thymine form two hydrogen bonds, which they establish with one another in the DNA backbone. There you have it! That is an example of learning to understand, not just to memorize.

Studying for Success

If you have been learning for success, then congratulations! You have already taken the most crucial step toward studying for success! Keeping up with the course material by understanding your assignments and making flashcards has been the cornerstone of this process. But with an exam fast approaching, it's time to switch gears and discuss studying for success.

Freshman year starts by preparing for your exam with more time than you need. I did not do this, and it was a whoopsie for sure. I began studying four days in advance for our first general chemistry exam because four days were plenty of time in high school. Boy, did I get creamed! I ran out of time to cover all the material and took no practice exams. It was a reckoning. Doing undergrad over again, I would start by studying two weeks in advance. I know, I know. Two weeks is a lot of time. But trust me – start with two weeks and then shave off time. You don't want to under-budget time and perform poorly on the first exam. A poor first performance will leave you scrambling to recalibrate for the remaining and final exams. Each time that the scramble happened to me, I did not recover. I got a B in the class. To recap: Start with overstudying (two weeks) and then cut down. You may be at one week of preparation time and maintaining your A by the third exam!

Working backward, from test day to day one of studying, let's go over what ground you need to cover to clutch the A. <u>This timeline is the ideal scenario</u>:

Test day (Day 0): No new material should be being covered; all practice exams should be completed and reviewed; relax, take a deep breath (or a beta-blocker), and do some review questions that will boost your confidence.

Days 1-4 before the test: Take all practice exams in a realistic setting (quiet, continuous, timed); review practice exams thoroughly and have all questions answered by classmates, Tas, or professors – you should be able to confidently solve all practice exam, quiz, and homework questions before test day.

Days 4+ before the test: Run through all your flashcards as many times as you need to recall the material off the cuff (Anki helps with this through spaced repetition). If you've been doing flashcards throughout the term, this shouldn't take much time; redo your homework assignments and any corresponding labs. Know how to answer every question in your sleep. If a question stumps you, go to office hours or email your professor/teaching assistants.

This schedule can be modified to fit your preferences. Again, I recommend starting with two weeks of total study time and then, if needed, reducing your timeline. ***It is important to stress that the practice exams are critical to this plan***. I dismissed practice exams for the first year of college because the professors wouldn't reuse questions. While questions weren't recycled, the concepts being tested and the *way* concepts appeared were repeated. The practice tests also presented the material at a higher level – the questions were advanced. They pushed the boundaries of how thoroughly you mastered concepts as well as your ability to make connections that you had not seen before on homework. Being introduced to this type of thinking before exam day to familiarize yourself with the difficulty level and train your mind for advanced problem-solving is optimal. Performance on practice exams can predict performance on the real deal. I typically did better on the actual exam than on practice exams (once I pulled my head out of the gutter and prepared with practice exams sophomore year). Heavy sigh.

Exam Game Plan

If academic accommodations are needed, ensure these are in place before your exam. If dealing with exam anxiety, try therapy for performance anxiety and ask your doctor about beta-blockers.

On test day, you will ideally master the material and have completed a comprehensive review of homework, labs, and practice exams. Time to build confidence! Redo practice exam questions and flip through flashcards. Go to the bathroom before the exam and bring extra calculator batteries and a water bottle.

Exam time. I like to sit toward the front of the class so I don't get distracted by others' nervous head popping and pencil clicking. Side note: Those of you who take *science* exams with *pens* are psycho — side note over.

Exams are all about points. Collect as many as you can in as little time as possible. Start with the easy questions. Mark questions you are unsure of, eliminate answer choices, and return to the question after completing the easy ones. Save the hardest questions for last. The hardest questions require the greatest amount of thinking and thus occupy the most amount of time (time being the limited resource in the exam). When I solved tough problems on our science exams, I often had to run through several scenarios to arrive at a correct or partially correct answer. I would do these last and work until the time was called. Also, glancing over all responses to catch errors is more important than squeezing every drop of energy into a hard question. Rare was the exam in which I did not make a stupid mistake. I cannot tell you how many points dumb errors have cost me because I didn't look over the questions before handing in my work.

Lastly, think twice before leaving exams early. Unless you have reviewed all answers to root out errors and literally are unable to solve the difficult questions, don't leave the exam room prematurely. Even if I do not know an answer to a difficult question when I first see it, surprisingly, it often works itself out in my mind 30 minutes later. If

I'm still sitting with the exam, I can write down my answer; if I've left when I have an aha moment, those are points left on the table. Final word – whenever I leave exams, I usually just snack and watch TV, so I'm not losing out on anything important by sitting in an exam for the full testing time.

ACING NON-SCIENCE CLASSES

For most of us premeds, non-science classes are often easier than science classes. While the material may not be our forte or superbly interesting, depending on the subject, the material is generally less complicated, and the exams are less rigorous.

Excelling in non-science classes is a great way to keep your cGPA propped up if you are struggling in a science course. This was the case for me. All of my non-science grades at WashU were some form of an A.

Don't slack in these classes. Do the work, study for the exams, ask for help when you need it, and you should be fine.

If you find yourself struggling with a non-science course, apply the same thorough preparation work that you do for your science courses. But please, stay away from known difficult non-science classes if you are already overwhelmed by your sciences. When I first took three four-credit science classes in one semester, I took Spanish pass/fail to ease into the heavy science transition and am so glad that I did. This was my only P/F class at WashU, and it was totally worth it because Spanish is challenging for me.

CHOOSING A MAJOR

We have all heard the advice – "*major in what you love.*" Yes, this could be great, but also maybe not. Let me explain.

If you are doing well in your core sciences (a.k.a. have a strong science GPA during freshman year and into sophomore), then yes. Major in whatever you are passionate about. Your strong sGPA will speak for itself, and you can enjoy completing your major in history, political science, business, film, or whatever wets your wagon!

Here's the caveat to "major in what you love." If you are struggling in the core sciences during freshman and sophomore year (thus you have a low sGPA), major in whatever science is easiest and most enjoyable for you. Hopefully, the easiest and most enjoyable are the same discipline, and if not, choose the easiest. By the end of my sophomore year, I had earned Bs in all core sciences courses. My sGPA was floating in the honey bucket's murky waters. I knew that my best subject was biology and that the upper-level classes were easier than the introductory biology courses. In my junior year, I officially declared a major in biology. Over my junior and senior years, I changed my study habits to the ideal ones showcased in the *Recovering From a GPA Blunder* section and earned As in all my upper-level biology courses. I took more upper-level classes than needed to complete the major to rehab my sGPA to a 3.56, which I graduated with. Respectable but not impeccable. But, my sGPA had a *strong* upward trend (FY: 2.96 ➤ SoY: 3.22 ➤ JY: 3.93 ➤ SY: 3.96). Since I took 3-4 science classes per semester during my junior and senior years, this gave a lot of credibility to my improved sGPA during my final two years of undergrad, even with a mediocre overall sGPA, particularly mediocre for the top medical school programs.

Feeling bummed that you might not major in what you love? Good news! There's a loophole! While it will still be important to major in a science to raise your sGPA and give admissions committees confidence that you will thrive in medical school, you can still earn a second major or a minor in your preferred subject. Psychology was my favorite subject, and it also became my second major. Yes, psychology is technically a science, but it doesn't factor into the sGPA or, alternatively, the BCPM GPA (biology, chemistry, physics, mathematics). So dumb that psychology is tested on the MCAT but doesn't count toward the sGPA. Am I right?

RECOVERING FROM A GPA BLUNDER

C+ or Lower

Retake these classes and earn an A- or above. You do not need to retake these classes right after earning your original grade. Feel free to get some distance from the subject. You may even choose to retake the class by itself during the summer. If the class was poorly taught at your institution or the professor is incredibly difficult, choose to retake the course at an easier school during the summer or after graduating. With science classes, try to avoid retaking these at a community college because some admissions officers will dismiss these grades.

B- or Higher

Do not retake a B- or higher. Instead, take additional science classes (ideally upper-level classes because these are often easier than introductory courses). These additional classes will raise your sGPA while showing admissions officers that you can indeed handle a medical school curriculum.

At WashU, I earned eight Bs – all in introductory science classes. The 13 As I earned in upper-division sciences allowed me to overcome this hurdle.

Magic of the Upward GPA Trend

Upward GPA trends really are magic. Floundering during your first year or two of college is normal and expected. Try not to let this floundering become too costly. Keep low grades at a B- or above and earn As in non-science courses to bolster your cGPA. Take it from me: I messed up the sciences during freshman year and sophomore year by earning all Bs. Recovering with all As during junior and senior years made up for these mistakes.

Here's my GPA breakdown:

- sGPA (a.k.a. BCPM): FY: 2.96 ➤ SoY: 3.22 ➤ JY: 3.93 ➤ SY: 3.96
- non-science GPA (a.k.a. AO): FY: 3.86 ➤ SoY: 3.85 ➤ JY: 4.00 ➤ SY: 4.00
- cGPA: FY: 3.39 ➤ SoY: 3.53 ➤ JY: 3.66 ➤ SY: 3.74

GPA (type)	Freshman	Sophomore	Junior	Senior
Science	2.96	3.22	3.93	3.96
Non-science	3.86	3.85	4.00	4.00
Cumulative	3.39	3.53	3.66	3.74

Note: These are my WashU GPAs – not counting organic chemistry and a dementia course, taken outside of WashU. My cGPA, including both additional courses, is 3.70.

Former classmates had similar stories. They improved over four years of college and ended up in one of the top 20 medical schools. GPA blunders early on did not hold them back. Please see *Appendix A* for a table of aggregate WashU undergraduate statistics (GPA and MCAT) based on where students matriculated to medical school. Aggregate data is from 2014-2018 matriculants (Washington University in St. Louis Undergraduate 2014-2018 Aggregate Matriculation Data).

AMCAS reports your GPA to medical schools in your primary application. In addition, some medical schools have their own systems of weighing your GPA, often giving greater weight to junior and senior year grades over freshman and sophomore year grades. Thus, many medical schools reinforce the importance of the upward GPA trend through their weighted GPA calculations.

POST-BACCALAUREATE PROGRAMS VERSUS EXTRA CLASSES

Perhaps you need to recover from a larger or more prolonged GPA blunder. Perhaps you want a slight boost to your GPA to move from 3.58 to 3.61, for example.

Post-baccalaureate programs are for those with significant GPA blunders or who did not recover with an upper GPA trend. Post-bac programs are also for those who decide to enter medicine late in college or after graduating. If investing in a post-bac program, put in every effort to succeed. These programs condense the introductory science coursework into a year or two, so it's worth setting aside all other activities to earn As. Prevailing in post-bac programs can make up for undergraduate GPA mishaps.

From what I understand, post-bacs, known as feeder programs into an associated medical school, often are not what they seem. For example, I know of one prominent "feeder" program where out of the 40 post-bac students, only one is admitted to the affiliated medical school. Research your program of interest to determine if this is the case.

Post-bac programs are not necessary if you want to raise your GPA on a smaller scale. Extra classes can be taken during a gap year. My friend took extra science classes after graduating from WashU with approximately a 3.5X cGPA and a lower sGPA (I don't know the exact number, but I would guess between a 3.1X-3.3X sGPA). She retook her introductory courses to raise both her sGPA and cGPA before reapplying after an unsuccessful application cycle. I also took an extra class during my gap year. My goal was to raise my 3.69 cGPA to a 3.70 cGPA while learning more about dementia. I took Intro to Dementia Care and Practice at Portland Community College. Not only did I learn about a disease that I am passionate about and that fit with my personal narrative, but I also raised my GPA over the 3.70 mark before applying to medical school. Yes, I see some of you rolling your eyes.

If taking extra classes for a marginal GPA boost, these can be taken at community colleges. However, if taking extra classes to make headway on a lower sGPA, check with your advisor if community college classes will be satisfactory. A four-year college might be more well-regarded in these cases.

CHAPTER 04

ACTIVITIES AND HONORS

Making yourself into a standout applicant – a shining star – happens through your activities. There is so much you can do to make a mouthwatering application! While there are many boxes to check off, remember to maintain a consistent and strong personal narrative throughout each of these activities, as discussed in the *Crafting Your Narrative* section. Longitudinal involvement with leadership in a few activities is greatly preferred to choppy involvement in many activities. Nitty gritty, here we come!

RESEARCH

Premedical students engage in four types of research during their undergraduate and/or post-baccalaureate years. Med School Tutors provides the following definitions for these research types: basic, translational, clinical, and non-science/non-medical research.

Basic research

Often referred to as "basic science" or "fundamental research," this type of research attempts to provide answers to the mysteries of modern medicine. Its primary goal is to deepen understanding of particular concepts, as niche as they may be. For instance, basic science experiments might explore how cancer cells replicate on a molecular level or how abnormal protein folding contributes to a congenital disease. Even more "basic" experiments could investigate how atom-atom interactions affect blood coagulation or even the electron-electron distance of an atom!

Translational research

Nowadays, translational research is a hot topic, and it seems everyone is doing a little bit of it. Translational research aims to take some knowledge of a particular biological phenomenon (that the basic scientists discovered) and translate it into something that might eventually be used in a clinical setting. Some examples of this include taking the knowledge of an enzyme's structure that a basic scientist discovered and synthesizing a drug that will bind to that enzyme and block its activity. Another might be finding a better way to deliver chemotherapy to cancer cells without exposing it to the rest of the body. A lot of translational research will take place using animal models. It can range in everything from mice to horses, providing a valuable tool for testing different therapies before moving into humans.

Clinical research

Usually, clinical research answers questions about human populations—and the key word here is human. In the context of basic to translational to clinical, clinical research is the last step in validating a new drug or therapy in real patients, looking at efficacy and safety, often compared to other gold standards for treatment. When methodically structured, these are termed "clinical trials." Clinical research in this regard is for the most practical, pragmatic, results-focused individuals. Clinical research can also include efforts at improving outpatient waiting times, decreasing emergency room waiting times, or decreasing patient hospital readmissions. These may not be "drugs" or "therapies" in the traditional sense but are interventions, nonetheless. Clinical research is rewarding because it is most directly related to the lives and health of human beings, and among the types of research, it is the most seemingly relevant.

Non-science/non-medical research

As the name suggests, this research is any research outside of the field of medicine and science. Many premeds gravitate toward public health research in this segment. Yet, non-science/non-medical research can be in any field (e.g., history, political science, English literature, etc.)

Choosing what type of research to participate in can be overwhelming. I would recommend finding a topic that interests you. Then, find out which professors at your school are conducting projects in this field or about this topic. Making a good choice of mentor and topic early on can save you from what's often called "lab hopping," which means frequently switching research mentors and projects. While some believe that working in multiple labs strengthens an applicant's profile, I beg to differ. Having dedicated myself to the same lab and working with the same mentor on numerous projects over 3.5 years, I was able to be published on multiple papers and form close relationships because of my dedication to the team. These close relationships allowed substantial, complementary recommendation letters to be written about my work. Of course, if you find yourself in an unhealthy workplace, please switch research groups. If you are awarded a summer research fellowship with a new team, take it! These are important exceptions. Among my classmates who frequently switched labs, they were not as invested in the projects, and their PIs had a harder time writing gleaming recommendations because they had only months or a year of shared work history rather than two, three, or four years to reflect on.

Though research isn't formally mandated for medical school admission, the increasing number of applicants boasting substantial, longitudinal research experience makes it an unofficial necessity, especially for the top research medical schools. Such schools are known research powerhouses, with many of their medical students engaging in high-level research – often resulting in publications. Notably, a number of these schools, like Northwestern (Feinberg), Yale, and Case Western, have research thesis prerequisites. According to AAMC data from 2016, 84% of matriculants reported research experience on their primary applications. MSAR's yearly data on matriculant statistics to each medical school shows that upwards of 90% of matriculants at the top 20 research programs performed research before medical school. At many research powerhouses, this number is closer to 98% of students conducting research prior to medical school. While there certainly are other ways to stand out as an applicant, from my experience, investigating a project that you are passionate about is one of the surest ways to get noticed by highly competitive medical schools. Why is this? Firstly, because medical schools love meaningful research experience. Secondly, most premedical students have not taken advantage of the numerous ways you can distinguish yourself as a student researcher, *even without the luck of being published.* We will dive into these overlooked tips after discussing how to choose a research mentor and project, as well as how to build your research schedule.

When To Start Research

Consider holding off on diving into research until after your first semester of college. While many eager incoming students might be itching to start building their experience immediately, initiating research in the second semester will still put you well ahead of the curve. I advise waiting a semester to nail down your academic routine, form strong friendships, and identify the research projects you want to get involved in. Spend the first semester finding research projects that match your interests and contacting project leads (PIs, mentors, etc.) about a position. You can interview toward the end of the semester and start research once you get back from winter break. I waited until my sophomore fall (i.e., one year into college) to begin research. Sophomore fall, I began working as a research assistant at the Holtzman lab - a lab led by Dr. David Holtzman at

Washington University School of Medicine in St. Louis that studies Alzheimer's disease and Parkinson's disease. Over my three years in the Holtzman lab, I was published as a co-author on two papers in notable journals and presented our findings at multiple regional and national research conferences. These three years with the lab were enough to make an impact because I invested my time and efforts into our projects as a research assistant.

Beginning research sophomore year is a perfect time to start. Like me, you will have three years with your lab. If you want research to be a highlight of your application, I would recommend *not* waiting until *after* your sophomore year to begin. Part of this timeline depends on when you want to apply to medical school. Taking no gap years means your application must be ready by the end of your junior year. As such, starting research second semester of freshman year is ideal. Taking one gap year means your application must be ready by the end of your senior year. Thus, beginning research by sophomore year is a strong target timeline. If you plan to take two or more gap years, beginning research during your junior year is not a problem if you want to transition to a research technician position or a formal research program (e.g., NIH post-baccalaureate program) after graduating.

Choosing a Research Mentor and Project

Research can be quite dull, especially if you're not genuinely passionate about your project. It is crucial to think about what topics interest you (e.g., congestive heart failure, food deserts and diabetes, psychological effects of bullying, health outcomes of different socioeconomic groups, etc.). Remember that your research does not have to be related to science or medicine. ***I am confident that medical schools are much more impressed by an applicant enthusiastically engaged in non-scientific/non-medical research than an applicant going through the motions with a health-related project.*** Additionally, if you choose a science/medical project, remember that threading this same topic through your volunteer work, shadowing, clinical experiences, and other activities makes for a compelling personal narrative. That being said, make sure you like your chosen topic/theme if it will become a centerpiece tying together multiple longitudinal activities in your application.

After identifying a topic that interests you, research which faculty at your college are investigating the subject matter. WashU has a database of faculty looking for undergraduate researchers that lists their projects and contact information. Your university may have a similar resource. If your college has an Office of Undergraduate Research, they may also be able to help with these resources. Next, see if the specific projects being worked on are to your liking. Perhaps a professor is researching Alzheimer's, but their focus is basic research investigating the apolipoprotein E gene rather than clinical outcomes (which you are more drawn toward). Also, note how frequently the lab is publishing. A lab churning out publications will give you a better chance of getting published yourself! A last point to note is *who* is being published on a lab's papers. Some PIs prefer to have few authors in publications, which means that undergraduates and research technicians may be cut from the author list even if they contributed to the work. Other PIs are committed to publishing everyone who contributed to a paper regardless of rank. Although a PI's papers may have a short list of authors, this doesn't necessarily mean that people are being left off. Make sure to ask in the interview if the lab publishes undergraduates as primary authors or co-authors if they add to a project. At the Holtzman lab, where I worked as an undergraduate, everyone who contributed was listed as a co-author. The harder you worked, the higher your name rose on the list of co-authors. I was listed as a third-author for my primary project under my mentor. I was thrilled as we invested months of continuous work, and the paper was published in *Neuron* – a highly regarded journal with a 2019 impact factor of 14.415 (Elsevier)!

I've noticed that I keep using the word 'lab' even though you may not be working in a lab setting. Clinical investigators often work in clinics or hospitals, while other researchers may investigate historical texts or conduct fieldwork. For simplicity, I will continue using 'lab'; however, please note that this term may not apply to the type of research you're considering. Now, back to the show!

Below is a sample email to send to faculty members you're keen on working with. I chose to have a concise email body and appended a more detailed cover letter elaborating on my enthusiasm for their projects. You'll find a sample cover letter below as well. I recommend that you do the same because potential mentors can get overwhelmed by super lengthy emails and may opt not to read them. When you begin contacting faculty, I would identify roughly ten people to reach out to. This was the number that I used. Of those ten, five people responded, and two of those five turned into interviews.

Sample email to targeted research mentor:

Dear [insert name of potential mentor and use honorific (e.g., Dr. Holtzman)],

Hope this message finds you well! My name is [insert your first name], and I just completed my [insert freshman/sophomore/junior/senior] year at [insert full name of university (e.g., Washington University in St. Louis, NOT WashU]. This [insert fall/winter/spring/summer], I am interested in beginning research, and while searching the undergraduate research website, I was immediately drawn to the work that your lab is doing with [insert topic]. It would be great to speak with you about a potential role in your lab. My resume and cover letter are attached for your reference.

Thank you for your consideration,

[insert your full name (e.g., Caroline Echeandia-Francis)]

Sample cover letter:

Dear Dr. Holtzman,

My name is Caroline Echeandia-Francis. I am a rising sophomore at Washington University planning to major in psychological and brain sciences - I am also a premedical student.

I am excited about the prospect of becoming involved in research during my undergraduate years. As I was looking through the undergraduate research website, your lab stood out to me as one I would be very interested in working in.

One of my passionate interests in medicine is Alzheimer's disease - one of the areas that your lab is currently researching. My grandfather suffers from Alzheimer's, so unfortunately, I have seen firsthand the illness's effect on one's mental abilities. My grandfather's case is advanced, and I have witnessed him experience mood changes, memory loss, inability to think rationally, difficulty performing ordinary tasks, and confusion.

I am particularly interested in new theories about the cause of Alzheimer's, such as one recently released from Harvard stating that the number of viral illnesses contracted during childhood may have a link to the disease. Significant research must be done to further understand the disease, identify treatments, and hopefully, develop a cure.

This past semester, I took a seminar class called Topics in Health and Community, taught by Professor Brad Stoner. In class, we discussed Alzheimer's disease. One of the points highlighted in the lecture was that severe memory loss and cognitive and motor skills deterioration are not a natural part of the aging process. This surprised me because of the large and growing number of people affected by aging disorders, especially those that impact memory and cognitive function. In my psychology class, we discussed both aging and the use of fMRI machines. Overall, researching the biomarkers of Alzheimer's disease is where I would love to dedicate my undergraduate years.

After graduating from WashU, I plan to attend medical school. I believe that research will help acclimate me to the world of medicine by discovering more about the diseases that affect aging adults. My lab experience includes two semesters of chemistry lab and one semester of biology lab. By the end of the summer, I will also have completed two semesters of organic chemistry lab. In the lab, I have sequenced DNA and worked with spectrophotometry machines and pH meters. I am a hard worker with meticulous attention to detail and strong analytical and observational skills. Additionally, I am a strong writer, as many of my college essays were used as examples for high school seniors. Overall, I am dedicated to my work and excited about the prospect of joining a research lab.

I would like to begin working in a lab this fall and continue this work through my senior year, including summers.

Please let me know if there is a position for me in your lab. I appreciate your time and consideration.

Yours sincerely,

Caroline Echeandia-Francis

When interviewing, keep these points in mind:

- **Seek a mentor, not just a project**. Your mentor will be one of your biggest advocates when applying for scholarships, honors, and medical school. A cheerleader who is dedicated to your prosperity and their own success can make a world of difference in your outcomes.

- **Ask if the person you will be working with has mentored other students and whether they have current mentees**. My mentor at the Holtzman lab had not mentored other students prior to me — I was his first mentee, and he did a great job. Being someone's first mentee is not a negative mark, but try to gauge if you think they'll have the patience and thoughtfulness to be a good mentor. Mentoring isn't for everyone. If they currently have a mentee, determine how much time they can allocate to guiding you. My mentor ended up bringing on a second mentee toward the end of my junior year. She is a very kind young woman, and I enjoyed her company. Yet, at times, it was tough sharing my mentor's attention with a new student.

- **Understand your potential mentors' work expectations**. How many hours should you spend in the lab per week to make an impact? Which days per week and what times each day are the best to spend with your mentor on the project? Are there opportunities to work for the lab full-time over the summer? Can you have flexibility with your schedule if you have an exam? Will you be working on independent projects or closely alongside your mentor?

- **Ask if the lab publishes undergraduates on papers if the student contributes meaningfully to a project**. As we touched on above, you want to join a lab that will give you credit for your work. Published papers — especially if you are a first-, second-, or third-author — carry a lot of weight in your medical school application.

Once you conclude your interviews, take note of any gut feelings that strike you. When considering mentors/projects, choose a team you can join for the duration of your undergraduate tenure and possibly during your gap year(s). I have heard the advice thrown around that it is good to work for a number of research groups rather than stick with one. While it is true that if your lab is a bad fit, you should make a change, I say investing long-term with one project rather than bouncing among several laboratories is better. Sticking with one group allows you to contribute considerably to the work. **Longitudinal involvement will increase your chances of being published** and earning a glowing letter of recommendation from your mentor and/or PI. Note: There is no issue if you work on multiple projects with the same mentor/lab. Multiple projects with your mentor are often a good sign that they trust you with the work and that the research is progressing efficiently.

Productive, Reasonable Research Schedule

Committing to a research project takes time. You are already a busy premed student working to ace difficult science classes. How can you balance academics, friendships, and activities with a productive yet reasonable research schedule?

This process all starts when registering for classes and thus building your class schedule. Before registering for the upcoming semester, ask your mentor what days and times are best for you to spend with them. My mentor liked large blocks of time and consecutive days of lab attendance because this worked best for our research. Because of this timeline, I scheduled my classes in the mornings, so I had the afternoons to spend in the lab. Of course, your schoolwork comes first – don't sacrifice taking a needed class just because it's at an inconvenient time for your mentor. Also, don't be shy about negotiating the best lab times with your mentor. You don't have to passively accept the times that are first offered if those times don't match with class schedules.

On the first day of classes (often known as syllabus day), note when quizzes, exams, and large assignments are scheduled. If you have a weekly Tuesday quiz in one of your classes, for example, you may choose not to go to the lab on Monday to complete your homework assignments for the week and prepare for your quiz. With the quiz and your homework out of the way, then perhaps you can spend Tuesday, Wednesday, and Thursday afternoons with your mentor stress-free!

Here are a few sample weekly schedules for research involvement:

Sample Schedule 1

	MONDAY	TUESDAY	WEDNESDAY	THURSDAY	FRIDAY	SAT / SUN
8:00 AM	Class	Class	Class	Class	Lab	
9:00 AM						
10:00 AM						
11:00 AM		Lab		Lab		

12:00 PM							
1:00 PM							
2:00 PM							
3:00 PM							
4:00 PM							
5:00 PM							
6:00 PM							

Sample Schedule 2

	MONDAY	TUESDAY	WEDNESDAY	THURSDAY	FRIDAY	SAT / SUN	
8:00 AM	Class	Class	Lab	Lab	Class	Lab	
9:00 AM							
10:00 AM							
11:00 AM							
12:00 PM							
1:00 PM							
2:00 PM							
3:00 PM			Class	Class			
4:00 PM							
5:00 PM							
6:00 PM							

Share a couple of schedule options with your mentor to see what will work best for the semester.

Publications

Juicy. Plump. Tasty. Just like a sugar daddy's wallet. Thick and ripe for the plucking. Mmm . . . who doesn't want a publication?

Having your name published on a research paper is a significant accomplishment. This accolade not only speaks to the time and investment you poured into your project but also signifies a promise that you will continue to immerse yourself in scholarly work as a medical student. Your research experience can still be incredibly compelling *without* a publication (we will get to that in a minute). In fact, the vast majority of medical students don't have a publication. Strong research backgrounds – either with or without a publication – are more common among applicants to the top research medical schools. These schools recruit a large proportion of students who will continue producing scholarly work as medical students and, beyond medical school, as physicians.

The author order was noted above, but I'll restate it here. The higher you are on the author list, the more weight your publication is given. First-, second-, and third-author positions are impressive. The more well-read journals the project is published in, the more weight the paper is given. Journals with impact factors above nine are especially notable.

Some universities even have student-run journals where students' work can be published without the high standards and costs associated with professional journals. These are great options for students, both with and without professional publications. Yes, student-run journals are seen as more junior-level by admissions committees. However, having your work in a student journal demonstrates pride in your research and commitment to sharing your discoveries with the broader academic community. I would have pounced on this opportunity had I known about WashU's student journal before I graduated!

Regardless of the field your research encompasses, admissions committees will look upon publications fondly. I believe that someone with one or more publications in non-science/non-medical work (e.g., English literature) can be favored above those with scientific or medical research with no publications. If your passion is not scientific or medical research, be confident pursuing research in your preferred field. Dedication to your project and intellectual enthusiasm are more important than the type of project.

However, gaining publication is only part of the battle. While being published is a remarkable accomplishment, you will be expected to know the ins and outs of your research during interviews. Background. Methods. Results. Real-world applications. Next steps. You will need to know it all. Some interviewers will ask in-depth questions about your project. To prepare for this, I made flashcards on each of my projects to ensure I had the information ready for recall. I also practiced explaining my mentor's and my work in simple terms, as I knew most interviewers would not be well-versed in the minutiae of Alzheimer's disease. The culmination of this preparation paid off during my third interview of the cycle, which was at Vanderbilt, where one interviewer asked numerous questions about my project. Instead of feeling nervous, I grew to look forward to the many research questions that were asked.

Not being conversant with your research can be detrimental to an interview. If you are well-prepared, you will have nothing to fear! Side note: I didn't have the answer to a particular methodology during my Vanderbilt interview. I had to make an educated guess, which ended up being correct (thank the Lord); however, I was upfront with my interviewer that I wasn't sure of my answer. And guess what? I was still accepted. So don't worry if you make a mistake!

Research was one of the strongest components of my application. When I submitted my primary **AMCAS** application, my name was published in four papers. Two were already in circulation – both of which were from my time researching Alzheimer's at the Holtzman lab. The majority of my time in the lab was spent on one project that was published in *Neuron* and where I was listed as a third-author. The other paper was published in *Molecular Neurodegeneration*. Because I spent less time on this project, I was the sixth-author. The other two publications came from working with a professor at WashU, Dr. Craig Smith. Dr. Smith teaches a popular advanced laboratory course for biology majors where his students work on a project analyzing protein structure during the semester. Most of the final papers end up being published, as they speak to novel insights on a particular protein structure involved in disease mechanisms. My student partner and I were co-first-authors on our paper that had not yet been published when I submitted my primary application. I listed this work as a pre-print since it was in line to be submitted. Dr. Smith also invited his students to work on another protein structure analysis paper with his colleagues at the University of Washington. Those who contributed ended up as co-second-authors on this soon-to-be-published paper. I also listed this work on my primary application as a pre-print. Lastly, during my application cycle, I learned that another project that I had contributed to at the Holtzman lab was published in the *Annals of Neurology*. Side note: I have been mispronouncing the word 'annals' for years. I bet you can guess how I mispronounced it – so embarrassing. My dad finally corrected me in *2021*. Delightful. Although this new publication was not on my primary application, I submitted updates to medical schools post-interview that included the publication. If anyone is curious, I was listed as the seventh-author, so I definitely was not a huge contributor to the project. How you write an update letter is important, and we will explore that topic in the chapter on interviews.

Ultimately, research was a significant part of my application. A lot of time was spent in the lab, and fortunately, these efforts resulted in numerous publications. In the next section, we will talk about the power of research presentations, which can – in many circumstances – be more impressive than publications.

Presentations

Undergraduate students widely overlook presentations and conferences. If students participate in research presentations, the experience is often limited to their university's undergraduate research symposium. Your school's symposium is a great introduction to research conferences. You stand out from your peers by pursuing additional opportunities to share your work.

Why do these presentations matter? One of the most important parts of engaging in scholarly work is sharing your findings with the greater academic community. Sharing your findings requires that you have learned something of note, understand it deeply, and are able to explain complex concepts to a wide variety of audiences. Without communicating our discoveries to the broader community, we are unable to learn from others' work and thus focus future investigations toward making novel progress into the unknown. These skills are vital to success as a medical student and physician who may participate in research. Demonstrating that you are actively improving your communication abilities through research conferences and actively seeking out these events will speak volumes.

How do conferences compare to publications? At the undergraduate or post-baccalaureate levels, research presentations can often carry more weight than publications in your application. Here's an example. One student (Student A) has a fifth-author publication and has worked in a lab for several years but is not too passionate about the research. Another student (Student B) has passionately taken part in the lab's research, and although this work has not resulted in a publication, Student B has presented their work at five conferences. Student B's continued strong participation in research conferences at this base level is more impressive than Student A's fifth-author publication (barring that Student A's publication isn't in *Cell*, *JAMA*, etc.). When an admissions committee member reads the two applications, the five presentations stand out with the backdrop of Student B's excited description of their research. If you are interested in your work, it will show in how you write and the way you speak in interviews. While Student A's publication is certainly consequential, a lack of interest in their project can undercut the significance of their paper. Because so few students present at conferences, to me, conference participation comes across as authentic enthusiasm about one's work. I believe admissions officers see it quite similarly.

Research conferences are offered at the local, regional, and national levels. If you are researching neuroscience, look up what conferences are offered in the neuroscience field. There will be plenty at all three levels – local, regional, and national. Additionally, ask your mentor or PI which conferences they recommend. Of course, conferences are also offered for the non-science fields! Next, make a list of when and where the conferences are held and the deadlines for submitting an abstract. Some conferences offer travel scholarships for attendees and presenters, so take note of the deadlines. Traveling to conferences, particularly those far away, can be expensive. Your university's undergraduate research office or even your PI may offer stipends to cover the expenses. The research fellowships that we will get into in the next section also often cover conference travel costs. Lastly, certain societies – such as Psi Chi (The National Honor Society in Psychology) – have grants that cover members' conference travel costs. Check if you can join similar groups that offer these benefits, like women in STEM or underrepresented in STEM societies. SACNAS (Society for Advancement of Chicanos / Hispanics and Native Americans in Science) offers scholarships for attendees and presenters at their annual conference.

Aside: if you do earn one of these travel grants or scholarships, it looks great on your application! A travel grant from Psi Chi was on my primary application, and the scholarship from SACNAS was an update for medical schools that I sent in September.

I had never written a grant essay before applying for a Psi Chi travel grant. Fortunately, guides from different colleges helped show how to outline an effective and compelling proposal. My essay is below, so you have an example of how to apply for these awards.

Travel Grant Essay:

> *If accepted to present at Rocky Mountain Psychological Association's 2020 convention, I will be thrilled to represent Washington University in St. Louis's Psi Chi chapter through my work researching Alzheimer's disease. The project I am presenting is one that I have worked on extensively as an undergraduate and was published in Molecular Neurodegeneration this fall. Psi Chi's student travel grant would help to alleviate part of the financial burden of attending RMPA, for which the registration, flight, and hotel stay totaled approximately $813. My university, unfortunately, does not have funds set aside to aid student expenses for research conferences, so it is imperative for me to secure outside financial assistance in order to attend the three-day convention.*
>
> *As a hopeful future MD-Ph.D. student in neurology, presenting a poster at RMPA would provide an excellent platform for me to introduce my research to others in the psychology field as well as an invaluable opportunity to incite discussion and build professional connections with experienced researchers in all stages of their careers. Moreover, as the former president of our Psi Chi chapter and our first Hispanic American president, it would be a privilege to be the first student from Washington University to represent both my school and my Psi Chi chapter at RMPA.*
>
> *Thank you to the committee for taking the time to review my application.*

Clearly, at the time, I thought that I would pursue an MD-Ph.D.. But it's all M.D. now, baby!

Another biggie: Awards for best posters and best oral presentation are given at most conferences. Earning these awards looks tremendous on medical school applications. You will have demonstrated both dedication to the research process as well as prowess in explaining complex academic work. While I was never so fortunate as to land a poster or oral award at the conferences where I presented, I wish you much luck in the endeavor! Although my posters did not win accolades, I still think that they were well done. Many examples of research posters are on the internet, but, if you want a reference, here are two of mine.

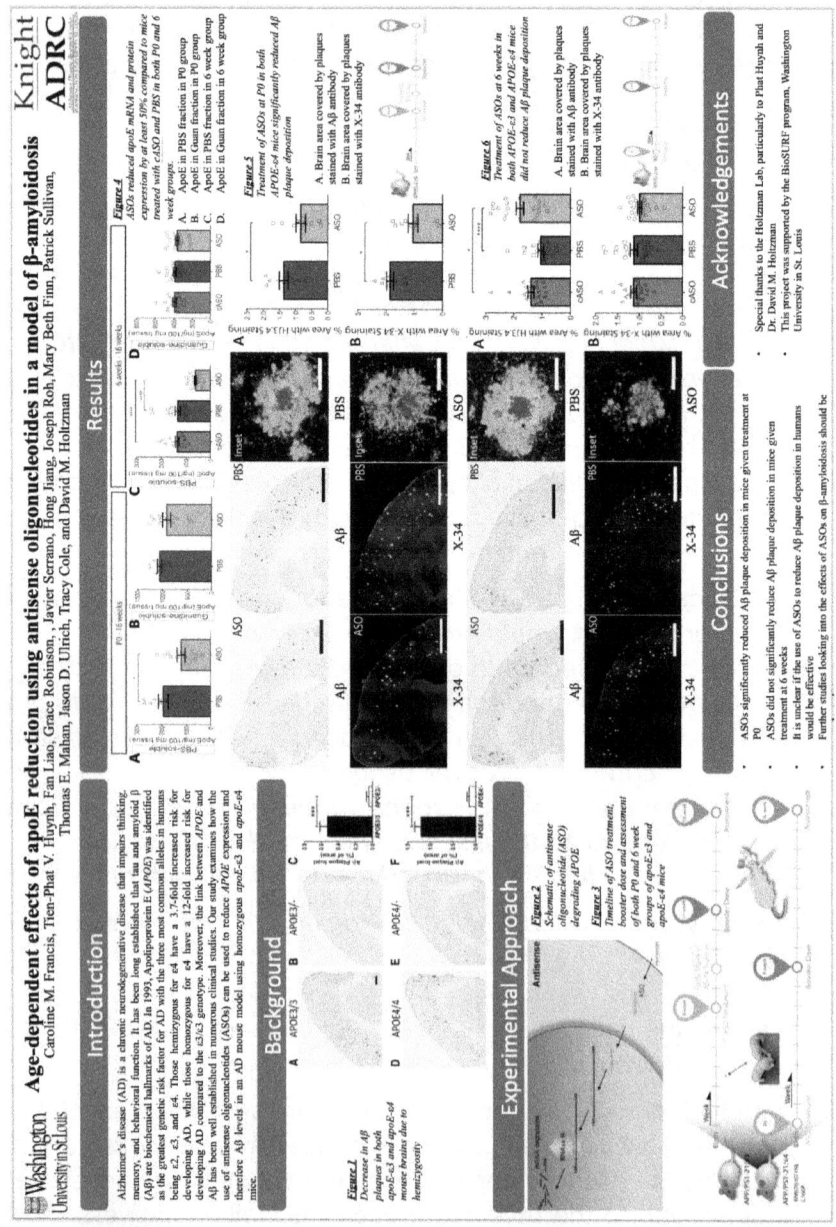

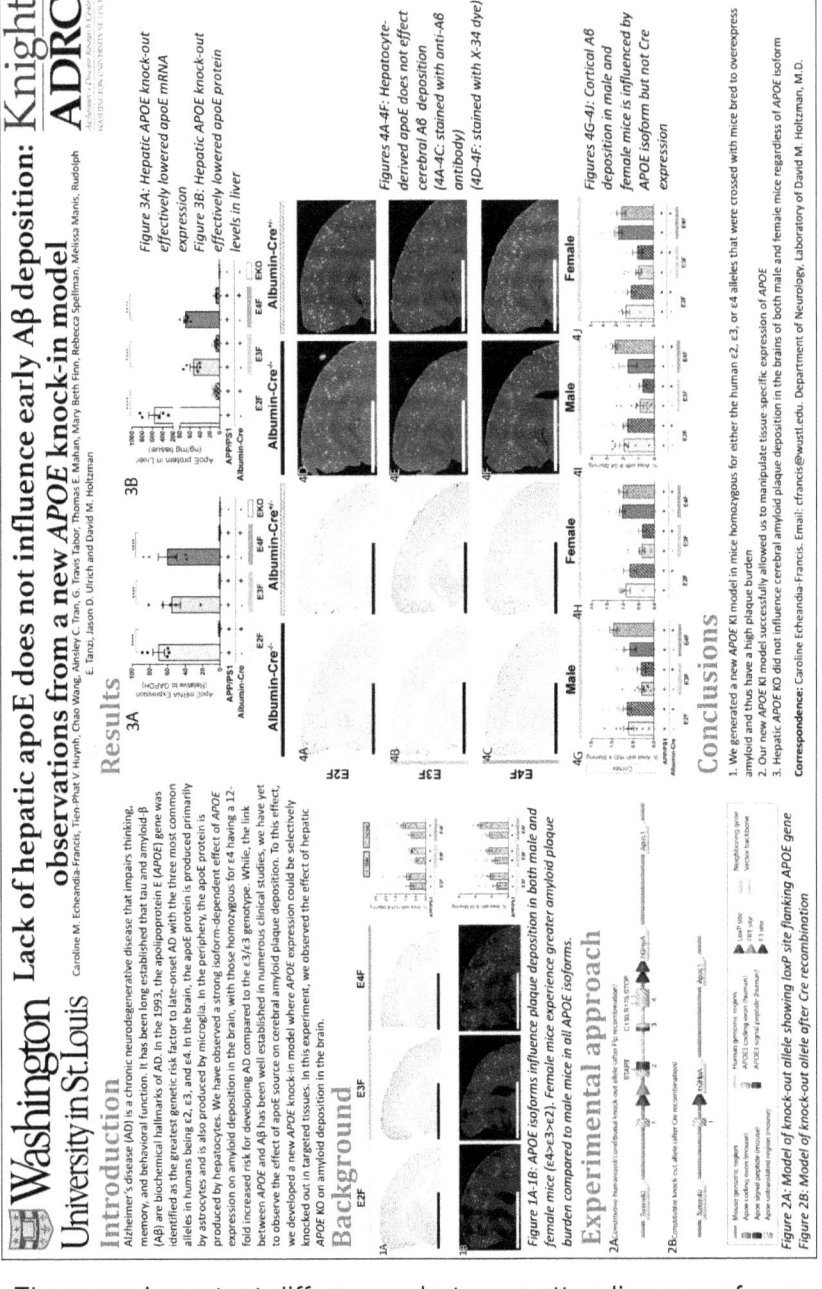

There are important differences between attending a conference versus presenting a poster versus delivering a research talk. Oral presentations carry the most weight in your application because few people are selected to give talks. Out of the seven conferences I attended, I gave talks at four (two required an oral presentation, and I pursued a speaking position at the other two). A poster carries the second most amount of weight. I had posters at six of the seven conferences that I attended — my group did an oral presentation at the one without a poster. Make sure that you have prepared a two-minute and five-minute walk-through of your poster. Some attendees want it quick and dirty, while others take their time. Finally, attending a conference is great for learning cutting-edge discoveries and making connections, but I'm not sure if attendance alone is compelling to admissions committees.

Okay, back to oral presentations. If your college's undergraduate symposium offers keynote speaker positions, ask if you can be considered for one of those spots. The keynote speaker appointment for WashU's symposium was the kickoff to 1) my six other conferences and 2) overcoming my paralyzing fear of public speaking. You, too, may suffer from public speaking phobia. I understand how suffocating it can be. So much as answering questions in a small class could scare me into silence. My class schedule used to be formed around classes with few oral presentations. In fact, several months prior to delivering the keynote address, I almost ran out of my Spanish class in tears when giving a talk that I was well-prepared for. My peers' thirteen sets of eyes terrified me. In order to avoid a meltdown when giving the oral presentation in front of two hundred symposium attendees — yes, *two hundred* people — my mentor and the symposium directors generously critiqued my talk. Then came the Godsend. My physician prescribed beta-blockers to ward off the fight-or-flight response that kicked in in front of audiences. These are the keys to the kingdom: tons of practice and beta-blockers (if approved by your doctor).

Quick tip for research talks — only put titles, photos, and citations (if necessary) on each slide. Three things — that's it! Almost everyone, including me, makes the mistake of putting text on slides. My mentor had me completely redo my slides for the keynote presentation, and I could only include photos (sometimes with labels) apart from one slide reviewing our findings where I used some text. People cannot listen and read effectively at the same time. Images enhance your presentation, keep things simple, and ensure that you will know your stuff inside and out since there are no words to read off of. Take my mentor's advice and use images, not text!

CLINICAL EXPERIENCES

Clinical experience is an indispensable component of a medical school application. Without it, you cannot get accepted. The best part about clinical experience is that it can double as work or volunteering. For example, if you are an emergency medical technician (EMT) or a scribe, you are both working and gaining clinical experience. If you give your time helping paraplegic children, you are both volunteering and gaining clinical experience.

As you choose which clinical engagement to pursue, consider the personal narrative that will tie your application together. The personal narrative is the theme of advice given in this guidebook because it is a little-known but extraordinarily powerful tool to make you a standout applicant. Using myself as an example, when I was looking to spend time with patients, I reflected on the activities that I was already involved in and my passions within medicine. At the time, I was immersed in Alzheimer's research and wanted my love of working with older adults to be the centerfold of my candidacy. This pretext led me to choose volunteering in memory care units as my clinical experience. When writing about my volunteer work in applications, I spoke about how my time spent with older adults living with dementia helped to inform my research. By engaging with aging adults, my research projects were directly tied to the patient population needing treatments and cures for dementia.

Each piece of my story came together in a clear, cohesive manner. My clinical experiences built upon my research and showed commitment to the population I am passionate about caring for through medicine. Because medicine is a lengthy, tiresome road, admissions officers look for those with a long-standing dedication to their endeavors. ***A themed narrative is a great way to achieve this objective.***

What are some of the most enriching clinical experiences to pursue? I'll break them up into paid clinical opportunities versus volunteer clinical opportunities.

Paid Clinical Exposure

EMT (Emergency Medical Technician)

Students can work part-time as an EMT during college or a postbac program. Many universities have a campus EMT unit staffed by current students. The student-run EMT unit was one of the most popular organizations at WashU, although the positions were unpaid. Gap-year students can pursue full-time EMT employment. What's great about working as an EMT is that you will gain exposure to a wide variety of patients – except service with an on-campus EMT squad where patients will mostly be students, faculty, staff, and visitors. With a diverse patient population, it is easy to discuss those patients, diseases, or injuries that fit within your personal narrative. You can also find the latitude of where to work as an EMT. Working on an ambulance versus a college campus versus a primary school versus a sports stadium versus a nursing home also allows you to control which patient populations you work with and thus control the molding of your narrative. Many organizations offer either accelerated or regular-paced EMT training. After course completion and passing certification exams, you are set to go. One downside is that the classes and tests are often expensive. Completing EMT training through your college's squad can help reduce costs. Also, scholarships may be available to cover expenses.

CNA (Certified Nursing Assistant)

Much like EMTs, CNAs can work part-time while in school or full-time after graduating. CNAs work alongside nurses to provide direct care to patients. The populations that you tend to can vary widely depending on where you pursue employment. Nursing homes, schools, hospitals, hospice centers, sporting arenas, rehabilitation centers, psychiatric facilities, you name it! You will be able to match your narrative to CNA opportunities. Another bonus about being an EMT or CNA: if you are interested in global health, mission trips often need EMTs and CNAs to join their teams. We will get into the dos and don'ts of abroad mission trips in a jiffy because these can either significantly add to or detract from your application. You have to be careful with work abroad! Again, similar to EMT licensing, courses, and a certification test is required to become a CNA. These can be expensive, so see if scholarships are available.

Scribe

Scribing has become incredibly popular among individuals taking gap years. Scribes work alongside physicians by taking notes in patient rooms regarding the doctor's discussion with the patient. Certifications are required for medical scribes. Scholarships may be available. Scribing usually takes place in healthcare facilities such as hospitals, clinics, and urgent care centers. Depending on your narrative, you could choose to work in the emergency department, a dermatology clinic, a pediatrics center, and a host of other specialized facilities. Scribing at a location that focuses on rural health, uninsured patients, or homeless individuals, to name a few, are outstanding options as well.

Volunteer (Unpaid) Clinical Exposure

Hospital/Clinic Volunteering

Simply put, this is volunteering that takes place in a hospital or clinic. Like DO! Examples include volunteer work in the emergency room, hospice, radiation center, pediatric oncology unit, etc. The one pitfall to watch out for with hospital or clinic volunteering is that you might be assigned administrative tasks with little patient interaction. These were the experiences of my classmates when they volunteered at Barnes-Jewish (the teaching hospital for Washington University School of Medicine in St. Louis). Barnes is so well-staffed that they typically do not use volunteers for patient interactions. The large exception to this was in the hospital's hospice center, where one of my friends spent time with patients who were in their last 72 hours of life. Talk about meaningful work. I've heard that smaller hospitals often allow their volunteers more patient contact, so check what is available in your area. I would also say that volunteering in pediatric units can offer lots of opportunities. Read to children, help with homework, have a finger-painting party – there's tons of creativity in how you can be involved! Think about your narrative (a.k.a. your medical and patient population interests), and then choose volunteer opportunities that fit your passion.

Other Volunteering

Helping children or adults with specific medical needs, such as students with autism, parents with multiple sclerosis, or older adults with Parkinson's, all fall into this grouping. There is such a large array of populations and specific illnesses or injuries that I can't list them all here. Your imagination is the limit. Again, reflect on your narrative and start searching for volunteer work that fits the people or disease you are invested in. As I have previously noted, I chose to volunteer in memory care units with older adults living with dementia. Even though our day-to-day activities revolved around exercising, discussing current events, playing brain games, and arts and crafts rather than medical matters, I was still working with my patient population of interest. That's what counts! Hotline volunteering is excellent and is often focused on suicide prevention, sexual assault and rape counseling, and domestic abuse support. These are heavy moments in people's lives that require outstanding support and delicate care, so know what you are getting involved in. Counseling is a similar option where you can train to speak with people – often peers – in need of help. Of course, much counseling requires master's or doctoral degrees, so the type of counseling you could be involved with – without these degrees – is limited. Your college may have its own hotline or counseling services that you can volunteer for. At WashU, we had S.A.R.A.H. (Sexual Assault and Rape Anonymous Hotline) as well as Uncle Joe's (face-to-face peer counselors). Both S.A.R.A.H. and Uncle Joe's members underwent over 100 hours of training before they could begin volunteering with WashU students, and both groups were extraordinarily competitive to join as student counselors.

Mission Trips

Mission trips can get dicey. There is a way to pursue mission work that is genuine and actually helps people. There are also ways to pursue mission work that are insignificant, possibly harmful, and more focused on providing participants with thinly veiled vacations as opposed to volunteer opportunities. Admissions committees will scrutinize your involvement and how you discuss mission trips to determine which side of the scale your work falls on. If you are found to be a sunbather wearing Mother Teresa's clothing, it will harm your candidacy and make admissions ask themselves why you would disguise a personal excursion as volunteer work. An important question to ask yourself before pursuing mission work is whether or not you think about posting pictures of your trip to social media. When I was in middle school, the fad of posting snaps with impoverished children during a week's volunteering became popular. I never understood how these Facebook friends did not see the showboaty and exploitative nature that lurked behind sharing this content. If you fantasize about sharing similar photos or writing public monologues for Instagram about the house you resurrected on a weekend, think twice about your motivations. You will likely fall into the trap of disingenuous mission work. On the other hand, volunteering abroad can be impactful. The solution to achieving moving, honest, benevolent mission work is having a continuous experience where you go back to the same place and do the same type of work over several years or have a long-term experience like a summer or semester expedition. My friend from WashU spent her junior summer in India, where she taught schoolgirls about reproductive health. Women's reproductive health was a love of hers, and it became her personal narrative. She was a hotline counselor with S.A.R.A.H. (WashU's Sexual Assault and Rape Anonymous Hotline), researched the reproductive field, and volunteered at a women's shelter. Her summer-long mission trip was heartfelt and, most importantly, consequential to the young women she worked with. Another WashU friend led Global Brigades' medical service trips to Honduras year after year. Although the group was only onsite for one week at a time, his longitudinal involvement and continued effort spent organizing the Brigades showed devotion to those he served. These two examples are how you ace medical mission trips. If you are invested in global health, abroad, service is an excellent demonstration of this commitment. Please note that volunteering abroad and mission trips can be expensive. Do not feel compelled to join these projects if it is a financial burden. There is plenty of impactful volunteer work to be done within our local communities.

Q: How many hours should I put into clinical work to be competitive for medical school?
A: When it comes to hours, I would say that 300 hours is great, and over 500 clinical hours is excellent. I always recommend shooting for excellence in our applications, so I would shoot for 500 hours. Now, 500 hours is a lot. How can we make that feasible with academics and other activities to attend to? Volunteering two hours per week during the academic year (about 32 weeks) over four years puts you at 256 hours total. Over half of your 500-hour "excellent work" goal and quite close to the 300-hour "great work" goal. Then, spending eight hours per week during the summer (approximately 16 weeks) over two years will get you another 256 hours. Voilà! You have reached the 500-hour "excellent work" mark. Note that if you cannot physically be with your patient population due to something like COVID, you can still volunteer for them from home, such as by making masks and sewing blankets. Those hours count! A high school student whom I interviewed for WashU undergrad had an incredible project where he made clear masks for those with hearing impairments. The clear masks allowed these individuals to read lips. One couple wrote to this young man and thanked him, as his clear masks allowed them to communicate in the hospital when the wife was giving birth to their first child. Without these masks, the couple would not have been

able to communicate during the birth of their first child. His work made a difference for these two (and then three!) people.

Q: How long should clinical experiences last?
A: So, we have our 500-hour goal. The timeframe to complete these hours is best organized over two or more years. Again, longitudinal involvement pulls greater weight than short, choppy activities. I spent only *one* summer in college volunteering with older adults (my junior year summer). Then, during my gap year, I knew I needed to beef up my clinical experience because one summer was weak sauce. Volunteering weekly at a local memory care unit occupied my gap year until the coronavirus limited visitors' accessibility. Then, I transitioned to sewing masks for the residents and the staff who cared for them. This work brought me more than 500 hours of total volunteering time. Yet, I would still say that I am not the model example of longitudinal clinical exposure. It would have been better to spend several summers in memory care units – not just one. I backloaded the vast majority of my clinical volunteering during my gap year because I knew it was my weak spot. Everything worked out, but I clearly didn't follow my own advice here. Do as I say, not as I do!

RESEARCH, CLINICAL, AND PUBLIC HEALTH FELLOWSHIPS

Fellowships for the academic term and summer are the golden eggs of undergraduate research accomplishments. Post-baccalaureate fellowships are equally prestigious. These fellowships are structured programs that fund your research, often travel to conferences, and provide immersive mentorship. Each program I am familiar with is competitive but incredibly enriching if you are selected. I was fortunate enough to earn two summer research fellowships – one through Washington University in St. Louis (my undergraduate school) and one through the Harvard T.H. Chan School of Public Health. I was also turned down from many more fellowships than I received (see the *Resume of Failures* section). It is common for universities to set fellowships aside for their own students. Apply to your university's programs as a jumping-off point – perhaps for your freshman or sophomore summer. WashU's Biology Summer Undergraduate Research Fellowship (BioSURF) occupied my summer following my sophomore year. The summer I submitted my medical school applications (the Summer of 2020) was when I participated in the Harvard Chan School's Biostatistics and Computational Biology Undergraduate Research Fellowship. This fellowship was for both undergraduates and post-baccalaureate students – I participated during the summer following my first gap year. The summer when you submit your medical school application is vastly underused among applicants. If you can squeeze a fellowship into those warm months, it will tie up your candidacy in a pretty bow. Personally, I am convinced that my final fellowship with the Chan School helped me earn interviews as well as admission offers to the top research medical schools. In my mind, these programs serve almost as pre-vetting that someone is a top applicant. Since both clinical and research fellowship programs are quite selective, admission to these programs is, effectively, a gold star on an applicant's candidacy – acting as its own voucher for the student. These "gold star" applicants thus become an illustrious and low-risk buy to the admission committees. Does that make sense? The same logic goes for prestigious scholarships like the Fulbright. These fellowships and scholarships have always seemed like stamps of pre-approval for an applicant.

One of the biggest benefits of presenting at research conferences is that presenting can help earn you one of these fellowships. Take it from someone who has been rejected from plenty of fellowships and accepted to two. The oral and poster presentations I gave legitimized my strong involvement and commitment to my projects. Since most students did not share my strong presentation background, this factor allowed my application to stand out. Everything ends up weaving together to make you one of the strongest research candidates in the application cycle. It takes time, but it pays off.

Research fellowships focus on just that: research. However, this research may be concentrated on basic science, translational, or clinical investigation. Plenty of research fellowships are offered outside of the sciences, but we will zoom in on health-related and science-related programs for our purposes. Clinical fellowships can span the realm of public health and advocacy and may intertwine with research or volunteer work. Civic service/public health fellowships are given their own category but often overlap with clinical work.

In *Appendix B*, you'll find a nearly comprehensive list of clinical and research summer fellowships. Additionally, for a far less comprehensive list, *Appendix C* lists post-baccalaureate and academic term clinical and research fellowships. These programs encompass clinical work, science- and medical-based research, as well as public health and epidemiological research. Don't hesitate to do your own searching, as there certainly were programs I missed - particularly post-baccalaureate and academic term programs.

Below are my application essays to WashU's BioSURF program and the Chan School's Summer Program in Biostatistics and Computational Biology so you can see what a successful submission looks like. Although I wasn't ultimately chosen for UCSF's Breast Care Center Internship program, I progressed far in the interview process. I will also include this application essay since it did move me through a few stages of UCSF's selection process. Your undergraduate research office may also have a stack of winning applications to these programs for you to view.

Application Essay for Washington University in St. Louis Biology Summer Undergraduate Research Fellowship:

I will be working in Dr. David Holtzman's lab under the mentorship of Tien-Phat Huynh.

Alzheimer's disease (AD) is a progressive, neurodegenerative disease that impairs memory and cognitive function. AD is characterized by amyloid-beta (A-beta) plaques and Tau tangles, which aggregate in the brains of AD patients. The apolipoprotein E (apoE) protein was first found to co-localize with plaques in the brains of AD patients in the early 1990s. Subsequent studies found different alleles (isoforms) of apoE to affect the risk of developing AD. Specifically, the E4 allele significantly increases the risk of developing AD, while the E2 allele is protective relative to the neutral E3 allele. Furthermore, individuals with one apoE4 allele are three times more likely to develop AD, while the risk increases to 12-fold for those with two copies of E4.

I will be working on a project that examines the effect of reducing apoE expression on the deposition of A-beta plaques in the brains of APP/PS1-21 mice, an established mouse model of amyloidosis. Reduction of apoE levels will be achieved by using antisense oligonucleotides (ASOs). Previous work has shown that APP transgenic mice crossed with apoE-/- mice had significantly reduced A-beta plaque deposition. Furthermore, our laboratory showed that APP/PS1 mice with only one copy of human apoE (hemizygous) have significantly fewer A-beta plaques in their brains compared to those with two copies. This finding was con-

sistent regardless of apoE isoform (E2, E3, or E4). Therefore, we hypothesize that lowering apoE in the adult brain using ASOs might reduce A-beta plaque deposition in this mouse model.

Twenty (10 male, 10 female) APP/PS1 mice carrying various isoforms of human APOE (APP/PS1/TRE) will be used in the study. These mice will be injected with ASOs dissolved in phosphate-buffered saline (PBS) in their right lateral ventricles at six weeks of age. At six weeks of age, the mice have reached adulthood, while A-beta pathology has yet to be detected. These mice will then be given a booster ASO dose at 11 weeks of age. There will be two control groups of mice. The control groups will be treated with either a non-specific ASO (nASO) with similar base length and chemical properties as anti-apoE ASOs or with PBS (vehicle control).

Brains from these mice will be harvested at 16 weeks of age when A-beta pathology is detectable. The right hemisphere will be used for immunohistochemical (IHC) studies, which stain for A-beta plaques. The left hemisphere will be used for PCR, western blotting, and ELISA assays. One-way ANOVAs will be used to determine the statistical significance of the study's findings.

We expect to observe at least a fifty percent reduction of apoE levels in the brains of mice treated with ASOs. This reduction should be consistent across all apoE isoforms (E3 or E4). Furthermore, we expect to observe a reduction of A-beta plaque in the brains of mice treated with ASOs.

If we do not observe lowered A-beta plaque formation in our mice, then this could be due to the different time points at which apoE is reduced via treatment in our study (6 weeks of age) compared to our previous study using the APOE hemizygous mice (day of birth). Consistent with this explanation, mice may need to be treated with ASOs earlier in their lives, as irreversible A-beta pathology may have already taken place at 6 weeks of age. To address this possibility, a separate cohort of mice in our study can be given the ASOs treatment at birth (at P0). Another explanation for non-mitigated A-beta plaque formation in our treatment group is that ASOs may need more time to work to reduce A-beta plaque levels in the brain. To test for this, the ASOs treatment can be extended for 20 weeks prior to analysis.

Application Essay for Harvard T.H. Chan School of Public Health Summer Program in Biostatistics and Computational Biology:

My brown butter cookies are famous. Well, famous among my family. I was shipping them off to be enjoyed back home, but I would not let the cookies crumble en route this time. I grabbed at the inky pages of The Wall Street Journal and then crumpled and stuffed them into the mustard yellow envelope containing my carefully constructed disks of flour and sugar. That's when it caught my eye. Printed on my impromptu cushioning was an article that would change what I saw myself investigating as a researcher.

The article, written by Professor Arthur Kleinman, who teaches medical anthropology at Harvard, discusses the two systems comprising the medical realm: the disease and illness systems. The disease system: all of the professionals and their facilities and treatment plans that tackle illness and injury when curable. But what happens to the chronic cases – those ill and injured who will not recover? They are swept into the illness system – a system that Professor Kleinman argues does not exist and is, at most, a shadow. He defines the illness system as a messy collage of in-home care, underpaid and overworked professional caregivers, hospice centers, nursing homes, and distressed, perplexed families trying desperately to navigate a system void of order and guidance.

Professor Kleinman and I were acquainted with the illness system through common tragedy. His wife and my grandfather quietly lost themselves to Alzheimer's dementia. And us losing them – standing watch, perfectly helpless.

For the past three and a half years, I have researched Alzheimer's disease at Washington University School of Medicine under the mentorship of Dr. David Holtzman – chairman of the neurology department. Somewhere in the mess of discarded pipette tips and fractured beakers, I discovered that I wanted to use research to help those with Alzheimer's and bring ease to families losing someone to dementia.

I thought wet-lab research was the only way for me to make a meaningful impact in the race to rectify dementia. After all, this was the only type of Alzheimer's-related research that I had been exposed to. That is until I learned about the power of bio-

statistics and how it could be used to create a scaffolding for the illness system first to exist and then flourish.

As my grandfather's memories faded and he became increasingly trapped in an inescapable past that now comprised his reality, my family waded wearily into the illness system. Like many others, we were left with instinct to guide us as nascent caregivers. We, like many others, had too many questions and too few answers.

When, during the course of the disease, do we take Grandpa's keys away? When can we no longer rely on his cognitive capacity to tell him when to take his medication and how much he is supposed to take? When is it no longer safe for him to live on his own?

According to the National Council on Aging, "falls are the leading cause of fatal injury and the most common cause of nonfatal trauma-related hospital admissions among older adults." Moreover, individuals with dementia are at especially high risk of falls, as the increase of falls rises as the disease progresses (Dementia and Geriatric Cognitive Disorders, Ballard et al., 1999).

Falling brought with it many questions. When during the course of Alzheimer's does falling risk begin to spike? Which subgroups are at higher risk for falling? How can we, as caregivers, prevent falls from occurring?

My grandfather died in November 2018 from a fatal fall that broke his hip.

During my senior fall semester, I took my first course in bioinformatics, taught by Dr. Craig Smith. I clumsily pecked at my keyboard while learning the basics of coding and soon discovered how statistical programs could be used to answer critical questions about disease. The following term, I begrudgingly trudged into statistics – the last place you would find a second-semester senior. I was stunned. Dr. Liberty Vittert, our statistics professor, was mesmerizing. Her ability to relate our lessons to solving real-world problems was exhilarating. I walked across the graduation stage three months later, wishing I had picked up a third major in mathematics.

The sum of these experiences has helped define my career goals and desire to earn a Ph.D. in biostatistics. My aspiration is to use statistics to answer the critical questions that caregivers — like Professor Kleinman, like my family, like millions of Americans each year — face when navigating the illness system and wanting to make the best choices regarding the care of their loved ones diagnosed with Alzheimer's dementia.

My aim is to not only provide answers using data and statistical models but also to make this information accessible to all people — not just those who wade through complex language and graphs in medical journals to find answers. I want to write a guidebook for caregivers that uses statistics to answer their most pressing questions and concerns, ultimately allowing them to make informed decisions regarding care. I want these informed decisions to be the ones that work best for their family and for their goals. Not everyone chooses in-home care. Not everyone chooses memory care facilities. Both choices have their merits and their drawbacks. But whatever choice an overwhelmed family makes when navigating the illness system, I want them to have confidence and comfort in these incredibly difficult decisions.

Participating in the Harvard Chan Post-Baccalaureate Internship in Biostatistics would be an empowering first step in this direction. Working with faculty such as Professor Milton Weinstein, Dr. Marcia Testa, or Professor Giovanni Parmigiani, whose research uses biostatistics to help individuals make informed choices regarding care, will allow me to learn from experts how I can use Alzheimer's research to accomplish the same objective. By engaging with other students who, like myself, are passionate about using biostatistics to solve health disparities, we will incite conversation that will be indispensable to my graduate study and professional goals.

I thank the committee for taking the time to review my application.

Application Essay for University of California San Francisco Breast Care Center Internship Program:

I aspire not only to be a physician but an outstanding physician. Yet, what defines those who are truly remarkable in the medical profession? Physicians are intelligent and possess a strong work ethic by nature. Many of the best physicians are empathetic, compassionate, dedicated to service, have integrity, and *listen and respond thoughtfully to their patients' questions and concerns. I would argue, though, that the remarkable physician does one thing that distinguishes her from her cohort: she pushes the bounds of the medical field. Interning at the UCSF Carol Franc Buck Breast Care Center would give me the experience to do just that.*

An individual can impact medicine in a number of ways: expanding current medical knowledge through clinical or basic research, providing care to medically underserved populations, or perhaps guiding communities in taking action to lower risks of chronic illness – currently the leading cause of death among our populous. The medical field is an indispensable asset in the United States and comprises the country's brightest minds. However, the innumerable ways medicine can transcend its current state to serve future generations better make the field particularly compelling to me.

UCSF and, notably, the Carol Franc Buck Breast Care Center embody the mission of what I consider to be pushing the bounds of medicine. The Buck Breast Care Center takes a three-pronged approach to bettering the current state of breast health. By advancing our current knowledge of breast cancer through research, providing less toxic and more effective treatments to patients, and preventing greater numbers of individuals from developing breast cancer through early screening and enhanced detection, the physicians at the BCC strive to perfect modern medicine. Furthermore, Dr. Laura Esserman has, throughout her career, worked to progress breast health and breast care. She has impacted clinical care through her efforts in both public policy and basic science. As an intern, I would seek and cultivate Dr. Esserman's mentorship along with the mentorships of all program faculty, as I am determined to follow in the footsteps of remarkable physicians.

For over a decade, the BCC Internship Program that Dr. Esserman founded has provided a standout opportunity for aspiring health professionals like myself to learn from and work alongside leading breast health experts and obtain an in-depth understanding of the gamut of medical specialties. This program is uncommon in that Dr. Esserman and her colleagues shape the careers of future health specialists markedly early in their professional journeys – something I see as critical to the mold-

ing of the outstanding physician. Few programs offer year-long or two-year-long patient care exposure to post-baccalaureates. Even fewer programs couple patient care with projects in basic science and clinical research, along with collaboration in decision-making processes to offer students a comprehensive medical internship. Learning first-hand how patient care, clinical research, and basic science work harmoniously to achieve improved health outcomes is a lesson that I find incredibly valuable, as thus far, my experiences in research and patient care, while enriching, have been separate.

For the past 3.5 years, I have researched Alzheimer's disease under the mentorship of Dr. David Holtzman – chairman of the neurology department at Washington University School of Medicine. Through this work, I have gained experience learning how to conduct and troubleshoot research experiments as well as how to effectively communicate my scientific findings to a breadth of audiences. Functioning as part of a team of physicians, post-doctoral fellows, and graduate students has been paramount to my success in the lab. Additionally, I work with individuals in the memory care units at two senior living homes located in St. Louis and Portland in order to gain a clinical perspective on the challenges faced by our aging population. As someone passionate about caring for older individuals, I see how age is critically linked to the risk of disease acquisition. Similar to AD, the risk of developing breast cancer increases as one ages. The majority of breast cancer diagnoses occur after age 50, with 80% of cases diagnosed among women aged 45 and older (Center for Disease Control). Even among men, the risk of developing breast cancer rises with age, with most male cases diagnosed between ages 60 and 70 (UCSF Department of Surgery). Providing outstanding medical care to our ever-growing aging population and addressing the novel medical challenges we confront as human beings live longer is where I choose to dedicate my medical career.

In addition to caring for the aging population, I am devoted to addressing the health of medically underserved individuals. Like St. Louis, San Francisco has a large and growing homeless population. This past fall, I founded Mission to Provide Nutrition (MPN) – an organization that responds to a crisis of hunger among St. Louis's homeless community by making and distrib-

uting nutrient-rich energy bites. I began this work in response to witnessing a rise in the number of individuals in need of resources surrounding the undergraduate and medical campuses at Washington University in St. Louis. MPN partners with three community organizations in St. Louis that provide shelter to those without housing to deliver energy bites to their residents. My work with St. Louis's homeless population has given me insight into the health risks posed to a medically underserved population – particularly those related to nutrition-related health risks. Furthermore, as a Hispanic American woman, I am acutely aware of the health risks posed to minority populations, such as their excess burden of breast carcinoma (American Cancer Society; National Cancer Institute). I have seen the consequences of these health risks play out not only in the St. Louis community but also among members of my family.

My experiences helping to advance medical knowledge through basic science, as well as working directly with the aging and medically underserved populations, have helped to define my career goals. As an aspiring future physician, my aim is to provide the best care to members of my community. Specifically, I am eager to work with aging populations of high need in order to address their higher risks of debilitating illness. I plan to accomplish this objective by confronting obstacles and questions as both a physician and a researcher.

Participating in the BCC Internship Program would be an empowering first step in this direction. As an intern, I would spend my year at UCSF becoming immersed in the multiple facets my peers and I will be exposed to of the medical profession – notably through patient interactions and our research projects. Working with and learning from the BCC faculty to gain insight into how clinical research directly impacts patient care will formalize my own research objectives when confronted with critical questions. Engaging with other interns who share my passion for caring for medically underserved populations will incite conversation and discussion that will be indispensable to our graduate study and professional goals. Ultimately, my year at UCSF prior to medical school will help build me into the physician I aspire to be – a remarkable physician capable of compassionate care, empathetic listening, and bettering the state of illness outcomes for future generations to come.

VOLUNTEERING

Volunteering comes in two varieties. Or two ~flavors~ as my former biology professor would put it. Shout out to you, Professor Duncan. The two flavors of volunteering are clinical and non-clinical. Clinical volunteering means working with people living with a particular illness or injury. Non-clinical volunteering is everything else!

We explored clinical volunteering in the *Clinical Experiences* section. Scoot your eyes upward for the goodies. Mommy's not in a repeating mood. Since clinical volunteering is completed above, we will just talk about non-clinical volunteering. Some of the most common types of non-clinical volunteering among undergraduates are tutoring, mentoring, and participating in programs like Habitat for Humanity and Relay for Life. What I love about non-clinical volunteering is that it's a great time to explore your interests outside of medicine, science, and patient care. Medical schools will be able to see that you're passionate about more than health through this type of work.

Mentorship was my biggest passion in this category. I served as a Washington University Student Associate for over 70 first-year students during my sophomore year. This role was a peer mentorship position where I worked with students to provide support and guidance through any personal or academic struggles. My sophomore and junior summers were spent planning and running one of WashU's orientation programs for our incoming students. Mentorship for our new students was an integral part of this orientation program. Although working as a teaching assistant was a paid position, I spent time counseling my students both in and out of the classroom. Guiding and cheering on others was a favorite way to give back to the WashU community. I was grateful for my mentors, who generously supported me in pursuing a career in medicine. Although this was not on my medical school application, currently I volunteer with WashU's Alumni and Parents Admissions Program, where we interview prospective students for WashU's undergraduate program. I plan to continue as an alumni interviewer for years to come, as I love meeting the incoming cohort of WashU students. Whatever you involve yourself in when volunteering in a non-clinical context, choose something that you truly enjoy, and feel free to stray from your narrative!

SHADOWING

Shadowing is another one of those boxes to check. But unlike your research, leadership, and volunteering, shadowing is rarely remarkable. Medical schools ask for shadowing to ensure their matriculants know what a physician's career looks like beyond the glamorized portrayals on *House M.D.* and *Grey's Anatomy*. Shadowing is much more of a box you can check than other activities where your involvement should be meaningful. Recently, some schools have eliminated hour expectations for shadowing after realizing that lower-income students have far less access to shadowing compared to middle- and upper-income students. Johns Hopkins has been quite vocal about these changes, and many schools have followed their lead (All Access: Med School Admissions Podcast).

On public forums, I have often seen the advice given that applicants need 50, 80, or even 100+ hours of shadowing physicians. These numbers are a gross overestimate. I applied to medical school with 31 shadowing hours, and no one batted an eye. Not my premed advisors, not the admissions officers, not my interviewers – nobody cared. Honestly, I think 20+ hours of shadowing is sufficient. Admissions officers know that shadowing is physicians doing *you* a favor. It's no great feat on the applicant's part.

Don't let not knowing physicians keep you from observing their work. Ask to watch any doctors associated with your research or volunteer initiatives. Request if your mentors can connect you to physicians. Even reach out to your own doctors to see if they have availability to bring you into the clinic. If all of these approaches wash out, a final tactic is to cold-call and email clinics and private practices. Do not get discouraged if you do not hear back or someone says no. Keep calling and keep emailing until you have made 100 contact efforts. Dr. Ryan Gray, founder of Medical School Headquarters, gives his students the "100 reach outs" advice; I think he is spot on. Pick up that phone and drop some lines!

Once again, think about your personal narrative when choosing who to shadow. If women's health is your jam, observe the work of OB/GYN doctors. If you enjoy surgery, ask to shadow within a few different surgical specialties. Since my narrative was grounded in geriatrics, I shadowed a neurologist (my PI) and a geriatrician (used my network to meet her). Don't feel pressured only to seek physicians whose work fits your narrative. Get a variety! I also shadowed in an emergency room as well as in a neonatology unit. Just be sure that at least one of the physicians you observe is doing something close to your interest. That way, medical schools won't be confused as to why you discuss your dedication to pediatrics but have only shadowed urologists.

VARSITY SPORTS

During my freshman orientation at WashU, one of our best premed advisors, Dr. Joan Downey, spoke to us about what it takes to get into medical school. Dr. Downey is a gifted neonatologist, a graduate of Harvard Medical School, and a former admissions officer at Harvard Medical School. She knows her stuff! In her talk, Dr. Downey noted that the *only specific* activity that correlated with a higher chance of admittance into medical school was playing a varsity sport (The Components of a Successful Applicant: Q&A Session).

Before you all grab your hockey sticks and tennis rackets, know that playing a varsity sport was only marginally helpful when examining matriculant statistics. Dr. Downey explained that admissions officers were impressed that varsity athletes were able to play a competitive sport while also succeeding in their premed endeavors. I think it is a feat to play a varsity sport, ace your science classes, and complete all of your other extracurriculars to the satisfaction of medical schools. At the same time, I believe that most premeds who try to compete in sports at a demanding level struggle and often fail to balance athletics, grades, and activities.

As a first year, I planned on playing varsity golf for WashU as a walk-on. Once I received our practice schedule, I soon began to understand that I would either need to sacrifice my grades or my golf career. I couldn't balance the academic rigors of WashU with golf. Some of my premed classmates who played varsity athletics couldn't balance science classes with their athletic schedule and ended up not pursuing a career in medicine. Other students whom I knew did, in fact, play four years of varsity athletics and went on to be admitted into top medical schools. The ability to balance athletics with the premedical curriculum depends on the individual. My one piece of advice is not to sacrifice your dream of becoming a doctor for a college athletic career.

I'll end this section by stating that chess is not a sport. Neither is video gaming. Disagree? Fight me.

GREEK LIFE

Gotta give props to Greek life. Sororities and fraternities make for strong friendships. I was never a part of Greek life at WashU, and at times, I regretted not joining when I saw how close women were to their sisters. Bigs and littles, grand bigs and grand littles. These were the types of friendships that I longed for. If you are considering joining a sorority or fraternity in college, it may be one of the best things you do. Or the worst. DUN DUN DUN! Kidding... toootally kidding.

On a more serious note, I want to touch on how Greek life affected a few of my classmates and their medical school prospects. The short of it is that sororities and fraternities with a lot of hazing, many required events, or those in which you are required to live in the chapter's housing can put a dent in your grades and ability to partake in other activities. This was the case for two of my promising classmates.

Both young men were nearly straight-A students at WashU from day one. An uncommon achievement. They both aspired to attend top medical schools and were on track to do so. Both men joined fraternities during their sophomore years and became heavily involved in the brotherhoods' social activities. Let's name these two men "Adam" and "Mick."

Adam's fraternity was big on hazing. Because of this, his grades plummeted to an all-time low during his sophomore fall. Intensive science classes, which Adam could once handle with ease, were soon out of reach. He struggled to get Bs. Beyond sophomore year, Adam's involvement in non-Greek life activities never recovered. When he applied to medical schools, the dreams that he had of attending a top research university were likely going to be unrealized. Adam matriculated to the University of Colorado School of Medicine. CU is an excellent medical school, yet it is not what Adam had hoped for and not what he was on track to achieve as a freshman.

Mick's frat was less into hazing but big into social events. Mick's grades did not take a hit in the same way Adam's did – overall, he remained a stellar student. Where Mick struggled was with his extracurricular activities. His fraternity's social events occupied most of Mick's weekly free time, leaving him only with summers to give notable energy to research, leadership, and volunteering. Although Mick secured an interview with Columbia (Vagelos), he was not admitted and matriculated to the University of Miami (Miller) School of

Medicine. Again, Miller is an outstanding medical school. However, it was not where Mick had aspired to attend.

I totally understand that some of you are scribbling "cry me a river" in the margins. Both Adam and Mick ended up at great medical schools — an incredible accomplishment considering how competitive the application process is. However, their anecdotes are something you should consider if your dream is to attend a top twenty medical school — just as Adam's and Mick's dreams were. Each organization we join takes up part of our time and thus limits what we can give ourselves to other activities. While Greek life makes for amazing friendships, it is not necessarily an activity that will significantly impact your application. Sometimes, I wonder if Adam and Mick wish that they would have set stronger bounds on time spent with their fraternities. What would they have done with this extra time? Would they have ended up at their dream medical schools?

With USLME Step 1 going pass/fail, those wanting to match into competitive specialties may choose to attend more prestigious medical schools since research and, possibly, school reputation may take more of a front seat with the vacancy left by Step 1 scores. My dad wanted me to title this section "Greek Life: Where Premeds Go to Die." This subtitle would have been hilarious, but I don't think things are all doom and gloom for pledged premeds. Plenty of my classmates who were in sororities are attending top medical schools. Their successes may have something to do with sororities at WashU not being housed while fraternities are housed. Physical separation from the sisterhood seemed to give these women more agency with their time and likely allowed them to build a more balanced schedule while maintaining their grades. I know fraternity members who went to the best medical school programs — yet, in general, men in fraternities seemed to have their premed ambitions more easily derailed than women in sororities. No matter what you choose with regard to Greek life, be sure to prioritize academics and other activities. Enjoy the friendships you will build — it sounds like a wonderful place to grow life-long relationships.

<u>Insider tip</u>: I've heard through the grapevine that applicants are advised to leave Greek life off of their medical school applications. The primary reason cited is that some admissions officers have perceptions of Greek life grounded in partying and drinking. Regardless of whether there is truth to that perception, I would check with your premed advisor if Greek life should be left off of your application.

Think about your personal narrative, too. Many chapters are involved in strong volunteer efforts, and you may have a leadership position within your sorority or fraternity. If this is the case, then you might want to include Greek life on your application. Check with your advisor and mentors. Greek life leadership certainly impressed Harvard Law School admissions for Elle Woods!

LEADERSHIP

Leadership is the siren song for the top 20 medical schools (a.k.a. the drooling sailors). Because top medical schools search for students who will become the next leaders in medicine, your past leadership experiences are given substantial consideration. In this section, we will chat about the different leadership options available to you.

Joining Clubs and Running for Leadership

Colleges today are home to a plethora of clubs. Activities fairs are crowded with dozens of tables teeming with enthusiastic students ready to greet and recruit any passerby. At WashU, we had clubs open to everyone and others that were selective with membership. I believe most universities have a similar mix of open and select clubs.

As a first year, I tested out several clubs that spoke to my interests: cooking, political discussion, and journalism. Soon, my time became crowded with studying, and I had to narrow these prospects. Because I was passionate about mentorship and enjoyed writing, I joined AcStart – a publication grounded in helping underclassmen. AcStart was a student-written guide to the introductory classes at WashU. The guide was intended to help students choose a balanced course load and aid them in succeeding academically in those classes. I believe, for many students, we achieved our mission.

AcStart was one of those clubs that you had to apply for. I submitted my application for a number of positions and was offered an interview with the co-founders. Now, there are two keys here that we need to address. First, put time and effort into the applications for selective clubs. Second, prepare for the interview, make sure you have questions to ask the interviewers and dress the part. Because of these tips, I was offered the co-Editor-in-Chief position and very much enjoyed the year and a half I spent with the organization.

Browse your university's clubs and try out several that excite you. Clubs do not have to fit within your personal narrative. Mentoring younger students made me happy, and it had nothing to do with aging adults and dementia.

While I was thrilled to join AcStart, I also want to acknowledge that there were many organizations that I applied to join but was not admitted to. Among them were Uncle Joe's (a peer counseling group), GlobeMed (a non-profit dedicated to global health), and Alpha Epsilon Delta (a pre-health honorary). There are plenty more clubs, scholarships, and awards that I tried for and didn't earn – we will go over these in the *Resume of Failures* section. Although there are many organizations to which I was not admitted, I was consistently invited to the final round of interviews. This is why putting effort into your applications and preparing for your interviews are essential. Sometimes, things will go your way, and other times, they won't, but the victory is in putting forth your best effort regardless of the outcome.

Transitioning to club leadership, I highly recommend running for these positions. My one experience with this was running for the President of Psi Chi (The National Honor Society in Psychology). Like many psychology majors, I was inducted into WashU's Psi Chi chapter during my sophomore year. Junior spring, our chapter's leadership invited members to apply for executive board positions. Although we had never considered running, my suitemate and I submitted our applications, interviewed, and were selected as chapter co-presidents. The dirty secret is that we were two of three people applying for executive board positions that year. We didn't know this when we applied, but that's one of the beauties about applying for leadership positions. More often than not, you may be one of two people vying for a spot. The process of running is certainly anxiety-provoking and intimidating since we are putting ourselves out there for critique and possible rejection. However, we learn to make ourselves better through the losses, and in moments of triumph, we truly rejoice.

Above, I noted that one of the clubs I tested out surrounded political discussion. Almost every campus seems to have similar organizations through College Republicans and College Democrats. Politics can be a lot of fun to join in on. Yet, when choosing which activities to list on your AMCAS application, it may be safer to leave political organizations off. Since the political divide in our country has grown distressingly wide in recent years, someone reading your application may have a bias against your perceived political affiliation. I wish we lived in a world where our differing thoughts and opinions weren't a risk to our education and careers. Still, I wouldn't want anyone sacrificing their chances at a medical school because of political affiliation. Check with your premed advisor regarding their advice on political clubs.

Starting Your Own Organization

The wide variety of clubs that exist on college campuses is a blessing. Students before you invested considerable effort into gathering their peers around a shared joy. There are times, though, when you may find yourself with a new idea for a group that does not exist. Beginning your own organization can allow you to address problems your community has not touched. Or perhaps, bring fans of hard fruit together for conversation and snacks. Yes, the Hard Fruit Club really does exist. One of my former classmate's brothers is a founding member at his university.

I founded no clubs as an undergraduate, but I did start a volunteer effort and an online service during my gap years. By describing how I began my own organization, I hope to inspire and guide you on starting your own initiative (if this interests you).

Here is the process by which I began a volunteer effort post-graduation. As I began spending more time off campus during my junior and senior undergraduate years, I noticed the stark rise in the number of homeless individuals needing food. I wanted to help these community members but didn't know how. Soon after graduation, I combined my love of baking with aiding the homeless crisis in St. Louis. It was then that the Energy Bite Project was founded. The idea was to make a delicious, nutrient-rich snack called an energy bite and deliver them to people in need of food. Energy bites can be left for two weeks unrefrigerated, so they were a useful option to give to those without homes. First, I reached out to over a dozen homeless shelters throughout St. Louis to see if they would be interested in receiving the energy bites. Three responded, and after a few rounds of correspondence, we moved forward as partners for the initiative. Second, I pursued funding for the Energy Bite Project from WashU's Gephardt Institute, which offered Small Change Grants. Despite meeting with Gephardt staff and pouring thought and intention into the application, I didn't receive the grant. The lack of funding was a setback, but it was important to continue the effort. For several months, I was able to fund the project myself since I had a job at the time. It was delightful meeting the people in charge of the different shelters, seeing their work, and meeting the men and women who lived there.

COVID hit in Spring 2020, soon after I had moved out of St. Louis and back home to Portland, Oregon. This was halfway through my first gap year. Since then, I have been able to send out several more rounds of bites via mail. Although I don't know what the future of the Energy Bite Project looks like, I am humbled to have made a small contribution to the hunger affecting our homeless community members in St. Louis.

Reflecting on how to make your own organization a success, pursue more funding opportunities than I did. Had I still been an undergraduate student, I would have sought funding from the robust Student Union Treasury budget, which supports nearly all campus clubs. Additionally, work on recruiting members to join your group. Offering leadership positions within your club is an effective strategy to attract new members. Being alone in St. Louis after graduation was not the most conducive environment to recruit people to join the Energy Bite Project. Again, had I been an undergraduate, I would've advertised the volunteer initiative and strove to get others involved. That way, once I left St. Louis, there would've been a team to keep the initiative running at high capacity.

Now, let's turn to how I founded an online service organization during my gap years. Returning to Portland in early 2020, I wanted to continue being involved with the well-being of older adults. I had just wrapped up my time at the Holtzman lab, where my mentor and I had researched Alzheimer's disease together since my sophomore year. Once more, I volunteered with older adults in memory care units. Speaking with the residents and their families allowed me to notice many people's confusion when making decisions surrounding eldercare.

Was it best for a family's loved one to remain in a long-term care facility? What were the risks of an aging adult living at home? How could caregivers mitigate the risks of at-home living if someone preferred to age-in-place?

These questions contrasted with the vast amounts of literature I was exposed to as an Alzheimer's researcher. I knew that useful information was out there regarding the health and care of our elders. Yet, this information seemed not to reach those who needed it most. It was this dichotomy that inspired my father and I to co-found

CaregiverZone. If anyone's wondering where my dad comes into the picture, he works in healthcare technology. Specifically, he focuses on developing technologies to help older adults age safely and successfully at home.

CaregiverZone, which I co-founded in 2020, is an online service dedicated to helping older adults and their loved ones make personalized, informed, and confident decisions surrounding eldercare (www.caregiverzone.com). By writing simplified, comprehensible articles on leading aging research, CaregiverZone brings our readers the vast empirical knowledge surrounding healthy aging. Our goal is to meet our audience where they are by boiling down dense and often inaccessible scientific findings into understandable insights. Helping answer the pressing questions that aging adults and their families are faced with regarding eldercare is our mission.

In addition to our website, CaregiverZone engages with our readers and leaders in geriatrics on Twitter. In 2020, CaregiverZone was humbled to be featured in Cambia Grove's Impactful Innovation Exchange (https://www.cambiagrove.com/caregiverzone). I plan to continue producing new content for CaregiverZone throughout medical school.

What are the takeaways from CaregiverZone, which is a much different endeavor compared to the Energy Bite Project? Beginning an online effort is quite manageable as it usually requires less funding than physically tangible projects. There is such a disconnect between the sea of knowledge available in academia and the everyday person. Starting an online advocacy group or resource is one way to help merge these disparate worlds.

Although I co-founded CaregiverZone only months before beginning my primary applications, imagine what progress and impact you could make if you began a similar effort during your freshman or sophomore year of college. Your work could turn into something outstanding and helpful to people.

Of final note – while CaregiverZone fit within my larger narrative of caring for older adults, the Energy Bite Project did not. Starting your own organization that sits behind your narrative is certainly compelling. Such an effort speaks to the definitive intention behind helping a particular population or those living with a certain illness or injury. No matter what you choose – either to begin a group related to or not related to your narrative – just be sure you are choosing something heartfelt. Your ardent devotion is what will make your organization stand out and will help it endure as years pass by.

Leadership is well-captured among those who venture out to begin their own initiative. Medicine, for all its glory, still needs fixing. Medical schools search for students who dare to pursue the foreign and unexplored. Therefore, leadership through entrepreneurship makes for a compelling applicant.

Teaching Assistant Positions

I'm curious to learn how teaching assistant (TA) positions are viewed at other institutions. At WashU, becoming a TA is highly coveted. In part, this may be because they are paid positions. Or perhaps because they make a resume sparkle. From most of the TAs I've worked with, it seems they pursued the job because they love teaching and helping fellow students learn.

Hearing from admissions officers, many medical school matriculants have worked as teaching assistants. What about serving as a TA makes an applicant compelling to medical schools, and how does the position relate to leadership? Both of these questions can be answered by thinking about what TAs do. If selected as a teaching assistant, it shows that you have mastered the subject matter. More importantly, the position shows a willingness and competency to communicate this complex academic information to other people. Medicine is all about experts teaching their students. The phrase is overused, but doctors really are life-long learners. **Admissions committees are enthusiastic about teaching assistants because medicine is grounded in teaching and learning.** The leadership required to guide students to further understand complex information is the same leadership required to teach medicine. Throughout our careers and even as medical students, we will teach ourselves, our own students, and our patients.

Senior year, I was fortunate to TA two classes – once each semester. In the fall of 2018, I TAed two laboratory sections of Principles of Biology II, the second course in WashU's introductory biology series. This position I applied for at the end of my junior year. To be considered, you must have earned an A in the class and explained why you were eager to help teach the course. In the spring of 2019, I TAed Introduction to Biochemistry. After seeing that I had done well in the course, one of my professors and mentors taught this class and asked me to work as his teaching assistant. No matter how TA positions are distributed at your school, message the professor of a course that you enjoy and have done well in to see if you can get the job. Some of my favorite students are those whom I met through TAing – I strongly recommend the role for you to consider.

Tutoring

Like TAing, tutoring is about helping others understand the information you have mastered. Tutoring can be either a job or volunteer work. One effective letter of recommendation to receive could be from one of your tutoring students. I'm unsure how medical schools view tutoring compared to TAing, but TAing holds a bit more prestige for me. Teaching assistants are selected by a professor who holds them to a standard of excellence. Perhaps I am biased because I have worked with a fair share of for-profit tutors who were not experts in their discipline, but I think tutors' competency range varies widely. A letter from a student you tutored may help establish your credibility. In short, tutoring is similar to working as a teaching assistant, and many medical school matriculants were also former tutors.

Mentoring

Mentoring students is a great way to give back to your university's community. As you have picked up by now, I was enthusiastically involved with mentorship as an undergraduate. My caring mentors had continuously supported me as a student aspiring to become a physician. Becoming that person to another student was my ambition following my freshman year. I served as a peer mentor to over 70 first-year students throughout my sophomore year. I and the other peer mentors were formally known as Washington University Student Associates (WUSAs for short). Everything from helping with roommate conflicts to brainstorming study strategies and helping students build their schedules to guiding those with academic infractions, I hold dear the time I spent with my first-year cohort. These students helped me feel grounded and purposeful, and I am thankful for their trust in me as their mentor. If peer mentorship is available at your university, it's a fulfilling way to contribute – definitely look into it. If peer mentorship is not available at your university, consider starting your own mentorship group! Prerak Juthani, a current student at Yale School of Medicine and YouTuber, started a peer mentorship organization years ago at UC Berkeley, and it is still running strong today!

Another two mentorship opportunities are volunteering with your college's orientation committee and working as a residential advisor. We will get into working as an RA below. Becoming involved with the orientation committee allows you to welcome new students and their families to campus. Students and parents alike are excited, anxious, and looking forward to speaking with current students. Being a part of the orientation team shows that you are an ideal representative of your university and value building a warm and welcoming community for your peers and their loved ones. During my junior and senior summers, I was an orientation counselor for our first-year students. Once again, I met some of my favorite mentees through acting as their counselor. Medical schools enjoy seeing that their applicants have given back to their peers and are enthusiastic about guiding others. So much of medicine is grounded in these two principles. Consider joining your college's orientation committee.

Working as a Resident Advisor

Resident advisors (RA) are a part of one's college life since day one. They welcome you and your family into the dorm and are notorious for shutting down popping parties. When RAs aren't narking on your hooch stash, you can find them guiding and helping their floor of students. Side remark: RAs are known as both resident advisors and resident assistants. Choose whichever term floats your boat. WashU calls them resident advisors, so that's what I'll use.

I am curious as to how sought-after the RA positions are at your university. At WashU, they are battled over like the last piece of crispy bacon at Sunday brunch. WashU students are obsessed with becoming RAs. There are the obvious perks of free housing and meal plans. Yet, I think most of my peers pursue the role for the rich connections they will build with their students.

A tremendous amount of responsibility is placed on resident advisors. They are responsible for the welfare of many younger students. They guide people through the academic stresses of beginning university, living conflicts, homesickness, institutional action, career dilemmas, and much more. Since RAs are carefully vetted to earn their positions, they are almost pre-audited for medical schools. It is known that former RAs can balance tremendous responsibility with academics and extracurricular activities. A strong recommendation from their supervisors will fortify these hunches. If you are considering seeking an RA position in college, it seems like a role that admissions committees love in their matriculants. RAs are proven leaders in their school communities. More than that, they are leaders who are invested in the success of younger students – a useful proficiency considering how much medicine revolves around teaching others. Just as when applying to all other activities that we discuss, put courageous effort into your essays and practice for your interviews.

Before you sign up to be an RA, be sure to understand the time commitments that are expected of you. Like with all activities, don't sacrifice grades or other essential premed extracurriculars in order to be an RA. Working as an RA is certainly impressive to medical schools, yet this accolade alone cannot overcome poor grades or lack of clinical engagement, for example.

Leadership in Research and Volunteering

I was going to end our leadership chapter with resident advisors as the last topic, but I thought I would say a quick word about leadership in research and volunteering. Exploring leadership within research endeavors and volunteer work is a worthwhile task. Medical schools, particularly the top research institutions, value academic investigation and community service. Any leadership you can secure will distinguish you from your cohort of applicants, especially considering that leadership positions in these two activities are not available often. I didn't hold leadership in either my work with the Holtzman lab or time spent volunteering with older adults, but I would have jumped at these roles. Be sure to take advantage of these opportunities are made available.

HONORS AND AWARDS

Dean's List

Each semester (or quarter or trimester), you are eligible to qualify for the Dean's List based on your term grades. Different institutions may have different names for the Dean's List, but nationally, it's a list honoring the school's top academic performers. The cutoffs change from college to college – you will likely have to earn a certain GPA while enrolled in a certain number of credits to qualify. At WashU, the cutoff was earning a 3.60+ GPA while enrolled in 14 or more units.

While qualifying for the Dean's List is common among applicants and won't make you stand out, it helps track academic progress. Graduating with honors in your major is a more notable accomplishment, and consistently making the Dean's List means you're trending well for honors.

Find out your university's requirements for making the List as you begin your first year. These requirements will be a good marker for academic success. Of course, always aim to earn the best grades you can, regardless of the List's cutoffs. From day one at WashU, I always strived for a 4.00, even though I fell below that mark in six out of eight semesters. Out of the eight semesters in college, I made the Dean's List four times: sophomore spring (3.71), junior spring (4.00), senior fall (4.00), and senior spring (3.94). I was below the GPA mark during my freshman fall (3.58), freshman spring (3.19), and sophomore fall (3.58). Junior fall, I was below the credit cutoff (3.90, but only 12 units were taken for credit – I took Spanish P/F). Clearly, you do not need to earn top grades every semester to crush the medical school application cycle. I am certainly a testament to this! As we discussed in the *Recovering From a GPA Blunder* section, the secret with grades is having a strong upward trend. Perfection from day 1 is *not* a requirement to earn a spot in top medical schools.

It is true that the Dean's List won't be the honor that gets you a spot in medical school. Yet, it is useful for earning other awards, scholarships, and honors along the way. As you apply to these other programs throughout college, your Dean's List honorary may help you secure these future scholarships, fellowships, awards, etc. The List is definitely something to strive for!

Senior Thesis

A senior thesis – also known as a capstone requirement – is an original piece of academic research conducted and written during a student's final year of study. It marks the culmination of study in your discipline. Some institutions do, in fact, require the completion of the capstone. The thesis is optional at other schools but may qualify you for special academic distinction or honors. A thesis is typically completed in one's major and under the guidance of a research mentor. Classes are often taken alongside the thesis to keep students on track with their progress and help them produce the final written work.

If you have been conducting research throughout college, one of your projects (or shared project with your mentor) can be the subject matter of your capstone. If you are in your junior year or early in your senior year and want to start a new project, a capstone can often still be completed. For those beginning in this later time frame (junior or senior year), it will be essential to speak with an advisor to plan a project that can be completed in the time remaining and find a mentor to help you through the process. Ideally, those beginning their thesis should start putting the pieces together over the summer before senior year at the latest.

Although I cherished studying psychological and brain sciences, I chose to complete my thesis through the biology department (I was a double major) because I had already completed significant biology-related research throughout my undergraduate years. My mentor and my primary project on Alzheimer's became the content for my capstone. The biology department did not offer a thesis class, so I looked up how theses were written and followed the guidelines. One benefit of completing one's capstone on previously finished work is that all you will have to do senior year is write the paper. This was the case for me, and it saved me considerable strife because of how many tough classes I was enrolled in! Some of my classmates, as well as my sister, chose to complete a new project over senior year and then write their paper. This took a lot of time but can be accomplished with determination.

A capstone was required to graduate with Latin honors – cum laude, magna cum laude, and summa cum laude – at WashU. If you strive to earn Latin honors or to do a thesis, look up what is required early in your academic career so you can be prepared and plan accordingly.

Awards are often given for the best senior theses. Overall best thesis and most innovative project were two of the honors the biology department gave. Students had to have their work nominated for these awards by their mentors, and then a selection committee would choose the winners. My mentor generously nominated me for the best thesis honor; however, it was awarded to one of my peers who discovered a new type of cell and wrote a first-author paper on it. He totally deserved the best thesis because his discovery kicked butt!

Completing a capstone in and of itself is certainly favored by medical schools. It shows devotion to academic research and competence in your area of study. Earning an honor for your thesis work is incredibly impressive and something that is extremely well-regarded by medical schools. Many students whom I have seen matriculate to top research medical schools have won awards for their capstone.

Look up if your university or department gives out these prizes and what the selection process is so that your work can be in the running!

The *Research* section explored what it means to be published as a premedical student and how publications impact your prospects as a medical school applicant. We touched on how publications are notably impressive at the undergraduate level, especially first-author papers. A benefit to completing a thesis is that you have an original work – possibly one that you and your mentor share – that may be able to be submitted for publication. Work with your mentor to identify a journal that could be compelled by your findings. Have several people who are experienced in research read over your work and suggest edits. After the edits are made, follow the journal's guidelines for submission. Even if you are still being considered by the journal by the time you submit primary applications, discuss a potential publication in your primary application. If your paper has been accepted to a journal but is not yet officially published, still include this information in your application. I did this with two papers – one first-author and one second-author work – that were in line to be considered for publishing. As the application cycle progresses, be sure to submit an update to tell your medical schools that your paper has been accepted (if this happens, of course!). Unless anyone directly asks you, there's no need to submit an update saying that your project was not selected for publication.

Many colleges also have student-run research journals that publish the work of the school's students. This can be a great avenue to submit your work and, likely, have it published quickly. If you are submitting to a professional journal, also submit to your student-run journal! That way, you have an egg in two baskets. While student-run journals are at a junior level compared to professional publications, they are still impressive and show initiative for sharing your discoveries with the academic community. WashU has one of these student-run publications and had known before graduation, I absolutely would have submitted several of my projects to the journal.

Graduating With Honors

Is completing a senior thesis required for graduating with honors at your school, too? Or was it just a WashU thing? I feel like other colleges don't make students complete a thesis to earn Latin honors. Anyway, this is the rule at WashU, so if you want Latin honors, you better get researching! There is a ~lesser~ prize for those who didn't do the grunt work of the thesis but had the grades to qualify for Latin honors. These kiddos graduate, instead, with college honors. When beginning college, check the rules for Latin honors at your institution. If a senior thesis is required, it usually takes preplanning and, most likely, the guidance of a research mentor, so you should start preparing at junior spring at the latest.

Latin honors are broken up into three distinctions. They are listed in order of increasing prestige: cum laude, magna cum laude, summa cum laude. Similar to the Dean's List, each school has different cutoffs for the three tiers of Latin honors. For example, you may need a 3.70+ GPA to qualify. Among those with a 3.70+, perhaps only the top 5% earn summa cum laude, the next 25% earn magna cum laude, and the rest earn cum laude. To make matters more complex, different majors might have different grade requirements to earn Latin honors. Unsurprisingly, this was the case for WashU. I decided to complete my thesis and thus qualify for honors through my biology major, not my psychological and brain sciences major. The biology department had its own guidelines for the thesis and for the grades needed to earn honors. Specifically, I needed a 3.65+ overall GPA, a 3.30+ subject-GPA in math, chemistry, and physics courses (this one almost killed me), a 3.30+ subject-GPA in biology courses, and a completed thesis. Yikes. I qualified by the skin of my teeth.

Be sure to check if there are requirements for your major to graduate with honors. Try to find this information early on to plan your class schedules accordingly. Before my last semester of college, I found out that I had below a 3.30 subject-GPA in my math, chemistry, and physics courses. Calculus III and statistics were crammed into my senior spring schedule so I could raise this particular GPA measure above a 3.30. Yet, I needed to earn solid As in both classes to do so. It was my most stressful and nauseating semester because each exam meant so much to me. More planning on my part could have saved me from panic attacks and crying episodes that speckled my final semester. So much for senioritis! In the end, I did end up graduating with cum laude Latin honors in my biology major. This is one of my proudest academic accomplishments, considering my rough start with science classes at WashU.

Phi Beta Kappa is the U.S.'s oldest academic honor society and is often regarded as the most prestigious one (*The Wall Street Journal*). Ten percent of U.S. colleges have Phi Beta Kappa chapters, which are led by professors who are members of the society. These professors usually nominate the top 10% of undergraduate and graduate students to join as members. Undergraduates can receive their invitations during their junior or senior years. Membership to Phi Beta Kappa is highly regarded among medical schools as it shows academic excellence. The society is a separate honor from earning Latin honors, yet there is tremendous overlap between Latin honors recipients and Phi Beta Kappa membership. If you are invited to join, I recommend becoming a member, as it will distinguish you from other applicants. Ask your chapter if there are funds to cover initiation fees if the price is not within budget. There are other academic honor societies similar to Phi Beta Kappa; however, I am unsure how admissions officers look upon these alternatives. As I sit at my desk writing this, I still await my Phi Beta Kappa invitation along with my invitation to attend Hogwarts. Don't worry, loves, I am patient.

University Awards

Universities give a wide variety of prizes to their undergraduate population. These awards are often granted throughout the four years of college, meaning everyone from first-years to seniors is eligible. Some honors are reserved for those in certain classes (i.e., there are awards just for freshmen, just for graduating students, and so on).

The most common awards are given to recognize those with superior academic performance, research (including the senior thesis), volunteer work and community service efforts, personal character, and leadership. Minority and first-generation students are likely eligible for honors that recognize their achievements, as the path to higher education for these two groups can often have its own set of obstacles not experienced by other students.

Nomination processes – by peers, faculty, or staff – are regularly used to determine who is awarded university prizes. Colleges may have a system where students can apply for the honors themselves. I believe that WashU operated primarily by the nomination system. Check to see what awards are available at your university and how candidates are selected. If you think that you would make a strong recipient, perhaps message a close professor, advisor, or mentor to ask for their nomination.

Admissions committees love university prizes. They are like receiving a gold star from your college. Similar to the other achievements we have discussed, many of the top medical school students

I know are recipients of these honors. Of course, if you are not a lucky winner, there is no need to worry. The closest I got to university recognition was being named WashU's first Researcher of the Week!

Academic Scholarships and Fellowships

Academic scholarships and fellowships are given out by universities and by outside organizations. As soon as you can, look up which scholarships your college offers so you can apply for those relevant to you. Most university-based scholarships are typically awarded to incoming first-years. Getting on top of these opportunities so that you can reduce student loan debt is the ideal strategy. Once in college, many schools still award funds to current students — look to see what is available at your school.

Incoming students are eligible for a plethora of academic scholarships given by outside organizations. Cities, states, small companies, and national and global organizations all support selected scholars annually. Websites like Scholarships.com and others can help narrow your search. Funds specifically for those pursuing careers in healthcare, majoring in STEM, graduating from X high school, practicing X religion, etc., are all common. There are so many opportunities that I cannot list them here, but a few hours of research should capture the majority of scholarships you are a great fit for! Make an Excel sheet to keep track of the scholarships, when they open, when they close, the award amount, and your progress.

Once in college, academic fellowships become available — mostly for juniors and seniors. These fellowships are often quite prestigious and are offered through outside organizations. I don't think WashU itself offered general academic fellowships (most were research- or civic service-related). General fellowships mostly fund post-baccalaureate study, and one of the most well-known programs — the Rhodes Scholarship — allows students to study at the University of Oxford following graduation. If you are considering a gap year, completing an academic fellowship is an incredibly impressive way to spend your time before medical school matriculation. The fellowship may take you outside of the United States, which would complicate your schedule for interviewing, but overall, it should be worth a few lost hours of sleep to interview from abroad! Several of my classmates joined the Fulbright Scholars Program during their gap years and seemed to have outstanding experiences!

A list of outside fellowships is often available via your college, as several of the programs require university nominations. If not available, an hour of research should allow you to find most opportunities out there. Once you have found which programs interest you, see if you can consult an advisor at your school to help put together a competitive application. WashU employed an advisor who was in charge of these large fellowships, as she would help match students to programs and guide them through the extensive application process.

Any scholarship or fellowship is an exciting opportunity that will distinguish you from your peers. Medical schools love seeing these on applications. As an incoming student at WashU, I was awarded their Thomas H. Eliot Scholarship and also brought with me the Andy Grove Scholarship from Intel Corporation. Post-baccalaureate fellowships are the most impressive among academic awards and are absolutely worth pursuing! Note that many require two gap years, so do some pre-planning if you want to apply. If research fellowships are gold goose eggs, academic fellowships are often platinum goose eggs. Being a Rhodes Scholar can get you an interview at nearly every medical school. At a number of my interviews with top research schools, fellow interviewees were Fulbright Scholars or recipients of similar fellowships. Halfway through my senior year, I thought I would only be taking one gap year before I realized two would work best for my application timeline. If I had known that I would be taking two gap years sooner rather than later, I would likely have applied for post-baccalaureate academic fellowships. Do better than me and think things out further in advance.

Research Honors, Scholarships, and Fellowships

Touched on in the *List of Research, Clinical, and Public Health Fellowships* section, research honors, scholarships, and fellowships are golden goose eggs of medical school applications. These give admissions committees great confidence in your prowess as a scholar and student researcher. Top research universities gravitate toward strong research backgrounds among applicants. Earning a research honor, scholarship, or fellowship gives a lot of credibility to your investigative credentials.

Where do we find these opportunities? All three – honors, scholarships, and fellowships – are available at most universities. Honors are typically given to graduating seniors and usually revolve around having a standout thesis. Thesis awards are discussed in detail in the *Honors and Awards* section. At WashU, a more casual honor was Undergraduate Researcher of the Week, where a recipient would discuss her projects with an interviewer, and then the interview write-up would be available via a university-wide publication. Yours truly was the first WashU student to be selected as Undergraduate Researcher of the Week!

Numerous colleges provide scholarships and fellowships to fund students' full-time summer research, although year-round awards can be available as well. One of the undergraduate schools that I was admitted to was Cornell University, and at the time of acceptance, I was awarded a research stipend for academic year research. Totally groovy. Unfortunately, I did not recognize the value of this stipend when I was admitted because I was a bit clueless. Heavy sigh. I learned with time! If you are awarded a similar stipend, either take it or ask another university to match it. I would enthusiastically say research fellowship programs are one of the best ways to spend your undergraduate summers. It is typically easier to be awarded one of your college's research fellowships compared to those of outside programs. At WashU, we have a number of fellowships reserved for entirely or mostly WashU undergraduates. I participated in the Biology Summer Undergraduate Research Fellowship (BioSURF) program during my sophomore summer. Becoming immersed in my mentor's and my project was fantastic and eventually led to a publication. Make sure to apply for these if research interests you. Have your mentor look over your application. These programs help make you competitive for top research medical schools.

Outside universities and larger organizations will also offer research scholarships and fellowships. The Amgen Scholars Program, The National Institutes of Health (NIH) Undergraduate Scholarship Program and the MARC U-STAR Scholarship program are three of the most notable around the country. However, there are plenty of these opportunities, which I have done my best to list to completion in the *List of Research, Clinical, and Public Health Fellowships* section. Each of these fellowships is outstanding and is, again, a golden goose egg worth pursuing. Completing one of these programs during your junior summer, senior summer, or during a gap year (perhaps after participating in your university's own fellowship) is excellent planning. I attempted to participate in Amgen during my junior summer (following my BioSURF sophomore summer) but wasn't selected. I got my comeuppance during my first gap year summer – a.k.a. one year after I graduated, a.k.a. the summer when I submitted my medical school applications – when I participated in the Harvard Chan School's Biology and Computational Biology Undergraduate Research Fellowship. Revenge was sweet.

If you are wondering what made me a competitive applicant for the Chan program when I was not selected for Amgen, I have a few insights. Firstly, when I applied for Amgen, I was only a psychological and brain sciences major and not yet a biology major as well. Since Amgen is geared toward people in the hard sciences, I don't think that I was taken as seriously with my psychological and brain sciences major. Two – my GPA was lower when I applied to Amgen (~3.50) compared to when I applied to the Chan program (3.74). Three – I had far more impressive research credentials when I applied to the Chan fellowship: four papers that were published or submitted for publication, five research presentations at regional and national conferences, and three and a half years spent researching Alzheimer's disease.

Looking back, what would I have done to make myself more competitive for Amgen? What can you do to make yourself competitive for any program? Publications and years of research experience are factors you have no or little control over. Focus on earning top-notch grades (especially if you are a non-hard sciences major like I was with psychology) and perhaps add a hard sciences major or minor if appropriate (like I did with biology – see the *Choosing a Major* section). Most critically, pursue research conferences. **Research conferences add a tremendous amount of validity to your background.** So few undergraduates know the impact of three or more regional or national conferences on your application because so few students seek these experiences. Beyond publications, one of the biggest factors that I believe helped me get into the Chan program was the conferences I had presented at. As an undergraduate, it is truly not difficult to be selected for these symposia if your work is well-written. For the love of Pete, please apply to present at symposia. Also, who is Pete?

Civic Service/Public Health Fellowships and Volunteer Awards

Similar to research fellowships, civic service/public health fellowships are golden goose eggs. From what I have seen, these programs are scarcer than their research counterparts. There still are a number of excellent opportunities available, but I would guess that research fellowships are more common simply because a larger number of students engage in research than civic service and public health work.

Where does one find one's shimmering egg? Both colleges and outside organizations offer civic service/public health fellowships, most geared toward summer work. If you are passionate about civic service or public health (or perhaps you are not hot and bothered about research), these programs are something to pursue. They are the research equivalent of strikingly distinguishing yourself from your peers in the world of public engagement. Note that these programs are quite competitive. If you are in the market to participate, it is best to begin crafting a compelling application as soon as possible.

How does one craft a compelling application? I am clearly not the expert here, as I have never been awarded one of these fellowships. However, I will give my insights from what I have observed among students who participated in these programs. First – find a public cause that you are dedicated to and become involved. This is how you begin to craft a strong personal narrative. Second – if possible, work with faculty on a project related to your public cause. This faculty member will serve as your mentor and advocate. Third – try to publish work related to your and your faculty mentor's project (even in your college's student-run journal) and pursue opportunities to present your work at conferences. Fourth – ask your faculty mentor for a strong letter of recommendation. I've heard from successful applicants to these programs that recommendation letters are heavily weighted in determining who earns a spot with the program. Fifth – write kickass essays highlighting your public cause efforts, how you will chase further progress toward your goal through the fellowship, and how you will continue to be dedicated to this work in your career. Make sure that your mentor or an advisor looks over your essays. These are critical application components. Sixth – polish your resume. Be sure to include your public engagement work as well as any publications and presentations. Of course, include all important resume criteria (education, volunteering, leadership, etc.). Seventh – see if your college or any local organizations have civic service/public health fellowships to apply to before seeking larger, more competitive fellowships. Eighth – apply to the big-name civic service/public health fellowships. You can apply to these well-known programs either while simultaneously applying to smaller programs or in the summer after completing a smaller fellowship. If you have completed a smaller program, you should become more competitive for the larger fellowships when applying the following summer.

The *Research, Clinical, and Public Health Fellowships* section includes civic service/public health fellowships among the list of research fellowships. The summer programs list is quite comprehensive, but the academic term and post-baccalaureate programs list is incomplete. Be sure to do your own research, especially pretraining to your own college's and local companies' opportunities in case I missed something. WashU's Gephardt Institute has several fellowships available for undergraduates: the Civic Scholars Program, the Goldman Fellows Program, and the Beuerlein Fellows Program. Check to see what your university offers! I know that WashU's Civic Scholars alumni went on to attend top medical schools, with many matriculating to Harvard. Crazy! These programs are without doubt highly respected – and also competitive among WashU undergrads.

You will see in my *Resume of Failures* section that I applied for a number of well-known public health fellowships and was not awarded any of them. How dare they! My experiences were definitely not tailored toward these programs – I was heavily embedded in wet lab research – which is likely why I was not competitive.

To wrap up, civic service and volunteer awards are given by both universities and the organizations that you are involved with. Most colleges give public engagement and community service awards to undergraduates, particularly graduating seniors. Nominations from peers, faculty or staff are likely necessary for consideration, but applications may also be available. Look into the processes for your school, and don't shy away from asking your mentor for a nomination! These honors are also often awarded by organizations that you work with. Impeccable leadership, unwavering dedication, unmatched work ethic, and innovative ideas are qualities that get someone noticed. However, please note that there are plenty of flaws when it comes to who gets recognized – many outstanding people are overlooked. Don't hang your self-worth on one of these distinctions. At the same time, awards honoring civic service or volunteer work are momentous accomplishments. They will, without doubt, help you emerge as a highly desirable medical school applicant, particularly considering that medicine is anchored in serving others.

Minority, First-Generation, and Women's Awards and Scholarships

Awards are increasingly popular to honor minority, first-generation, and female students. Most, if not all, U.S. universities have awards and scholarships for these three groups of students. Scholarships likely need an application and may be available as soon as you matriculate. Awards can either be applied for or require a peer, faculty, or staff nomination. Be sure to research which awards and scholarships are given by your university as well as the requirements so that you know what to pursue. Earning these distinctions at the university level is remarkable and will be great for your medical school candidacy!

Scholarships for minority, first-generation, and female students are also available at the local, regional, and national levels. States have specific awards for high school seniors in addition to current college students. Large corporations similarly award tuition funds to incoming and current students on an annual basis. Many scholarships are out there, and more opportunities are constantly being made available. Research which scholarships you would be a good fit for and apply away! There are so many that I cannot list them all here. Not only will these funds help to reduce loan debt, but, like all distinctions, they are prized by admissions committees.

CHAPTER 05

RESUME OF FAILURES

Throughout much of this guidebook, I have shared my successes and recommendations to give a sense of what my application looked like. My intent is that this detail has been helpful in showing you what an accepted profile contains. Is that cringe? My goal is not to sound braggadocios – just to give clear, precise information about a process that can be clouded with confusion.

This chapter focuses on my resume of failures: all of the pursuits where I have not triumphed since I began college. Prerak Juthani – a YouTuber and current student at Yale School of Medicine – inspired this idea by sharing his resume of failures with his YouTube audience!

Below is my own resume of failures - divided up by academic scholarships that I wasn't selected for, research and clinical fellowships that I didn't earn, general research-related 'no's' that I received, and student groups to which I wasn't offered membership.

- Academic scholarships: WashU's Danforth Scholars Program; WashU's Annika Rodriguez Scholars Program; WashU's University Scholars Program in Medicine (now discontinued)

- Research and clinical fellowships: The Barry Goldwater Scholarship; Amgen Scholars Program with UCSF, Harvard, WashU, MIT, and Columbia; WashU's ENDURE summer research program; The Gephardt Institute's Small Change Grant; UCSF Breast Care Center Internship Program; The UCLA Public Health Scholars Training Program; Columbia's Summer Public Health Scholars Program

- General research-related opportunities: five+ labs that I applied to as an undergraduate and didn't hear back from; a number of research conferences that I submitted my abstracts to and wasn't invited to present at (SACNAS - Society for Advancement of Chicanos/Hispanics and Native Americans in Science - was one of these conferences); WashU's Spector prize for the best Undergraduate Research Thesis in biology

- Student groups: 2016 Presidential Debate Student Volunteer; The First Year Center Executive Board (FYX) member; Uncle Joe's Peer Counselor; GlobeMed; WUSTL's Missouri Gamma chapter of Alpha Epsilon Delta (U.S. health preprofessional honor society)

Pretty hefty, eh? That is the intent – to show you that we all have failures ... and it is okay. **Behind every successful person is a sea**

of failures or 'no's.' (My mom doesn't like the words 'failure' or 'rejection' because they're a bit harsh. Sorry about the chapter's title, mama!)

My resume of failures has taught me that it can take many no's to have a few impactful yes's. This may be the second or third most important lesson I learned since beginning undergrad (the first most important lesson being the value of hard work). I've received many no's – more no's than yes's, to be exact – and, yet, I would have never earned the distinctions that helped me get into medical school without the failures, too.

A recent example is from the Spring of 2020 (the spring before submitting my medical school primary application) when I applied to four fellowships. The UCSF Breast Care Center Internship Program, The UCLA Public Health Scholars Training Program, Columbia's Summer Public Health Scholars Program, and the Harvard T.H. Chan School of Public Health's Biostatistics and Computational Biology Undergraduate Research Fellowship – I applied to them all. Out of these four programs – I was not accepted to three of them. My one acceptance was to the Chan School's Fellowship – my golden goose egg. This program was likely the most prestigious accomplishment on my application, and I believe it made the difference in earning me interviews and acceptance to top research programs. It took three no's to get this one impactful yes. The rejections were more than worth it. Plus, I was accepted to the program that was the best fit for my background experiences and future goals!

Another example. This example is meant to show how silly some rejections are and why not to take them personally. In my junior year, I applied to WashU's Alpha Epsilon Delta (AED) chapter – a pre-health honorary recognizing academic excellence and personal achievement among pre-health students. My friend, the President of AED, encouraged me to apply. After submitting a written application, I was invited to interview with members of the chapter. Now, there were a few things that caused this interview to get off on the wrong foot: 1) my roommate had a mental health crisis the night prior, and I had to call the police to help search for her after she ran out of our dorm building in distress, and 2) the interview was suddenly moved to a new location the moment it was supposed to begin meaning that I and a bunch of other applicants had to rush to another location on campus. We were totally flustered when the interview began (we had no notification that the interview had changed location).

My first interview was a series of choosing between two random things (e.g., ice cream and pie) and then explaining why I chose one over the other. I don't know if this was an attempt to relax us, but I've never been a fan of cutesy questions in a formal interview setting. Everything was going fine until the student asked me to choose between cats and dogs. As a lover of both and owner of two kitties and one puppy, I simply could not favor one of my pets over another. They are family to me! I told the interviewer that I had to pick both because I have two cats and a dog and love them equally. My interviewer, deciding to take his role too seriously, told me I had to choose. As a woman of principle, I told him I couldn't do that. He was clearly displeased with my answer when he moved on to the next question. His behavior is something that I want to emphasize: many people, especially young people, can power trip and get hung up on the marginal and momentary authority that they have over you. Instead of this student simply understanding that these were supposedly fun questions and allowing me to pick both cats and dogs, he decided to put his foot down over something trivial. I knew at that moment that my answer would likely cost my membership to the organization based on how he was behaving, but it was more important to me to stick with who I was than pretend to favor one of my pets over the other. I totally understand that this may sound dumb to some of you. Why not pretend to like cats over dogs to get into the honorary? One of my principles is loyalty to my loved ones – pets included – and not acting in ways, even momentarily, that cross my own boundaries. This means that I don't bad mouth my family members, and I don't claim to love one family member over the others. My principles may not be yours, and maybe your values don't extend to pets. However, I do encourage you to think about your values and stand by them even when lapses may be easy. Years later, my principles would be tested again in a medical school interview. Again, I chose to stick with my morals. It cost me an acceptance. We will get to this story later. In both cases, I am proud that I stood by my beliefs.

After the first messy AED interview, the remainder of the conversations were in a small room crammed with applicants who were answering more questions. These interviews also went downhill. I wasn't in the best state of mind because of the stressful circumstances preceding the interviews, which were compounded by the unpleasant first student whom I spoke with. My performance was not ideal, and I take complete responsibility for this. What also didn't help was that I couldn't hear the questions because the noise level in the room was high. The whole day was a flop. I was unsurprised when I wasn't offered membership. My friend, who was the President, was supportive of me throughout the ordeal.

I was never a member of WashU's pre-health honorary – a group that selected those with promise in healthcare. Part of this was due to my own poor performance, and part was due to a young man who was a lousy interviewer. But here's the kick: even if this group didn't think much of me as a premedical student, the medical schools thought differently. Nineteen interviews. Ten acceptances. Offers to top research programs. As far as I know, not one member of AED who interviewed me has achieved these statistics. **Your wins and losses don't define your worth. Neither do your peers.**

Use the losses (and, at times, people who treat you unfairly) as motivation. Years later, guess who gets to revel in the sweet satisfaction of being a kick-ass medical student even if AED couldn't see it? Me! There's irony in the things that work out in life versus those that don't. Find humor in the irony, allow it to motivate you, and then let it go.

Power and authority are enticing. Moving from an underclassman to an upperclassman, pursuing leadership, and involving yourself in different activities will sometimes give you leverage over other people. While testing the bounds of authority may be attractive, I urge caution. I could tell countless stories of big-headed TAs, arrogant club leaders, and conceited student government members who were unfair and even cruel to the people they temporarily held power over. I can also tell countless stories of when that behavior came back to bite them. You never know where your peers will end up. They may one day be your boss, on a hiring committee where you seek employment, a connection that would help your son get a job. I've never understood why people treat others contemptuously without reason. My mother once shared that this is called "common cruelty." Don't fall to the temptation. I've only seen treating people poorly make the bullies themselves miserable. If you are the victim of common cruelty, I always advocate standing up for yourself, using their behavior as a motivator, and, perhaps, seeking vengeance when justified.

Rejections are always a disappointment. However, I have found that the more no's I receive, the less they impact me. During my freshman and sophomore years, I remember the devastation that came with failure. My worth seemed to decrease with every unmet goal, and I did what I could to avoid that feeling. Avoidance came in the form of not pursuing opportunities or not putting full effort into my candidacy. About the same time when I began to really try in school was the same time when I stopped letting losses rule my behavior and attitude. Today and for the past several years, rejections truly roll off my back. Yes, I am bummed to not earn something that I wanted. Nevertheless, my mental state and self-worth are no longer affected. Just recently, I was waitlisted at the Mayo Clinic – a medical school I loved. Bummed at the outcome? Yes. Thinking less of myself and wallowing in misery? No! **Have the courage to chase failure.**

> *"It is not the critic who counts; not the man who points out how the strong man stumbles, or where the doer of deeds could have done them better. The credit belongs to the man who is actually in the arena, whose face is marred by dust and sweat and blood; who strives valiantly; who errs, who comes short again and again, because there is no effort without error and shortcoming; but who does actually strive to do the deeds; who knows great enthusiasms, the great devotions; who spends himself in a worthy cause; who at the best knows in the end the triumph of high achievement, and who at the worst, if he fails, at least fails while daring greatly, so that his place shall never be with those cold and timid souls who neither know victory nor defeat."*
> **- Theodore Roosevelt**

CHAPTER 06

PLANNING YOUR SUMMERS

Housekeeping! A.k.a., a few housekeeping items to address. Throughout this chapter, I will refer to freshman, sophomore, junior, and senior summer. Just for clarity, freshman summer is the summer that follows freshman year, sophomore summer is the summer that follows sophomore year, and so on.

With that housekeeping out of the way, let's get into content! This chapter is dedicated to helping you make the most of your summers. The three to four months you have off from school are essential to molding you into a compelling applicant and keeping you ahead of your peers. Summers should generally be spent taking organic chemistry (if necessary), conducting research, volunteering, exploring public health work, engaging in clinical experiences, completing fellowships and internships, and studying for the MCAT.

The structures of your summers will heavily depend on when you want to apply to medical school. A table showing two possible paths for summer planning in order to take zero, one, and two gap years is at the end of this section. The earliest cycle when you can submit your applications is junior summer. If you want to take one gap year, apply during senior summer. So on and so forth. Whenever you choose to apply to medical school, there is one critical rule to follow: make an informed decision about when to apply and then stick to it. Following this rule will ensure that you are prepared for your chosen cycle. If you suddenly find yourself unprepared for a fast-approaching cycle that you had planned for, it is better to wait until the following cycle than wade through the chaos of becoming a reapplicant. Now, it's time for the summer strategy specifics!

FRESHMAN SUMMER

Anyone out there terrified of organic chemistry? I was! Not only is it a hard class in and of itself, but it's also a challenging course to take with a full schedule of classes. WashU's organic chemistry series is particularly terrifying. Students earning eight points out of 100 on some exams can get a C. *Eight points out of 100!* Students with 20 points can end up in the B range. Those with 40 points get an A. Is that crazy, or what? There are a bunch of super smart kids who are earning one to three points on organic chemistry exams at WashU. And that's considered normal...

Our professors wanted the exams to be challenging. However, challenging to these professors apparently means not testing if anyone learned the material because the questions are mind-bending vortexes. Every year, there is one student I have fondly named "Spock" who gets 80 or 90 points on these exams. Spock is not human. Well...duh! If you are in a similar cluster **** at your ~~asylum~~ university, consider taking organic chemistry over freshman summer. For anyone totally freaked out about WashU, organic chemistry is the only science that I have heard of that is like this. Every class that I took was completely normal.

The downsides of taking organic chemistry over the summer include only getting a marginal break from academics (on the scale of weeks rather than months), spending coin on a class that you are already paying for at your university, and loss of opportunity to engage in research, volunteer work, and other meaningful activities. Upsides of taking organic chemistry over the summer: it's easier to earn an A because you can fully devote your energy toward the one class, and the course can and should be taken at less rigorous college (more on that in a minute), you may be able to take the MCAT earlier and possibly avoid an extra gap year, you can live at home and bond with family while taking the course, and you still can participate in smaller volunteer work or extracurricular activities while taking o-chem.

How do you know if taking organic chemistry over your freshman summer is the right decision for you? For those attending a school where organic chemistry is super difficult and if you've struggled in other science classes (you are in need of an sGPA boost), I would highly recommend taking o-chem during your freshman summer. You can take it at your college if the cost is reasonable and the exams are not soul-shattering like they are at WashU (bonus points if you can live at home and save money on housing). Alternatively, take o-chem at a school near your hometown where getting an A is much more feasible. I would stay away from community colleges, as some medical schools are picky about prerequisites taken at junior colleges. My friends who took o-chem close to home and at an easier school aced the course! Stay focused when you take the class to make sure that you succeed. Once you are settled in, start volunteering for a few hours each week to strike a balance in your life. Also, begin investigating who you can do research or clinical work with at your university if you didn't begin these activities during your freshman year. Toward the end of the summer, reach out to these faculty members and set up interviews so you can hit the ground running in sophomore fall.

A critical piece of advice: do not be tempted to pay a buttload of cash to take organic chemistry at a prestigious university. This is a terrible idea. How do I know? Because I made this mistake myself. During my freshman year, I heard that a bunch of my classmates were taking o-chem over the summer at Harvard. Yes, Harvard. In my full intellectual glory, I thought joining them would be a good idea even though I had yet to earn even an A- in any science class at WashU. I was literally coming off of a 3.19 semester GPA freshman spring. It is painful to write this. My classmates and I had heard that organic chemistry was easy at Harvard, and having a Harvard A on your transcript looked great. We got screwed.

The easy professor stopped teaching the course the year before us, so we got in bed with two maniacs who made the class incredibly difficult. I am cringing typing this. A bunch of my classmates and I paid a bucket of cash to earn Bs in o-chem at Harvard. How dumber could we get? Very few people I knew in the class squeaked out with an A. Even if I had earned an A, I would still say this was the stupidest decision ever. I could've simply lived at home, taken organic chemistry at Portland State University, earned an A, spent time volunteering, saved a ton of money, and no one would have cared! Please do not repeat my idiotic mistake. Yes, I got into great medical schools, but my goodness, I am still so mad for making this decision – especially because it cost too much money. UHH! WHY, LORD!? Worst summer of my LIFE!!! Worst academic decision I have made in the last six years! I'm disgusted to this day. Rant over.

For people attending a college where organic chemistry exams are not horrific, who can handle taking o-chem along with other courses, and whose sGPA is already strong, there's no need to spend your time and money taking organic chemistry over the summer. One exception is if you want to invest more of your time in activities during the school year, you may want to take o-chem over the summer to free up your academic term schedule. Another exception is if you are spacing out your prerequisites; taking o-chem over the summer may help you avoid an extra gap year because you can take the MCAT earlier. To be clear, though, I don't think you need to have taken o-chem to crush the MCAT. Watch Khan Academy videos on the foundational organic chemistry reactions; that should be enough for the MCAT.

So, for those not taking o-chem during freshman summer, what are your options? This may sound coo-coo, but if you have a strong grasp of the basic sciences and want to apply to medical school at the end of your junior year (a.k.a. take no gap years), consider taking the MCAT over freshman summer. You will still have your sophomore and junior summers to engage in activities that will go on your AMCAS primary application. If you achieve a killer MCAT score, this may be the move in order to matriculate to a top medical school straight out of college.

Don't want to take the MCAT? No problem! Those conducting research or clinical work can continue those pursuits and keep building a strong application. Full-time summer involvement can lead to compelling publications. Even if you haven't begun these activities during your freshman academic year, the summer is an excellent time to start! Research labs, especially, would love to train you when you're working full-time as opposed to over fragmented hours during the school year. Look into any clinical or research fellowships to apply to! Some of these fellowships are reserved for or geared toward underclassmen - it's a great time to secure yourself one of these golden goose eggs while your classmates are asleep at the wheel. Lastly, see if you can start volunteering a few hours per week or month in order to begin meaningful, longitudinal service to your population of interest.

In case anyone's wondering, I used o-chem to abbreviate organic chemistry because it makes more sense when written, but I say 'orgo' when speaking. The o-chem versus orgo debate can get a bit feisty. I'm definitely on the orgo side despite what I wrote in this chapter.

SOPHOMORE SUMMER

Suns out, buns out? More like suns out, pipettes out! Sophomore summer is the time to invest in research and clinical experience. Fellowships are ripe for the plucking. These fellowships should be applied for during your sophomore year (October-March is the typical application season) so you can participate during the summer. It is often best to start by applying for your own college's fellowship programs for sophomore summer because they tend to be less competitive than national programs. Junior summer and senior summer, you can focus on the larger programs. My sophomore summer was spent completing WashU's Biology Summer Undergraduate Research Fellowship (BioSURF) program, which funded my research full-time in the Holtzman lab.

If you aren't selected for a research or clinical program, don't worry! Continue your research or clinical experience full-time, as this will help your odds of becoming published. This is exactly what I did when I wasn't selected for a fellowship for my junior summer. Additionally, apply for conferences where you can present your work. Remember, conference presentations separate the girls from the women in medical school applications and will help you earn fellowships for the following summer.

Volunteering is a great activity to pursue for a couple of hours each week or each month while immersed in a larger activity. A few hours of community service here and there can build up to a dedicated, authentic effort by the time you submit medical school applications. This long-term investment can also earn you a robust recommendation letter from the organization where you volunteer.

Let's say that you completed considerable research or clinical work during your freshman summer and still want to go straight to medical school out of college (a.k.a. applying at the end of your junior year). If this is you, you might want to take the MCAT over your sophomore summer. A sophomore summer MCAT will allow you to complete the exam with sufficient study time and at a more feasible pace compared to testing during the academic year or trying to squeeze it in during junior summer when submitting applications.

To elaborate, waiting until you're in the mix of junior year to take the MCAT is risky because your grades may suffer. The MCAT is a black hole. It takes a ton of time and effort to prepare properly. I do not recommend that most students – especially those at rigorous colleges –take the MCAT during the school year. I have seen that either people's grades fall, their MCAT score is not as high as they wanted and were capable of achieving, or both grades and the MCAT score suffer. **Rare is the unicorn who can juggle both grades and the MCAT during the school year.** Also, please be careful about trying to jam in MCAT studying over winter break. Do you remember Nyra from the beginning of the guidebook? Sweet Nyra tried to prepare for the MCAT over winter break and earned a 508. Now, she is studying properly and consistently scoring 520+ on practice exams.

The issue with postponing the MCAT for junior summer is that waiting for your score will delay your application review by admissions committees. Again, this is only if you are applying to medical school at the end of your junior year. Applying late within an application cycle (e.g., late within your junior summer) can completely derail your prospects. Even worse, if you earn an unideal MCAT score, there's no time for a retake if you already applied late that year. Lastly, managing MCAT studying during the summer with writing primary and secondary application essays would be a headache - save yourself the Advil runs and take the exam earlier.

JUNIOR SUMMER

Suns out, buns out? More like suns out, books out! Any laughs? No? Okay, I'll stop. Much like sophomore summer, junior summer is all about research and clinical experience - two key extracurriculars for the stellar medical school applicant. Let the fellowships fly, baby! Your junior academic year is the time to apply for both your university's fellowships and the highly competitive outside fellowships so you can participate in the programs over the summer. October through March is the usual application season, so ensure that you are prepared to begin planning for junior summer months in advance. Both clinical and research fellowships are regarded as prestigious academic opportunities by medical schools - that is why they are worth applying to.

No tears if you are not selected for a fellowship. I wasn't during my junior year. Continue to work full-time with your research or clinical mentor, just as I did. Pursue symposia presentations. Keep volunteering for a few hours each week or each month. Look at your GPA and assess if there are any weak spots. You may want to take a class in the mornings or evenings if your grades could use a boost. This can be taken at an easier college to save moolah and take a break from academic exhaustion. If your sGPA is suffering, take an advanced science elective (these tend to be easier than the introductory courses). If your cGPA is struggling, take any course that you will enjoy and do well in. It can even be taken at a community college. I did this during my gap year when boosting my 3.69 cGPA to a 3.70 cGPA. At Portland Community College, I took Intro to Dementia Care and Practice because it focused on caring for older adults – my population of interest! Work that narrative, girl!

Any eager beavers out there? If you plan on applying to medical school at the end of your senior year (i.e., one gap year), then you probably want to get a jump on writing your personal statement. Other important essays to write are the diversity essay and the overcoming challenges essay, among others. See the Essays chapter for specifics. These essays are critical, so taking the time to write outstanding responses over the summer is an excellent use of time. During my junior summer, half of my personal statement poured out of me in the library one day. It was totally worth the unexpected writing bonanza to have my personal statement in the bag way ahead of when I applied. Over your senior year (for those taking gap years), continue to polish and complete essays for the primary and secondary applications. This pre-writing will save you from a world of stress when you apply. **Submitting essays first will also put your application at the top of the completed pile and thus increase your odds of securing an interview.**

More MCAT talk. Are you wanting to apply to medical school at the end of your senior year (a.k.a. take one gap year)? If yes, then roll up your sleeves and break out the pocket protector! It's study time! Most of my classmates wanted to take one gap year, so they studied for and took the MCATs over junior summer. In retrospect, I probably should've made the move only to take one gap year and not two. Studying for the MCAT is a full-time job. I studied part-time over my junior summer and planned to study throughout my senior fall to take the exam in January. Did this happen? No. As I said before, studying for the MCAT while enrolled in college is super difficult. I couldn't pull it off. Rather than get a poopy score, I rescheduled my test date. Expect to spend two to four months of focused, intentional studying to achieve a top MCAT score. If studying correctly, these months are enough time to earn a 518+. Learn more about studying in the MCAT chapter.

An address to the gunners applying to medical school over their junior summer: You are bananas. Also, I am jealous that you don't have to take any gap years. I feel like an old hag entering medical school at 25. By the time you are applying (this summer), what should be completed is stellar grades, sparkling recommendation letters, a sultry MCAT score, sterling extracurriculars and leadership, and standout essays. These are all the adjectives that I know that start with the letter "s." My entire vocabulary lies before you. Your junior summer should not go to waste just because you are applying to medical school. Few people recognize that the summer when you apply can still be written about on your AMCAS application. If you can squeeze in another fellowship or a new clinical experience, do it! And, of course, add it to your activities section on the primary. The summer when I applied was when I participated in the Harvard Chan School Fellowship. It went on my application and is a big reason why I think that I got into top research schools. My little goose egg came through! So can yours! While completing your activities, be sure to prewrite *all* of your secondary applications and begin preparing for interviews. You read that right: prewrite *all* of your secondaries. More to come in the *When to Write* section.

SENIOR SUMMER

Buns may actually be out this summer. Hike up those cheeky bikinis, gentlemen. You graduated! Take time to celebrate! Go to the beach, go to the mountains, go to Disney, go to Japan. Do something memorable to celebrate this achievement.

Your senior summer will either be filled with submitting your medical school application (one gap year track) or studying for the MCAT (two+ gap year track). The third option is that you've already been accepted to medical school because you applied last summer. If that is you, have a blowout. Throw a rager. You've worked hard. You earned it. Check out Getting to Know Your Medical School Options for tips on researching your new medical school. If you are vying for a competitive specialty, begin to search for mentors. Research might be essential for matching into your specialty. If you don't know what specialty you're interested in, start investigating. Shadow physicians. Falling in love with a competitive specialty should happen sooner rather than later. The sooner you know what you want to do, the sooner you can prepare and the more competitive you become.

GAP YEAR(S)

Mortals, attention! Time to discuss you muggles who are not going straight to medical school following college graduation. Admittedly, I'm a muggle too. A super muggle, considering that I took *two* gap years. Those submitting medical school applications during senior summer will be slammed. Recommendation letters should be submitted, your personal statement and the activities section should be written, and transcripts should be sent in. These need to be completed before May 1 – the approximate date the AMCAS application opens. From May 1 onward, prewrite secondary applications for each medical school to which you are applying. Prewriting takes a lot of time, but it is more than worth it. Then, begin preparing for interviews. Interviewers will want to know what you are doing during your gap year. Whether it is a job, an abroad experience, volunteer work, a fellowship, or your Hollywood debut, be sure not to lay on the sofa all year. Since prewriting and interview preparation takes so much time, I recommend not beginning your gap year plans full-time until August or September.

Poor suckers like me are taking two or more gap years. Senior summer is MCAT summer. Senior summer was *my* MCAT summer. It was kind of a bummer to graduate college and then begin studying for the hardest exam of my life. But I had no distractions, and my patience paid off. The *How to Study* section details how to effectively ace the MCAT. Sit for the exam in August or early September. Then, transition to your gap year endeavors. The *What to Do During Your Gap Year* section explores gap year opportunities. A huge benefit of taking two or more gap years is that during your first gap year, you can take time to prewrite your personal statement, activities section, and all secondary essays. Putting in the proper effort should result in high-quality essays since you took time with your writing. This is another trick of the trade that we will talk about in more detail: most applicants flop on the essays. Phenomenal essays will add to the irresistible quality of your application. My final words of advice are ones that you've read above. The summer when you submit your AMCAS primary is not to be squandered. It is the last summer you can add a compelling accomplishment to your activities section. Not to beat a dead horse for those reading the guidebook all the way through, but for those skipping around, the summer when I submitted my primary is when I participated in the Harvard Chan School's Undergraduate Research Fellowship. Quite a bang to end my academic career with. Follow my lead, youngster.

Possible Summer Schedules For Different Gap Year Lengths

0 Gap Years		
Academic Year	**Path 1**	**Path 2**
Freshman summer	Research or clinical work; volunteer part-time	Research or clinical work; volunteer part-time

Sophomore summer	MCAT	Research or clinical work; volunteer part-time
Junior summer	Submit applications; research or clinical work	Submit applications; MCAT
Senior summer	Relax before medical school	Relax before medical school

1 Gap Year		
Academic Year	**Path 1**	**Path 2**
Freshman summer	Organic chemistry	Research or clinical work; volunteer part-time
Sophomore summer	Research or clinical work; volunteer part-time	Research or clinical work; volunteer part-time
Junior summer	MCAT	MCAT
Senior summer	Submit applications; research or clinical work	Submit applications; research or clinical work
Post-grad summer	Relax before medical school	Relax before medical school

2 Gap Years		
Academic Year	**Path 1**	**Path 2**
Freshman summer	Organic chemistry	Research or clinical work; volunteer part-time
Sophomore summer	Research or clinical work; volunteer part-time	Research or clinical work; volunteer part-time
Junior summer	Research or clinical work; volunteer part-time	MCAT
Senior summer	MCAT	Begin a 1-2 year fellowship or grad program (e.g., Fulbright, Master of Public Health)
Post-grad summer 1	Submit applications; research or clinical work	Submit applications; continue fellowship, grad program, or clinical work
Post-grad summer 2	Relax before medical school	Relax before medical school

CHAPTER 07

LETTERS OF RECOMMENDATION

HOW IMPORTANT ARE THEY?

To understand how important recommendation letters are, consider what information is available to medical schools looking to make a decision on your candidacy. There are primary and secondary applications – both self-descriptors of your character. There are grades and MCAT scores – both of which are systematized and quantitative views of your academic achievement. There is an interview. The interview is a single day when current students and faculty get to ask questions about your professional aspirations and personal history and fit with their program. Yet, they ask questions to a polished, rehearsed you, not you in the raw. How can admissions committees obtain a third-party glimpse into your values and work ethic, untainted by rehearsals and self-bias? This is where recommendation letters become important.

Letters of recommendation are incredibly important. Testimonials by professors, researchers, mentors, employers, patients, and volunteer and clinical supervisors speak to who you are day-to-day. What is the attitude that you carry? How do you work on a team? What contributions have you made to your team? How have you changed over time? While we all bring refined versions of ourselves to professional environments, concealing our nature and personality over time is hard. Recommendations may be the most honest evaluation of an applicant's disposition and integrity available to admissions committees. Because of this, **recommendations hold tremendous sway over your candidacy**.

Below is a chart showing admissions officers' evaluations of the importance of different admissions criteria (AAMC, The Evolving Medical School Admissions Interview). Note the weight held by recommendations – particularly after the interview. Post-interview, recommendations become one of the most important factors in determining your final candidacy decision: admittance, waitlist, or rejection. A color version of the table can be accessed via https://www.aamc.org/media/5916/download.

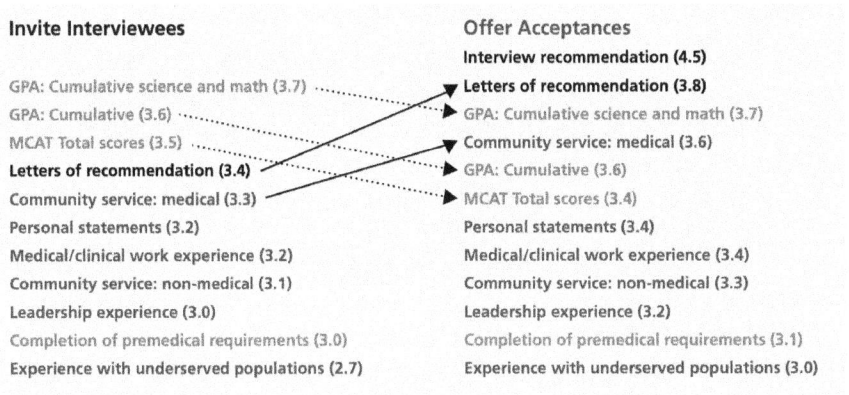

Figure 1. Importance of Application Data to Admission Officers at 113 Medical Schools in Their Decisions to Invite Interviewees and Offer Acceptances

Invite Interviewees
GPA: Cumulative science and math (3.7)
GPA: Cumulative (3.6)
MCAT Total scores (3.5)
Letters of recommendation (3.4)
Community service: medical (3.3)
Personal statements (3.2)
Medical/clinical work experience (3.2)
Community service: non-medical (3.1)
Leadership experience (3.0)
Completion of premedical requirements (3.0)
Experience with underserved populations (2.7)

Offer Acceptances
Interview recommendation (4.5)
Letters of recommendation (3.8)
GPA: Cumulative science and math (3.7)
Community service: medical (3.6)
GPA: Cumulative (3.6)
MCAT Total scores (3.4)
Personal statements (3.4)
Medical/clinical work experience (3.4)
Community service: non-medical (3.3)
Leadership experience (3.2)
Completion of premedical requirements (3.1)
Experience with underserved populations (3.0)

Note. Mean importance ratings are shown in parentheses. Application data are presented in descending order of importance to admissions committees' decisions about which applicants to interview and accept into medical school. The admissions data presented standard deviations ranging from 0.9 to 1.7, indicating variation in importance across medical schools. Data about the importance of "interview recommendations" were not collected at the "invite interviewees" stage. See supplemental material for a complete list of application data rated, mean importance ratings, and standard deviations.

Color Scheme
Red = Academic data
Blue = Experiential data
Green = Demographic data
Black = Combination of multiple types of data

Rating Scale
5 = Extremely Important
4 = Very Important
3 = Important
2 = Somewhat Important
1 = Not Important

WHO TO ASK

The first question surrounding who to ask is who you *need* to ask. Most medical schools have requirements for who can write letters on your behalf. Most programs require at least three letters. From a quick internet search, it seems like many schools are getting rid of specific requirements regarding *who* should act as a letter writer. To be safe, two or more letters should come from science professors. If you conducted research, your mentor and/or PI should write one of your letters. Recommendations from employers, non-science professors, those you've volunteered with, and clinical supervisors are all outstanding options. Feinberg School of Medicine requires at least one recommendation from a science professor who taught you, and then they give flexibility on the other two letters. Obviously, family and friends cannot recommend you – professional relationships only. Yale School of Medicine's website states: "Letters should come from individuals who are in a position to comment knowledgeably on your accomplishments, abilities, experience, and/or personal qualifications." Five or six letters is usually the maximum.

Day one of college is when you start searching for potential recommenders. Clean off those binoculars and keep your eyes peeled. Most universities have large introductory classes. The sheer size of introductory courses makes it difficult to make personal relationships with the professors primarily because class time is geared toward lecturing and not discussion. Students participate in lectures through questions rather than sharing insights. A strong relationship with a professor teaching a large course can, of course, be achieved. To do this, sit in the front of the classroom and attend office hours regularly to ask questions (if you think you don't have questions, think harder – you are not all-knowing in the subject). If the professor is not annoyed by in-class questions, feel free to ask a question in the lecture every other week or so. Make sure the question is on topic. Showoffs annoy everyone. If you earned an A or A- in the course, apply for a teaching assistant position with the same professor. We will discuss this more soon, but taking a class and working as a TA is an outstanding strategy for forming a genuine connection with faculty. If you are interested in the professor's research, perhaps you can work on her projects – another method of building a genuine connection.

I'm unsure if any of your universities have this setup, but at WashU, there was a special end-of-year soiree for students in the top 10% of general chemistry. No, I'm not kidding. The party is real and is where faculty woo top students to become chemistry majors. I believe the social is limited to the top 10% of the class, but it may be the top 5%. Don't quote me on the exact percentage. Your college may have similar functions – do some digging! In addition to being invited to wine and dine, the top general chemistry students were also invited to apply to lead weekly learning workshops for the next group of students taking general chemistry. These workshops were called Peer-Led Team Learning (PLTL). PLTL sessions allowed current general chemistry students to work through a problem set together under the guidance of a PLTL leader who aced the course. PLTL leaders were the general chemistry professors' best former students. Being selected nearly guaranteed you a glowing letter of recommendation. Regular TAs for general chemistry were relegated to grading quizzes and exams. Check if your university has a program similar to PLTL. If you can, pursue a PLTL-esque position. With my two Bs in general chemistry, I did not serve as a TA or PLTL leader for the class!

Upper-division courses are where you can get down to business. These classes are typically smaller and more discussion-based. This gives professors the opportunity to get to know how you problem-solve and think critically. These intimate (any ewws for using the word intimate?) learning environments are a Petri dish for securing influential recommendation letters. Hike up that mini skirt, whisk on some mascara, and start strutting those high heels. It's seduction time! Okay, yes, unfortunately, I'm kidding. But it is time for an ~intellectual~ seduction. How do you best stand out in small discussion classes? Come to class prepared every day – complete the assigned work and write down at least five insights or questions. Make a point to actually share those insights or ask your questions during each class. In other words, engage in class discussion at least three times per day, if appropriate. Once per day, commentary means that you are just checking a box. Zero comments will give off the impression that you are uninterested in the subject. You may, in fact, lack interest in the material but fake it until you make it, sweet cheeks. Attend office hours, especially to receive help on assignments and big projects. When a large project presents itself, schedule a meeting with your instructor to discuss ideas or a rough draft. When you receive a grade on papers or presentations, ask for additional feedback on improving your work or clarifications on suggested improvements. If TA positions are available, apply for one. If you want to join your professor's research efforts, ask to do so.

Reflecting on my letters of recommendation, three were from science instructors (two who taught me and one who I TAed for during her first year), my PI and bench mentor co-wrote one, and one was from my supervisor, where I volunteered. How did I get to know each of these people to feel comfortable asking for a letter?

Example one. Dr. Smith taught me in a small advanced laboratory course. My class partner and I worked on a paper together that Dr. Smith is currently working to publish (he tries to publish most papers by students in this particular class because we examined the structure of proteins that have yet to be discussed in scientific literature). He invited the class to work with him on another paper, and I joined in. Dr. Smith also asked me to work as his teaching assistant, which I gladly accepted. From seeing how I work as a student, a researcher, and a TA, Dr. Smith was able to comment on my candidacy for medical school from multiple perspectives. We also got to know one another personally from office hours, which allowed him to reflect on my character.

Dr. McCommis (example two) briefly taught me in an advanced science course. This is likely surprising, but he only taught our five-person section for three weeks. How did I get to know him in this short amount of time? Each class was about three hours long, so there was plenty of time for discussion. I and the other four students gave a presentation every class, so there was a lot of individual evaluation. Through email, I spoke to Dr. McCommis about improving my presentations, as well as the research I was involved with at the medical school. During that same semester, I gave a research talk at WashU's symposium and invited him to attend. While he wasn't able to make it, we were able to connect over more than just course material. We continued to discuss research over the semester – after he had finished his three-week rotation with our section. At the end of the semester, Dr. McCommis invited me to join his laboratory. While I was unable to juggle his position with my current role in the Holtzman lab, I was flattered by the offer, and we continued to stay in touch. It was through a sincere connection – grounded in more than just grades – that I was able to ask for a letter from Dr. McCommis.

My final science instructor letter came from Dr. Lambo – our third example. Dr. Lambo was one of two instructors I was assigned to TA during my senior fall semester. The class was the laboratory section of Principles of Biology II – this was the first course Dr. Lambo taught, as she was new to WashU. I was fortunate that Dr. Lambo wanted to work with me to teach the course. She knew I had done well in the class a year prior and relied on me to provide insights into how experiments would be conducted if instructions were unclear. We would often stay late to help answer student questions. Dr. Lambo fostered a collaborative teaching environment among herself, myself, and the current students. I think Principles of Biology II, being her first class at WashU and my first time TAing the laboratory course, allowed us to lean on each other and bond. One thing to note is that not all teaching assistant positions will necessarily lead to a recommendation. Dr. Cruz taught the other section of this laboratory course. He was the head of the entire course and literally wrote the laboratory experiment manual himself. Although I tried to provide extra help and connect with Dr. Cruz, he seemed more comfortable with me sticking to grading and assisting students. The relationship was not naturally close, and it would've felt forced to pursue a closer bond. Because of this, I chose not to ask Dr. Cruz for a recommendation. He is a very kind man and a talented professor, yet we did not get to know one another. A letter from him would not have highlighted my best attributes.

Student researchers must ask for letters from their mentor and/or PI. It looks sus not to have a recommendation from one of these two people. This brings us to example four. My PI, Dr. Holtzman, intimidated me, yet I still asked him for a letter. To be fair, my bench mentor, Phat Huynh, wrote a lot of the content, but Dr. Holtzman gave it the sign-off and added a little flair. PIs and bench mentors speak to an applicant's intellectual curiosity and diligence in pursuit of new knowledge. The mission of many medical schools – particularly the top research schools – is to train their students to push the current medical knowledge forward through basic science, translational, and clinical research. These schools are not simply training doctors but forming tomorrow's leaders in science, policy, and entrepreneurship. As a student researcher, your PI's letter will carry magnitude in making a final decision on your candidacy. The best way to get a first-rate letter from your mentor is to show up ready to help and move the project forward. Consistently bringing a positive attitude and willingness to learn, as well as respectfully suggesting your own ideas, will impress those you work with. Keep this up, eagerly present at conferences, and regardless of publication record, your letter will glow.

Volunteering was the source of my final letter - example five. Halfway through my first gap year, I wrapped up my projects with the Holtzman lab and returned home to Portland, OR. This was in January 2020. After finishing my research, I looked for new activities to become involved in. It would still be 1.5 years before I matriculated to medical school. Assessing my application made it clear that I was lacking in clinical experience. Previously, I had spent a summer volunteering with older adults in memory care units. Yet my intentions to continue volunteering were interrupted by a full course load involving research and numerous extracurricular activities. In Portland, I again began volunteering with older adults in memory care units. COVID hit a few months into my volunteering, and I was able to transition from visiting residents in-person to making and delivering masks to the senior care facility. Over the course of the spring and summer, I was able to deliver hundreds of masks. Abigail Green, the Life Enrichment and Wellness Director who oversaw my volunteering, was thrilled with the masks. Her close friend, a freelance journalist, wrote an article about the masks I made for Touchmark Senior Living. This article, published in the *Oregon Faith Report*, became the subject of one of my update letters to medical schools. The overall time spent with Abigail and the adults living at Touchmark prompted me to ask her to write me a recommendation letter for medical school. Abigail was able to speak to something none of my other recommenders could capture: my ability to engage with the older adults whom I hoped to, one day, care for as a physician. The perspectives that those we volunteer with can give medical schools a glimpse into who we are as caregivers. Our other letters speak to who we are as learners, leaders, and teachers. But letters stemming from clinical experience are different from those – in fact, they may show the most human side of you. Volunteering happened to be my form of clinical engagement. Whatever your time spent with patients looks like, consider asking for a recommendation. It will soften your application's resolve, giving heart and warmth to the sterile process of sifting through thousands of medical school hopefuls.

How do you respond if a letter writer asks you to read what they've written on your behalf? Read their letter! That's how you respond. So many people seem thrown through a loop about the morality of reading a recommendation. Clearly, you shouldn't break into someone's office at 3:43 AM to get a sneak peek into your professor's thoughts on your work ethic. However, if someone wants your feedback, by golly, give it to them! You are not breaking any ethics rules. Two of my recommenders showed me their letters, and I was overwhelmed by their kind sentiments. More importantly, I was able to correct a critical error in one of the letters. My recommender thought that her letter was being submitted to *one* medical school. She addressed the letter to that specific school and referenced them at the end, not realizing that it was being submitted to all 35 programs I applied to. Who knows, this error could have gotten me the boot at the other schools! Moral of the story: Do not feel guilty about reading your reference if asked, and don't feel shy about sharing suggestions to make the letter stronger.

Closing this section on how to ask for recommendations, I want to share a story about an unexpectedly powerful letter written on one student's behalf. This story was told to me and a handful of other students by one of WashU's best premed advisors, Dr. Joan Downey. Dr. Downey is an incredibly gifted neonatologist, pediatrics professor, and Harvard Medical School (HMS) graduate. Before coming to WashU, Dr. Downey sat on Harvard Medical School's admissions board for, I believe, over 10 years. At her home in St. Louis, Dr. Downey recalled the story of the best recommendation letter the committee received during her time at HMS. The letter came in an envelope. It was neatly written on lined paper. In broken English, a gas station owner described his employee – a young man who now sat before Harvard's admissions board asking for a seat in the incoming class. An older woman would drive up to the station every few weeks to fill her car with gasoline. She was frail and struggled to maneuver the pump from its stand to her tank. On each visit, the youthful attendant would greet his customer. He walked over to her station and filled the older woman's car himself, saving her from the discomfort of struggling to pump her own gasoline. This duty was not part of his job. He was not compensated for his assistance. His actions were entirely his own – a reflection of his truest character. Through this repeated act of kindness, the gas station owner knew that his employee would make a remarkable doctor. Harvard's admissions board agreed.

HOW TO ASK

Asking for a recommendation can be a bit awkward. It's always been tough for me to ask a favor of someone when I don't have much to offer in return. My parents always scold me when I bring these feelings up. "It's what people do! They will be happy to write you a letter. Not every relationship is about parties doing equal favors for one another." I know that there is truth to my parents' words. Still, anxiety around "the ask" lingers.

One way to quench the nerves around asking for letters is by asking the right people. Discovering *who* to ask for references was detailed in the previous section. General tips are to ensure that you've gone out of your way to build a relationship with this person and that you feel like they can speak honestly and positively regarding your nature and assiduity. Asking people who don't know you or haven't observed you in the best light can backfire. I personally know of one doctor who described having to write a less-than-enthusiastic recommendation on behalf of a medical school applicant. One of my high school teachers once wrote to a college saying, "Dudley asked me to write this reference four hours before the deadline. That is all you need to know about him." Ouch!

Not only is it important to ask the right people, but it is also critical to deliver your ask with grace and gratitude. Freshman year, I made the mistake of simultaneously asking my Spanish professor to consider rounding up my A- to an A for the semester and asking if she would recommend me for a study abroad program. Not my brightest moment. She was displeased with this particular combo. I made sure not to make the same mistake of asking for both a grade boost and a favor moving forward. She did, however, write me a letter for the abroad program, even though I ended up withdrawing my application a few months later. Nothing bad happened: I realized that a semester overseas wouldn't fit with my particular academic plans.

Several times, I have been asked to write recommendations for a student or coworker. While most of these have been lovely asks, there was one instance that flopped. One of my former coworkers had asked for several references that I was more than happy to provide. Yet, when it came time for him to ask for a third reference, he didn't think it was necessary to let me know that he had listed me as a recommender. I began receiving a flurry of reminders to submit my evaluation on the day that the reference was due. Not once was I contacted by my former coworker in the weeks or months leading up to the deadline to let me know what was expected of me. It seemed that he thought he could simply list my name and email address, and I would acquiesce. I waited for his frantic text to ding my phone, stating that he had forgotten to inform me to fill out the reference form. His text never came. I never submitted my evaluation. That is how *not* to ask for a recommendation.

Rather than tell you how to write a recommendation request, I thought I would show you. My own recommendation request emails are below. A few important things to note are 1) to request a meeting to discuss the *possibility* of a letter, 2) to state how the potential recommender's class/laboratory/clinic has impacted you, and 3) to show interest in the relationship and not just the recommendation itself. I hope my emails can serve as a template for your reference requests.

Recommendation Request Email:

Dear Dr. McCommis,

I hope this email finds you well!

I just completed my undergraduate thesis for biology, and as I was writing the acknowledgments section, I was reflecting on professors who had supported my research during my time as an undergraduate. I ended up naming you, Dr. Smith, and Dr. Lambo, specifically, and I sincerely thank you for the advice and interest you showed in my research last spring.

Although my time learning from you was brief relative to other classes, your insight into research and guidance in presenting experimental findings in PBL stands out to me as one of the most impactful learning experiences during my undergraduate years. I so much appreciated and valued your engagement in my project and being able to discuss the nuances of effectively presenting research with you. What I learned through PBL and your teaching has significantly impacted and improved my undergraduate research and is something that I will continue to incorporate throughout my career.

I attached a copy of my completed thesis above and, additionally, wanted to ask if you had time to meet to discuss the possibility of you writing a recommendation to support my application to M.D. programs.

Let me know if you would be willing to meet, and if so, what times would be best for you. I hope you are enjoying teaching PBL this semester and that your students enjoy the course as much as I did!

With appreciation and gratitude,

Caroline Echeandia-Francis

Now that we know the language to ask for a recommendation, the final piece includes supplemental documents for your letter writer to reference. When your recommender agrees to write on your behalf, be sure to send them your resume/CV and personal statement. Your recommender will be able to pull details from these documents, and it will also allow them to know who you are outside of being their student, employee, volunteer, etc. Simply put, the resume and personal statement will help to humanize you by putting your life in context for someone who may know you only through a single lens.

POLITE FOLLOW-UP FOR YOUR LETTER WRITERS

Your relationship with a recommender doesn't end once your letter is received. This continued bond doesn't mean that the two of you are breaking bread at each other's tables once a month. It *does* mean that you don't disappear from their lives like a wandering ghost following the receipt of your letter. Someone who recommends you for medical school has the potential to become a lifelong mentor and friend. This person believes in your abilities as an aspiring physician – that says a lot. You respect your recommender's expertise in her field and opinion of you – that also says a lot. Maintaining a relationship with your letter writers does not have to be time-consuming. However, taking the time to check in with your advocates once a year or maybe once every few months is entirely worthwhile.

Ghosting your letter writers can cause them confusion. Keep the ghosting for your Tinder dates, sparky. At the very least, do two things: 1) thank your recommender when he submits your letter, and 2) let your recommender know the outcome of your application cycle. Whether you are admitted or need to reapply, informing your advocates of the outcome and thanking them again for their efforts is an important step. It gives them closure for a result that they care about. If you need to reapply, your recommender may be eager to work with you to improve your candidacy and update your letter. I know it stinks to tell someone you weren't selected for a program, but it's better than leaving them hanging. I've told many a recommender that I was not awarded a scholarship or chosen for a fellowship. It's a bummer, but they will still support you regardless of a committee's decision. The coworker whom I spoke about in the last section was both accepted to and denied two internships that I recommended him for. In both cases, he never told me what had happened. Years later, when I ran into him and asked direct questions, I finally knew how everything had worked out. Full confession: I have definitely made the mistake of not telling my letter writers the outcome of an application. With time, sweet Caroline has learned.

A favorite example of excellent follow-up came from one of my students. When she began her sophomore year of college, I advised her to run for a leadership position in Psi Chi (The National Honor Society in Psychology). She was a psychological and brain sciences major who struggled with confidence in pursuing leadership positions. Being an international student made her feel like an outsider, even at our university. These feelings gave her some hesitancy in assuredly pursuing positions that she was well-qualified for. Two years after our conversation in which I had encouraged her to run for Psi Chi's board, my former student texted me to celebrate her being selected as the President of Psi Chi. I was thrilled for her and honored that this young woman remembered our conversation from years ago.

Struggling to come up with thank you messages and update emails for your letter writers? At a loss for words? The check-ins that I sent to my recommenders are below for you to use as guidance. Additionally, people love baked goods – send your advocates cookies! Also, last December, the brilliant idea that struck me was to send my recommenders our family Christmas card. It was a hit! Consider doing the same.

Update email to recommender 1:

Dear Dr. Smith,

I hope you are doing well! I wanted to share with you that I was admitted to the University of Michigan Medical School today (your alma mater)! My application cycle has been going amazing so far, and I look forward to keeping you updated! How has everything been at WashU? Have you and your wife decided to get a dog yet? Sending wishes for a merry Christmas! Go Blue!

Caroline

Update email to recommender 2:

Dear Dr. Smith,

Hope you are enjoying the beautiful spring weather! I wanted to share with you the exciting news that I have made my final medical school decision. This summer, I will be matriculating to Yale School of Medicine to join the Class of 2025! I'm so thrilled to share this moment with you, as your mentorship has been such a gift to me.

It was an incredible honor to earn acceptance to WashU and UMich (your alma mater!), among others, and it was a very difficult final choice, but I am eager to apply to Barnes-Jewish and Michigan for residency. As always, thank you for everything that you have done to support me in becoming a physician - this is our shared victory! In August, I'll be switching over to my YSM email and want to give you my new Outlook address - [redacted for privacy] - so we can continue to keep in touch. Please let me know your updates - I am excited to hear them!

Warmest wishes,

Caroline

CHAPTER 08

MCAT

TESTING ANXIETY

Testing anxiety can cripple performance potential. We discussed testing anxiety in the *Testing Anxiety* section in the chapter on college academics.

As a refresher, if you think you're suffering from testing anxiety, speak with an advisor or a physician. Beta-blockers made a world of difference during my senior year when I would freeze during calculus exams. The medication helped ease my panic so that I could focus on the questions rather than my fear. When it came time to take the MCAT, and I was shaking in my boots, beta-blockers, again, helped me quash my nerves. Those not wanting to take a prescription can look to natural meditation and cognitive therapy to overcome testing anxiety. Speak with a professional to learn more. Don't suffer in silence.

MCAT ACCOMMODATIONS

For those who needed testing accommodations in college, it is smart to pursue testing accommodations for the MCAT. The MCAT is likely the hardest exam that you will have taken at this point in your life. The quantity of material that is covered is overwhelming. The questions are difficult. The format is designed to test how you manage limited time. The length of the exam requires notable stamina. Take all the help you can get – accommodations included. The exam will push you to your limits, allowing you to trace your hands along the rough edges of your capabilities. Even if you thought college testing accommodations were unneeded, you will want them for the MCAT.

When To Begin Planning for Accommodations

Submitting an initial request for accommodations takes up to 60 days to review. In other words, it may take two months to get a 'yay' or 'nay' regarding your request. This timeline is directly from the AAMC - AAMC: Review Cycle and Important Dates. If you are displeased with the board's ruling on your accommodations decision, reconsiderations take up to 30 days to process and receive a response. So far, you need to budget months ahead of your test date to properly pursue accommodations.

To understand the pre-planning needed to make an accommodation request prior to submitting the formal paperwork to the AAMC, we have to look at what kind of accommodations are offered. Extra time, food and drink, separate testing, and nursing mother and pregnancy-related accommodations are all offered by the AAMC to test takers (MCAT Exam with Accommodations FAQ: What types of conditions or impairments might need to be accommodated?). Individuals applying for extra time need to be evaluated by an appropriate professional. The professional works to determine if extra time is required for equal opportunity performance and how much additional time is recommended due to a person's circumstances. For example, if your evaluator is assessing you based on a learning disability or ADHD, the evaluation needs to take place "no more than three years prior to the anticipated MCAT date." If you are being assessed for a psychiatric disability, your evaluation "should have been administered no more than six months prior to the anticipated MCAT date" (An Overview for Applicants: What Does My Evaluator Need to Do?: How Current Must the Evaluation Be?). A full list of specific accommodations and their processes for applying for exam adjustments can be found here on the AAMC's website: MCAT Exam with Accommodations - Submitting Your Initial Application.

Taking this pre-planning into account, to obtain appropriate evaluations, you may have to begin preparing a full year before your test date to be considered for accommodations. To me, this wouldn't be as absurd if the cost of getting a professional evaluation wasn't so high. When I applied for extra time based on my own disability, evaluations that provided my original diagnosis had long expired according to the AAMC's expiration window. I had to get diagnosed (as if I had somehow grown out of my disability) by another professional. The professional we found (someone who was in St. Louis and approved by the AAMC) had an assessment fee of well over one thousand dollars. This is exactly where I think the AAMC has made a wrong turn with regard to its stringent evaluation rules. Only families of a certain socioeconomic status can afford these professional assessments. For an association claiming to strive for diversity in medical school students, diversity is repressed when looming financial hurdles prevent fair competition among applicants. It is true that the AAMC awards up to $800 to aid those who qualify for their Fee Assistance Program (FAP) in paying for evaluations (MCAT Exam with Accommodations: Accommodations Financial Benefit). Yet, plenty of applicants do not qualify for FAP but still cannot pay for such a pricey assessment. Until the AAMC changes its requirements, I only advise starting planning early for accommodations and seeing if you qualify for FAP.

How To Apply for Accommodations

With pre-planning underway, it's time to start understanding the accommodations application itself. Here's what's involved. Most, if not all, accommodations will require proof that adjustments are necessary. For learning disabilities, as we discussed above, one form of proof comes from the professional evaluation that you are required to obtain. Prior documentation is also requested for learning disabilities (MCAT Exam with Accommodations: Submitting Your Initial Application: Academic and Medical Supporting Documentation). This documentation comes in the form of previous evaluations that expired according to the AAMC's rules, accommodations that were requested for the SAT or ACT, as well as accommodations that you have used during college, secondary school, and primary school. SAT or ACT scores, in addition to your college and high school transcripts, are asked to be submitted. Finally, you have to write a personal statement addressing which accommodations are being requested, why adjustments are needed, and why such measures will give you equal opportunity on the MCAT (Submitting Your Initial Application: The Personal Statement). There also may be a number of short answer questions. Gathering these documents and writing your statements takes time to do properly. Make sure you get started ahead of time and put your best effort into your writing. It is difficult to have accommodations – especially for extended testing time – granted by the AAMC. Putting together the strongest case on your behalf will give you the best chance of approval by the accommodations board. Remember, if they do not approve your request or do not grant the specific adjustments that you were hoping for, it takes a maximum of 30 days to hear back with a petition to reconsider.

Below, I've included the cover letter (now called the personal statement) that I wrote to the board when I requested accommodations for my learning disability. My disability has been well-documented since primary school (three total evaluations, including the last evaluation that I had to get before the MCAT). I had used extended time on the SAT, SAT Subject Tests, AP Exams, and throughout high school and college. All of this paperwork was submitted as part of my application. I hope my cover letter can provide some guidance as to how to make your case to the AAMC. Of course, my experience is only through applying due to a learning disability, yet from speaking to others, I know how difficult it can be to get time adjustments approved by the AAMC.

AAMC Accommodations Request Cover Letter:

Dear MCAT Accommodations Board,

My name is Caroline Echeandia-Francis. I am a senior at Washington University in St. Louis, double-majoring in biology and psychology, who is planning to take the MCAT this spring. As per the MCAT Accommodation Board's request, I was retested for my learning disability this past November by Dr. Martielli of the Neuropsychology Center of St. Louis. In summary, Dr. Martielli diagnosed me with a specific learning disorder with impairment in reading. Her assessment report is included in the paperwork provided. Overall, I am seeking double time on the MCAT to have equal opportunity to perform on the exam to the best of my ability. Below, I summarized my medical history and diagnoses relating to my learning disability and explained how my disability affects me both inside and outside of the academic environment. Thank you for your consideration of my case.

I was born with a bilateral branchial cleft cyst that likely was the cause of the numerous, prolonged ear infections I experienced throughout infancy and childhood. As Dr. Martielli discusses in her report, these ear infections may have stunted my early language acquisition development and thus affected my auditory processing, reading, and spelling abilities.

My deficits in language development went largely unnoticed until the fifth grade when I scored markedly lower on state standardized achievement exams than expected. I was tested for learning disabilities, and, as the report states, I was diagnosed with a slow processing disorder and was suspected of hearing loss.

My disability did not noticeably hinder my academic performance again until I took the PSAT. Again, I scored much lower than expected for a high school student with a 3.95 GPA.

After consultation with my pediatrician, I was referred to Dr. Stephanie Verlinden from the Diagnostic & Treatment Clinic – Children's Program. Through Dr. Verlinden's testing and evaluation, I was again diagnosed with a learning processing disorder, NOS (slow processing speed), and mild ADHD.

I received 1.5 X time accommodations on the SAT and AP exams. My scores improved from scoring at the 25th percentile on the PSAT to the 99th percentile on the SAT. On my AP exams, I scored 5s (highest score) during my senior year with accommodations compared to 3s during my junior year without accommodations.

In Fall 2015, I began college at Washington University in St. Louis and was unaware that testing accommodations were available for college students. As such, I waded into my courses without this assistance. I believe my experiences in my first and second biology courses at WashU perfectly demonstrate how my slow processing disorder (now diagnosed as a specific learning disability with an impairment in reading) affects my academic performance.

I took my first two required biology courses at Washington University without testing accommodations. As I opened each of the three semester exams, I flipped through pages of increasingly complex problems. They required me to synthesize numerous principles that we had learned in class to reach an answer. I knew I could solve these questions, so I began answering the questions I knew first and strategically skipping the problems that I was unsure of. I worked as efficiently as I could but could never finish my exams. Pages of questions that I could solve were left blank. I earned Bs and Cs on my exams and ended up with a final grade of B- (the lowest grade I've earned at WashU).

While I was aware of the Disability Resources Center at WashU, I did not consider my slow processing disorder a disability. However, during a discussion with one of my professors, she told me that the Center assisted students with learning disabilities and encouraged me to reach out to them. After reviewing my situation and assessing clinical reports, I received time accommodations on all university exams. These accommodations were made to provide equal access to testing to address the way in which I processed information.

I was hopeful that testing accommodations would finally allow me to demonstrate my full academic capability to myself and to my professors. I knew the answers to the complex exam questions, but I needed more time to synthesize the material in front of me. After receiving testing accommodations from the University, my academic experience changed.

I was dreading the second biology course in WashU's two-semester biology sequence. I wanted to be a successful student. I *didn't want to disappoint myself like I had in the biology course prior. Despite knowing that I had extra time on the first biology exam, I was incredibly nervous when I sat down for the test. I opened the exam and again was confronted with complex questions that were unfamiliar to me. But ones that I knew I could solve. I had spent hours after class making flashcards from my notes. I spent the week before the exam taking every practice exam that our instructors made available to us, reviewing our lab reports, and asking our TAs and professors every question that I could not answer on my own.*

I lifted my pencil and started answering every question I could, strategically skipping the ones I was unsure of. I finished every question I knew on the exam, and for the first time at WashU, I had time to turn my full attention to the questions I had skipped over. I answered those questions to completion as well. I handed in my exam feeling hopeful for the first time since high school - at last, I had regained control over my testing and education.

Two weeks later, all exams had been graded. Our professors stacked 600 exams at the front of the lecture hall organized by last name. I tentatively took mine from the looming pile and stuffed it in my bag. My friend Amelia turned to me, "You have to look at what you got! You studied so hard. I know you did well."

Even though I was able to finish my exam, the memories of the semester prior flooded back into my mind. A pit in my chest would form as I looked at the scores of exams that I had spent countless hours preparing for, only to receive average grades. But I knew that Amelia was right. I needed to see if extra time was the change that had finally made a difference in my academic performance.

I opened my exam, and my eyes rushed to the bottom of the page. I earned an 87. The mean of the 600-person class was a 67. I scored 20 points higher than the mean, putting me in the top 5% of the class. Only eight students had scored higher than I had, and my letter grade was nearly an A+. The second exam came and went. The mean was a 67. I earned an 81.5 – another A. The third exam came, and I earned a 90.5 – the mean was a 75. I earned high enough As on all three exams that I did not have to take the final to keep my A in the class. This was the first time I had earned an A in one of WashU's most challenging premed courses.

With my academic success matching my effort, my confidence soared. I took one advanced biology class after another – earning As and A-s in all of them. I declared a second major in biology – something that I would have never imagined possible after earning a B- in my first biology course at WashU. This semester, I just learned that my grades have qualified me to graduate with Latin honors in my biology major upon completing my senior thesis. I was offered a position TAing the introductory biology course, in which I earned my first A, and offered a second TAing position in biochemistry, in which I earned an A+.

Currently, I just completed my first semester of my senior year at WashU and have a 3.71 GPA. I've earned 4.0s during the past two semesters and haven't earned anything lower than an A- since my sophomore year. As I began practicing for the MCAT with standard time, I was scoring below the 50th percentile. By my third practice exam that I took with extended time, I scored above the 90th percentile, indicating, to me, how my specific learning disability with impairment in reading affects my MCAT performance – particularly since it is a reading-based exam.

Without the timing accommodations on my practice MCAT exams, I was confronted by the same problems that I faced on my first biology course exams. I knew the answers to the majority of the questions, but I ran out of time reading, thus forcing me to leave large sections of the exam blank. It was too large of an issue to be bridged by timing and testing strategies. With double time, I was able to read the exam material and pace myself to answer the corresponding questions.

As per the MCAT Board's request, I was reevaluated for my learning disability by Dr. Tammy Martielli of the Neuropsychology Center of St. Louis. She explained to me that slow processing disorder (my previous diagnosis) was now understood to be a symptom of something larger, and we needed to figure out what that something was. It was through her testing, as can be read in detail in her report, that my diagnosis was reclassified as a specific learning disability with impairment in reading.

Outside of the classroom, my learning disability still affects my life. It takes me longer to search for the right words when I speak to someone, and it takes me longer to retrieve simple information from my mind, such as my age. It may only take me a second or two longer than the normal person – not slow enough for anyone to notice – but I can still feel my brain racing while my motor churns as quickly as it can to keep up with my mind so that I can communicate effectively with other people. My learning disability only becomes a severe hindrance when the questions I'm asked – such as the ones on exams – become inordinately complex, causing me to take minutes longer, rather than seconds, to reach an accurate answer.

I love myself for the way I am. My brain is not perfect, but it is capable of incredible things. I wouldn't exchange my mind with anyone else's because my brain – impaired reading ability and all – has made me a successful undergraduate researcher and an accomplished student and leader. One day, my brain will make me an outstanding doctor.

I am requesting extended time while taking the MCAT so that my reading disability does not hinder my performance on such an important exam. I seek an equal opportunity with my peers to perform well on the MCAT to demonstrate my intellectual capabilities to medical schools. I spent three months preparing for the MCAT this past summer and have continued to study through this fall. I will spend several more months preparing before taking the exam in May. I am incredibly excited to take the MCAT and submit my application to medical schools.

I am confident that I will be a caring and capable physician, and I strongly believe that receiving testing accommodations on the MCAT will help me convey this message to medical schools. Thank you for your time and consideration of my request.

Caroline Echeandia-Francis

Possible Results

There are three possible outcomes when applying for AAMC accommodations: 1) you are approved - either with adjustments to your request or with no adjustments, 2) the board requests additional information, or 3) your request is denied (MCAT Exam with Accommodations: Information on Reconsiderations, Appeals, and Extensions). The first time I submitted my paperwork, the board asked for additional information. My professional evaluation had expired, and I hadn't read the instructions closely enough to know that a new evaluation was needed. After getting re-evaluated and submitting the results, my request for extended testing time was approved, but with a catch. This catch was one that I've noticed is common among those requesting extended testing time. The board granted half the time extension that my current and previous evaluators had advised. Throughout high school, college, and other standardized exams, I was always given 1.5X time. I was surprised when the board had only approved me for 1.25X time. One of my friends who also had a well-documented learning disability was, similarly, approved for half of her normal extended time. It's frustrating that the board asks you to be evaluated by professionals and submit years of documentation only to decide how much time you "actually" need. Why do the board's doctors – who have never met any of us test-takers – know better than the evaluators who tested us? Why are professional evaluations needed if the recommendations are going to be ignored?

There was an option to appeal the board's decision and ask for the full 1.5X time that I was used to. However, I was not confident that my request would be approved and was worried that they may even take away the 1.25X time I was given. I decided not to petition for reconsideration and make my merry way with a 1.25X time extension.

Do I think that being approved for 1.5X time would have made a difference on the MCAT? Yes. I think my normal extended time would have made a difference because I ran out of time on the CARS and Chemistry/Physics sections. Yet, the difference would likely not have caused a massive jump in score. Perhaps one or two points at most. Each of these points certainly matters on the MCAT. However, practicing with whatever accommodations you were granted can help you perform best on test day. Leading up to the exam, I took my practice tests under 1.25X time conditions. Honestly, I think that I could've finished CARS and Chemistry/Physics on the actual exam if I wasn't as nervous. The beta-blockers helped with my nerves, but anxiety was still there.

If you have been granted adjustments that will not work for you or your accommodations request was denied, I recommend fighting for the testing circumstances you need rather than underperforming on the exam. I'm unsure what the process is like when asking the board to reconsider and how successful these cases are. Consult with your premed advisor or your professional evaluator when wanting to contest the board's ruling. From my understanding, extended time is one of the hardest, if not *the* hardest, accommodation to obtain. Those with mobility limitations, nursing mothers, etc., should have a much easier time having their needs met. It seems that the board fears students with no learning disability taking advantage of extended time to get an unfair benefit in the exam. For this, I do applaud them for their strictness. The SAT has extraordinarily loose regulations for those granted extended time, which is truly to the detriment of students with learning disabilities, like myself. Instead of an equal playing field, those with inside knowledge benefit from extended time when it is not actually needed. However, as I mentioned before, if a student's request for extended time is legitimate, then I see no reason why the full amount of extended time shouldn't be granted. Commie bastards!

CHOOSING WHEN TO TAKE THE EXAM

There are several options for when to take the MCAT. At the earliest, freshman summer is a viable option, but I would only suggest this timing for those with specific circumstances. We will dive into the details in a few minutes. At the latest, senior summer is ideal for more traditional applicants. Senior summer is long gone for non-traditional applicants, and the exam can be taken whenever you feel most prepared. The difference between traditional and non-traditional applicants is usually defined as the following: traditional applicants take a maximum of two gap years between college graduation and medical school matriculation, while non-traditional applicants take three or more years between finishing college and medical school matriculation. These are the widely accepted definitions in 2021. As gap years become more common (possibly becoming a soft requirement for medical schools), I expect the definitions of traditional and non-traditional applicants to change. For now, this is what we'll work with.

Freshman summer is quite early to take the MCAT. This should only be done for those committed to taking no gap years. If you need even one gap year, your score may expire at some schools by the time you apply, thus forcing you to retake the MCAT. Yuck. We like to avoid retakes. Right gang? A freshman summer exam is also only appropriate if you have a strong scientific foundation. Perhaps you are a super genius and took biology, chemistry, and physics all freshman year. If you did well in those courses, getting the MCAT out of the way may be a good idea while the information is still fresh. Alternatively, maybe you just took chemistry freshman year but have a strong grasp of biology and physics from high school. This is also a circumstance in which you may want to take the MCAT sooner rather than later. Personally, I don't think I've met a soul who has taken the exam this early. But it is something to consider for those with the no gap year objective.

Sophomore summer is another ideal option for those wanting to take no gap years or one gap year. By this time, you've had more classes under your belt and more time to adjust to the rigors of college exams. One of the best benefits of exposure to difficult college exams is that they prepare you for the difficulty of the MCAT. You strengthen your critical reasoning skills and stamina to perform well on MCAT test day. Those wanting to take no gap years will be submitting their medical school application over their junior summer. For these applicants, freshman or sophomore summer is your best bet for acing the MCAT. We touched on this in the Planning Your Summers chapter, but taking the exam while enrolled in classes is extremely difficult to achieve. There are some superhumans who can pull it off. Yet, these individuals are rare. For us mere mortals, freshman or sophomore summers are our golden ticket for top MCAT scoring. Many students will try to squeeze in the exam during winter break. Do you remember Nyra? Precious Nyra attempted a winter break exam. It totally flopped. She scored a 508 when she had the potential to score a 520+. She was not admitted to medical school during her first cycle and is now taking three gap years in order to retake the MCAT, boost her grades, and deepen her research experience. Silly Nyra! Why cause such chaos? The only person I know who has successfully pulled off a winter break exam was another WashU student. She was a verified superhuman who aced WashU's daunting medical school prerequisite courses. Let's call her Molly. After Molly's girlfriend broke up with her before the semester ended, she dealt with the pain of the breakup by spending every waking moment of winter break in the library. Molly poured over practice questions and exam content to distract her from the loss of her girlfriend. Studying was a much-welcomed distraction from the grief of her relationship's conclusion. Molly's intense preparation paid off, as she scored nearly a 528 on the MCAT. Please do note that Molly is an exception, not the rule. Moreover, she was an exception, working at peak capacity to avoid the pain of love lost. Make sure you are a Molly before you attempt a Christmas miracle.

Junior summer is the final summer to take the exam for applicants wanting to take only one gap year. Almost all of my classmates tested during their junior summers. Yes, technically, those planning to take no gap years can take the MCAT during junior summer. But this is a risky move. Taking the exam too late during the summer when applications are submitted can delay your application's review by admissions committees and thus lower your odds of earning an interview. Furthermore, if you do not like your score, you have no time to retake the MCAT for that cycle. I would wait to test until senior summer or beyond for those planning to take two or more gap years. The three to four months of your junior summer are better spent immersing yourself in research, clinical experiences, volunteering, and other impactful activities, especially while your university's resources are still at your disposal.

Senior summer is the perfect MCAT testing time for those looking to take two to three gap years prior to matriculation. With graduation having just passed, you are still in university mode. You have yet to fall into the more relaxed routine of the gap year. Couch surfing, barbequing, making your own line of cheeky bikinis – ah, the gap year! Just kidding – I know most gap years are busy to the brim. It's a bit of a bummer to celebrate graduation and hop into studying, but I didn't mind it. After a family celebration in Florida, I returned to my apartment to study. I saw taking the MCAT during my senior summer as the culmination of my undergraduate work. Everything that I had been practicing and perfecting in the classroom – from sharpening my problem-solving to building stamina during four-hour physics exams – led to these moments. While the studying was exhausting, I actually enjoyed the routine. I had forgotten much of the chemistry and physics I learned during my freshman and sophomore years, so relearning everything was a nice way to pay homage to the hard sciences. I'm such a dork. I know. I never really mastered chemistry and physics in high school or college, so it felt great to nail down these disciplines through the MCAT. The downside of taking the MCAT during senior summer is largely that you – like me – may have forgotten much of what was learned during your prerequisite courses. In reality, I don't think most of this information is completely forgotten, but rather, the specifics have faded into shadows. The shadows will be resurrected into fully-formed ideas with a bit of review.

A note about taking the exam at the *beginning* of summer: Suppose you want to apply to medical school during the upcoming summer but have yet to take the MCAT. You may think to study for your exam during the school year and then sit for the MCAT at the beginning of summer. Many WashU students had this plan. Similar to my worries about taking the test during the academic year, your classes and extracurricular activities may make it difficult to prepare for the exam during the spring semester properly. When finals end, and your test is weeks or a month away, you can easily find yourself scrambling to catch up on preparation. Delaying your test date is certainly preferable to taking the MCAT when not ready. However, delaying your test date will hold up your entire medical school application, assuming you are applying during the same summer. Avoiding application hold-ups to increase your chance of being invited to an interview is best. The WashU students I knew at the beginning of the the summer testing plan could not sufficiently prepare during the school year. They either needed to delay their exam or did not perform as well as they could have. If you want to effectively pull off the beginning of summer testing plan, take a light course load to master exam material like a pro.

Beyond senior summer is when non-traditional applicants will be taking the MCAT. This may mean that you are studying for the exam during a post-bac program while working, completing research, etc. Whatever your circumstances are, give yourself the time to reach your maximum score. Consider taking time off to study for two to three months if possible. If time cannot be taken off, it will likely take more time to prepare. With no time off, your study schedule may be extended to six months rather than two or three. That is perfectly fine! The most important thing is you earn the score that you are capable of – the score that will make you the best candidate for medical school. It is far better to take more time rather than to retake the entire exam. I personally know of people working full-time who took their time studying for the MCAT and achieved a 520+. They are rock stars! I am confident that you can follow in their footsteps.

HOW TO STUDY

The *How To Study* section will be broken down into choosing your target MCAT score, the materials necessary for kicking MCAT's butt, and how to prepare for each of the four exam sections. There will be brief comments on post-MCAT anxiety and blues, as they are common among test-takers. Note that these are the recommendations that helped me achieve my score of 517. Had I executed better on my plan, I am confident that I could've scored a 520+. Nyra, who we've mentioned throughout the guidebook, scored a 508 on her first MCAT due to a lack of a well-thought-out study plan. After I received my MCAT score back, I spent about two hours with Nyra on the phone, helping her craft a game plan for her retake. Much of what I shared with her was my own preparation strategies and is what I will share with you below. I will also disclose what study strategies didn't work for me and what I would've done differently if I were to take the exam again. From what I have read on the MCAT subreddit, these study strategies have been successful for students across the world. Many extraneous MCAT preparation resources are not needed, besides poor advice that can lead someone astray. Fear not! These testing strategies are built with exam domination in mind. Sharpen those pencils. Erasers at the ready. Let's get studying!

Choosing a Target Score

My advice for choosing a target score is straight and simple. **I believe everyone's target score should be a 520**, with the lowest subsection score being a 128. Do you need help picking your jaw up off of the floor? Let me explain why I think you should shoot for the stars. First, a 520 will not keep you out of any medical schools. In fact, it will open doors where a lower GPA may have kept you from getting an interview. Harvard, Perelman, NYU, Yale, WUSM, UCLA – they are all within reach with a 520. Second, if you prepare for a 520 and fall short of this mark, you will still likely be in excellent shape. It is rare to prepare for a 520 and then have your score fall to a 510. AAMC practice exams are an extraordinarily accurate predictor of your test day score. A ten-point drop is truly rare and is usually due to unusual test day circumstances (you are sick, some lunatic is tapping their foot incessantly, etc.) or, alternatively, you did not take your AAMC practice exams under proper test conditions. What is far more likely is a two- or three-point drop where you would end up with a 518 or 517. These outstanding scores will also not keep you out of *any* schools. Third, from what I have seen, the score we prepare for is often the one we get. While studying for the MCAT, I targeted a 517 and earned a 517. My roommate targeted a 514 and earned a 514. Our target scores set up expectations in our minds for what we will achieve. Our targets give us mental parameters of our capabilities. Because people are naturally lazy, our brains subconsciously cling to achieving the score that we aim for. Therefore, if your target score is a 510, but you are really hoping for a 514, it is risky to rely on luck alone to get you those four extra points. Shoot for the stars. You just might reach them. Fourth, studying for a 520 isn't a tremendous amount of work compared to studying for a 510. Suck it up, buttercup. It's worth it. Fifth, if you are aiming for a competitive medical specialty (dermatology, ophthalmology, interventional radiology, radiation oncology, etc.), you will need to kill USMLE Step 2, so long as it doesn't pass/fail. You will also need to ace your shelf exams unless you go to Yale, where shelf exams aren't counted into our clerkship grades. Might as well get used to dominating standardized tests and boost your confidence by crushing the MCAT. Am I right, or am I right? Sixth, I am quite confident that you are capable of achieving a 520+. Have we met? No. But I used to be a terrible standardized exam taker. Literally, my elementary school and high school counselors scheduled meetings with my parents because my standardized exam scores were so low compared to my classroom performance. This is actually how we found out about my learning disability. However, learning disability or not, I know plenty of naturally poor standardized exam takers who have learned to get top scores. This exam is so much more about thorough preparation and well-practiced strategies than raw intelligence. Raw intelligence does carry you to the higher scores (think the high 520s) along with luck. But a well-executed strategy alone should get you to at least a 515.

If you are truly opposed to aiming for a 520, here is the alternative plan. Make your school list (*How Do GPA and MCAT Affect Your School List?* Section) and compile the highest *average* or *median* MCAT scores for schools on your list. Perhaps the highest average score is a 510. In that case, yes, you can choose 510 as your target score. However, your chances of earning an interview will be helped by aiming for a higher score, so you might as well try for a 520. There is one exception where a high MCAT score may actually harm you. Let's say that your dream schools have average MCAT scores of 513 on the high end. If you come strutting in with a 3.9 GPA and a 520 MCAT, you run the risk of being yield-protected out of the school. Let me first explain yield protection (fondly referred to as Tufts Syndrome). Yield protection is the act of turning away top-tier applicants who are not expected to matriculate to the school due to their tremendous caliber (Yield Protection, a.k.a. Tufts Syndrome: Everything You Need to Know). Is this a phony legend, or does yield protection actually exist? We only have anecdotal evidence to go off of until someone does a proper study. From the anecdotes that I've gathered, yield protection very much exists. Personally, I had a much easier time getting interviews to the top 20 medical schools than I did to the mid-tier and lower-tier medical schools. Many other applicants whom I've spoken with have shared my experience. Mayo, Mount Sinai, Vanderbilt, and Northwestern are all over them.

Less competitive schools don't acknowledge their existence. Therefore, if you are aiming for a mid- or lower-tier school, a 514 MCAT rather than a 520 may be the way to go. I've seen too many people who have the scores for a top 20 program (3.8+ GPA and 520+ MCAT) paired with mediocre activities. They are too often ignored by mid- and low-tier schools but are also stiffed by the top programs because their activities are lackluster. Overall, aiming for a 520 is ideal, but exceptions exist for those in this particular high statistics, mediocre resume circumstance.

Materials and Preparation Strategy

<u>There are four materials that you absolutely need to ace the MCAT:</u> **the UWorld MCAT QBank, the AAMC MCAT Official Prep Section Bank, the AAMC MCAT Official Prep Question Packs, and the AAMC MCAT Official Prep Practice Exams**. These four pillars alone can get you a 520+. These are the four thicccc daddies. Thickies unite!

If you've surfed the internet without a VPN in the past year, Big Brother has probably told Big Tech what you're up to (i.e., applying to medical school). This means you've likely met the spiffy Princeton Review guy sporting a bow tie and thick daddy, rimmed spectacles on YouTube. Princeton Review, Kaplan Test Prep, and Examkrackers are a few companies offering classes, preparation books, and practice exams to MCAT takers. As someone who took a Kaplan MCAT course, read their books, completed their question pack as well as took their practice exams, I can say these resources are mostly poop with a few exceptions. I took a Princeton Review class for the SAT, which was incredible for helping boost my score. The MCAT courses, on the other hand, simply cannot cover all of the information on the exam. Mine was very much a waste of money and time. The books and question banks these companies offer do not hold a candle to the information in UWorld. There are so many UWorld QBank questions – literally thousands – (and I recommend doing UWorld twice) that you do not realistically have time to complete UWorld properly, along with another question bank. The books that the test prep companies offer do, in fact, cover a lot of standard material, but there is an easy shortcut for you to take to cover your content bases. To nail down the basics of each of the three science MCAT sections, the Kaplan MCAT Quicksheet is sufficient. The Kaplan MCAT Quicksheet is a highly condensed version of the fundamentals of chemistry/physics, biology/biochemistry, and psychology/sociology - simply search Kaplan MCAT Quicksheet on the internet to find the publicly available PDF. Know the Quicksheet like the back of your hand, and you will be set up to score a 510+ with that knowledge alone, plus practice exams. It really is that simple. Please do not waste months of time like I did reading the Kaplan MCAT books cover to cover. Make flashcards from the Quicksheet and use the rest of your time on UWorld and the AAMC's materials. This is critical advice that people can be hesitant to take. Yet, it is imperative to use your time as wisely as possible. I estimate it will take about a week to turn the Quicksheet information into flashcards and other forms of practice material. Other practice material includes fill-in charts for learning amino acids or fill-in-the-blank graphics for learning the Citric Acid Cycle. After creating flashcards and practice material, spend two weeks nailing down the basics. The timelines I will give are approximate - adjust them for your learning needs.

Concurrently with the Kaplan MCAT Quicksheet studying, you also want to mix in the AAMC Question Packs. The Question Packs include 720 questions spanning each of the four MCAT sections. These questions are known to be a good way to get down your basics – the questions are straightforward and cover high-yield material. In other words, the Question Packs are not too challenging (apart from CARS). The most important part of the Question Packs is CARS, which can be purchased separately in case you don't want the entire bundle. The CARS questions have the same level of difficulty as the real exam. The questions from C/P and B/B are more standard, but if you want some question preparation before diving into UWorld, the Question Packs are like dipping your toe in the water before plunging cannonball-style into the deep. Yah feel?

UWorld is the holy grail of MCAT preparation material. God bless the creators of UWorld. If you haven't heard of the UWorld MCAT QBank, it is an epic question bank. The questions cover everything from high-yield to low-yield testing material. The questions are at or slightly above the difficulty of the actual MCAT exam, making it an outstanding source of practice material. Mastering UWorld is how you get to scoring a 520+. All of the knowledge you need to get a near-perfect score is in UWorld. Their explanations of why certain answers are right and others are wrong are the best in the industry.

After mastering the Kaplan MCAT Quicksheet and the AAMC Question Packs, I would start doing UWorld like a mothertrucker. (I'm trying to reduce my swearing.) UWorld is divided into seven primary disciplines: behavioral sciences, biochemistry, biology, critical analysis and reasoning skills, general chemistry, organic chemistry, and physics. The seven disciplines are further divided into subsections (for example, biology contains ten subsections, one of which is circulation and respiration). Spend the next six to eight weeks of a full-time study plan, mastering UWorld. That should give you enough time to thoroughly go through each question. Each day, I would wake up and review your Quicksheet information and then turn to UWorld. I would start with whatever section of the MCAT is most challenging for you (for me, this was C/P) and do a question set. Then, review your flagged and wrong answers. Repeat this with another MCAT section (CARS, B/B, or P/S). Keep going until you've gone through all four MCAT sections. You may want to structure your day to do larger question blocks (maybe 50 or so questions at a time) and thus do the four sections once per day. Or you may prefer smaller question chunks (~ ten questions at a time) and choose to cycle through each of the four MCAT sections several times per day. Whatever your rhythm, make sure that you understand why you got questions right and wrong on UWorld. This will set you up for MCAT supremacy. Truly, the value of UWorld in their superbly clear and detailed explanations when examining potential answer choices. Take advantage of these explanations to know why you got questions right and wrong.

About 75% of the way through UWorld, consider taking AAMC MCAT Practice Exam Four. Doing a practice exam at this stage gets you used to the exam format and shows you where your weak points are. Perhaps you earn a 130 on CARS but a 126 on P/S. This information will inform your focus the final weeks of your preparation on P/S. Do not get too hung up on your score. With this being your first practice exam and without having seen the AAMC Section Bank, you are missing experience with challenging AAMC material. AAMC MCAT Practice Exam Four is the newest, which is why it is the best one to use for preliminary practice. Although you don't want to be emotionally swept away with your score, take time reviewing incorrect and flagged questions. Make sure to completely understand why a certain response was right, and the other answer choices were wrong.

Once you are in your final four to five weeks before your exam (a.k.a. Kaplan Quicksheet is mastered, the AAMC Question Packs are finished, your first thorough pass at UWorld is complete, and one AAMC practice exam has been taken as a benchmark), it's time to turn to more AAMC materials. Just for a timeline reference, I discovered UWorld only about a month before my MCAT exam and was able to complete most of the questions over the four weeks when I used it. Tragic! I wish that I would have discovered it earlier. If I had done UWorld the way I am advising you to, a 520+ would have likely been my outcome. The low-yield material in UWorld is what gets you from a 515 to a 520+. Okay, enough gushing about UWorld. Let's discuss the AAMC Section Bank and the remaining three AAMC Practice Exams.

In your final four to five weeks before your exam, begin with Monday through Friday spent working through the AAMC Section Bank as well as your second pass of UWorld. The AAMC Section Bank contains 300 questions in total – 100 questions for each science subsection (C/P, B/B, and P/S). These 300 questions are more challenging than the AAMC Question Packs but are great preparation with comparable difficulty to the actual MCAT. With the goal of completing the AAMC Section Bank in the first two weeks of the last ~month of studying, plan to do 40 total questions per day plus review. Feel free to step up this question load if you would like to finish earlier. Spend your first Monday through Friday completing the first 200 bank questions. On Saturday, take AAMC MCAT Practice Exam One. On Sunday, review the exam and rest. Rest is not to be underestimated. Resting is not a waste of time but rather a necessary recharge. Whatever your weak areas were on your practice test, spend extra time fortifying those subjects during the upcoming week. Extra time is time when you are not doing the Section Bank. Tailor your UWorld review and Kaplan Quicksheet flashcards to your weak areas. Soon, we will talk about the specific conditions under which to take the AAMC MCAT Official Prep Practice Exams. For now, getting back to the schedule, spend the next Monday through Friday completing the AAMC Section Bank, reviewing your answers, and improving on your weakest subjects from AAMC Practice Exam One. On Saturday, take AAMC Practice Exam Two. On Sunday, review and rest. Get the rhythm? After this, you should have a good idea of where you are set to score on exam day, with about two to three weeks remaining before the real deal.

With these two to three weeks remaining before test day, spend the first week or two completing your second pass through UWorld and re-reviewing the AAMC Practice Exams and Questions Bank, all with the goal of strengthening areas of weakness. This is where

Kaplan, Examkrackers, and Princeton Review material may become useful. Specifically, if you are struggling with CARS, I can testify that Kaplan CARS is close to what is on the actual MCAT. Check out the reviews on other companies' CARS material and get in as much practice as you can to score well on this section. Warning: Avoid taking full practice exams from anyone other than the AAMC during these final weeks. Outside companies' exams – especially Kaplan and Princeton reviews – tend to deflate scores. I took several of Kaplan's practice exams. The C/P section is incredibly difficult and unlike the real MCAT. CARS is pretty realistic. P/S is the next most similar section to the real MCAT. B/B is somewhere in the middle but not very useful. When taking the Kaplan exams, I could not break a 508. My C/P did not move beyond a 125. These exams were crushing my confidence that I could ever achieve my target score of a 517+ on the MCAT. I stopped taking Kaplan exams during my preparation and focused just on studying. Admittedly, I had more studying under my belt by the time I took an AAMC Practice Exam, but my first AAMC practice exam score was a 516. I believe my C/P score was a 128. The AAMC practice exam was much more representative of a range of easy to difficult questions. Kaplan's C/P was skewed toward challenging material. Moreover, I knew of one student who took Princeton Review's practice exams right when he was taking the AAMC Practice Exams, and he scored a 505 on Princeton and a 520 on AAMC. His real MCAT score was right where the AAMC Practice Exam scores put him. You have been warned. Please be careful with outside companies' exams. They might just crush your soul. Avoid them, especially when close to your official testing date.

With one week to go before your exam, take AAMC MCAT Practice Exam Three between five and seven days out from the real deal. This will give you time to review your answers and shore up any weak areas. Do not take the last AAMC Practice Exam a day or two before the official MCAT. This can spook you if you don't score where you want to. You can also hurt your stamina by sitting for a ~7-hour practice session right before the ~7-hour test day. Over the final days before your actual MCAT, take it easy. Review your weaker areas with flashcards and other preparation materials. Avoid difficult questions like those on UWorld that may deflate your confidence. Go into the MCAT after a full night of sleep and know that there are plenty of dumber nuts than you who have aced this exam. If they can do it, you can do it. No offense intended.

Running through your mind may be the thought: "I want more than the four practice exams offered by the AAMC. You told me not to use outside exams. What should I do?" Oh buddy, do I have a solution for you! As we have established, UWorld is da bomb. Did you know you can make your own practice exams out of UWorld questions? If you are familiar with their platform, you will know that you can select how to form your question blocks. You can choose ten questions about amino acids, 15 questions about reproduction and cell growth, and five questions from critical analysis and reasoning skills in order to create a tailored question block. This is one example of countless combinations to fit your study needs. To make your own practice MCAT exam, choose the appropriate number of questions from each testing category. Select 53 critical analysis and reasoning skills questions and 59 questions from each C/P-, B/B-, and P/S-related section. Set the appropriate time limit – 375 minutes of total *test-taking* time under standard time conditions. This breaks down into 95 minutes for C/P, B/B, and P/S and 90 minutes for CARS. Naturally, if you have been granted extended time accommodations, account for the adjustment. Abracadabra! You have additional practice exams at your disposal.

An important note is that these UWorld practice exams will be most realistic if you have not seen the questions before. Therefore, before diving into using UWorld, calculate how many questions you may want to leave unseen for a potential practice exam or two. The last point of attention is that UWorld will not give you an MCAT-style score. You won't be given a score of 118-132 on the subsections or a total score of 472-528 on the total of all four sections. UWorld will only tell you how many questions you got right and wrong. From there, you can look at a conversion sheet showing how many correct questions translate into a certain score. Fifty correct CARS questions may result in a 130, for example. This will be a rough translation, but it can give you a sense of where you stand. Finally, account for the fact that UWorld is a bit more difficult than the actual MCAT. Don't be devastated if you had 49 correct B/B questions on your UWorld mock exam. Forty-nine correct B/B questions on UWorld would likely translate into 54+ correct questions on the MCAT—food for thought.

Speaking of practice exams, let's gab about under what conditions to take these practice runs. The skinny is that you want to take your practice exams under near-identical conditions to the actual MCAT. Near-identical conditions are replicated by following these guidelines. Begin your exam at the same time your actual MCAT starts. If you have an 8:00 AM start, then guess what, papa? You're practicing for the test at eight. Beginning your exam on time will train you to think critically and problem-solve during the morning hours. Hardcore students can go through the ritual of waking up before their start time to take a shower and get dressed in their lucky t-shirts. Take the exam in a quiet room. Once again, the hardcore homies will perhaps find a room in an unfamiliar place (a library, for example) to replicate the unfamiliarity of the testing center. Have your snacks made ahead of time like you would on game day. Secure a pair of headphones, earplugs, and a small whiteboard and an erasable marker. These are the supplies that you are given in the testing center. Use them like you plan to during the real exam. A desktop computer will be most similar to the computers in the testing center. If one is available, it is a better simulation compared to a laptop. Also, be sure to take any medications that you will need during the MCAT. Beta-blockers, Adderall – whatever your cocktail is, bottoms up! When you begin your practice exam, you will be able to set the time conditions. If you are testing under standard time, do not give yourself extended time in practice. If you are testing with extended time, test with the same extension during the sample exams. Sometimes, the time extensions will mean that you will take your MCAT over two days – if this is the case, follow the two-day procedure in these mock trials. Be sure to take the breaks given to you in practice, as you will likely need them for a bathroom stop, snack, or mental rest during the actual MCAT. Each of these steps will help replicate what you will experience during your official MCAT exam. Following this procedure will give you the most realistic score on practice tests to gauge your realistic score on test day.

What's all the hype with the AAMC MCAT Official Prep Practice Exams? They are truly the best resource to estimate your score on the actual MCAT. Right now, there are four practice exams that the AAMC has released. Each of them is an official MCAT exam that has been taken out of circulation. While these exact passages and questions will not end up on your actual MCAT exam, similar questions, especially the high-yield problems, will be on your MCAT. Take all of these AAMC Practice Exams over the timeline that we discussed above. Review your flagged and incorrect answers to completion. These exams are gems. When taken under test-like conditions, they are excellent predictors of your score. For example, my AAMC Practice Exam scores were 516 for exam one, 516 for exam two, and 518 for exam three. I scored a 517 on the actual MCAT (95th percentile), which is essentially an average of my practice exam scores. We will get to this a bit later, but the actual MCAT was incredibly harder than my practice exams. Why, then, did I score similarly to my practice scores? Because the curve was much more lenient on my official MCAT to account for the more difficult questions. My score breakdown on the actual MCAT was 129 for C/P (92nd percentile), 128 for CARS (90th percentile), 129 for B/B (90th percentile), and 131 for P/S (98th percentile). The official score report is inserted below. Part of the reason that I know my official MCAT exam was a harder version is because I've seen other MCAT versions where a 128 is the 78th percentile (in CARS, for example) and a 129 is the 83rd percentile (in B/B, for example). It's crazy how much fluctuation there is in percentile! Rarely an official MCAT does not match your AAMC Practice Exams. If this happens to you, a few important questions to ask are the following. Did I take my practice exams in exam-like conditions? Were my practice exams taken within a month or so of my actual MCAT? Did something unusual happen at the testing center, like another test-taker tapping a pen the entire time? Did you have a panic attack? These reasons are some of the most common to explain a discrepancy between AAMC Practice Exam scores and your official MCAT score. If none of these apply, speak with your counselor to understand what happened on official test day.

Official MCAT Score Report:

Section	Score	Confidence Band [1]	Percentile Rank of Score [2]	Score Profile [3]
Chemical and Physical Foundations of Biological Systems	129	128–130	92%	
Critical Analysis and Reasoning Skills	128	127–129	90%	
Biological and Biochemical Foundations of Living Systems	129	128–130	90%	
Psychological, Social, and Biological Foundations of Behavior	131	130–132	98%	
MCAT Total	517	515–519	95%	

The section *MCAT Retakes* will address why retakes happen for so many students. One of the best ways to avoid a retake is by delaying your official MCAT if you are unprepared. To be clear, you will never feel 100% prepared for an exam like the MCAT. There is simply too much information to know. The best indicator of heading down the path of a retake is sitting for the official MCAT when your AAMC Practice Exam scores are not up to par with your goal score. If I had been scoring around a 514-515 on my practice exams, I would have delayed my test day to scooch myself up to the 517+ range. Setting yourself up for a score you will not be happy with is a huge indicator that you will become a retaker.

Another question that may be bouncing around your noggin is why I haven't mentioned the famous Khan Academy psychology/sociology review document. This is a mega document created and added by students who have made their thorough psychology/sociology review available to help current test takers. The version that I downloaded from Reddit was 280 pages! By the time you read this guidebook, the document has likely grown in size. Here is perhaps my unpopular opinion on the Khan Academy P/S review document. The review is extraordinarily detailed, and knowing everything on the document will no doubt earn you a 131-132 on P/S. Why not use it then? The biggest issue with this review document is that it's *super* long, and most people who read it will likely forget much the material. Reading is a passive form of studying – no good for locking information into long-term memory. Unless you are Lexie Grey from *Grey's Anatomy*, of course. Damn your photographic minds! If by the time you take the MCAT, someone has turned the Khan Academic P/S review document into flashcards, then by golly, do those cards! If not, other practice materials will put the same P/S information into your long-term memory more effectively than reading the massive transcript. Perhaps the best way to use the Khan Academy review is to use UWorld and the AAMC materials to their fullest and then skim the Khan Academy document to see if any holes were missed. Study those holes with the Khan Academy mega sheet, and you will be ready to rock P/S!

Goodness! That was a lot of information! To condense everything that was written in the *How To Study* section, I've made a study schedule below for easy reference. Make adjustments as needed. Happy studying sucka!

Detailed Three-Month MCAT Preparation Schedule:

3 Month MCAT Prep Schedule	
Days 1-7 T minus 13 weeks	• Turn Kaplan Quicksheet into Anki flashcards • Make fill-in charts for learning amino acids; types of enzymes and substrates, etc. • Make fill-in-the-blank graphics for learning the citric acid cycle, gluconeogenesis, etc. • Complete preparation of all study materials
Days 8-21	• Study entirety of newly made preparation materials (flashcards, charts, graphics, etc.) and become comfortable with the information • Complete 720-question AAMC Question Pack while working through preparation material • You do not need to know everything perfectly by this point but feel like you are gaining familiarity and working towards mastery
Days 22-51; 54-63 Start: T minus 10 weeks; End: T minus 4 weeks	• Continue reviewing and mastering preparation material • Complete all UWORLD questions • Make new flashcards from UWORLD information that is absent from your other preparation materials (much of this will be low-yield information that is critical to scoring within the top 5% of MCAT scorers) • Use explanations for both correct and incorrect answer choices on UWORLD to make these new flashcards • Review UWORLD flashcards
Day 51	Take AAMC MCAT Practice Exam Four; closely mimic the testing conditions of the actual MCAT
Day 52	• Thoroughly review AAMC MCAT Practice Exam Four • Make new flashcards for information that is absent from current prep materials
Days 64-68; 71-75; 78-82 Start: T minus 4 weeks; End: T minus 1 week	• Complete 300-question AAMC Section Bank • Complete second pass through UWORLD or complete UWORLD incorrect questions • Review preparation materials that are not yet mastered • Use Kaplan, Examkrackers, or Princeton Review CARS practice passages if in need of more CARS practice • Take one day to rest
Day 69	Take AAMC MCAT Practice Exam One; closely mimic the testing conditions of the actual MCAT

Day 70	• Thoroughly review AAMC MCAT Practice Exam One • Make new flashcards for information that is absent from current preparation materials
Day 76	Take AAMC MCAT Practice Exam Two; closely mimic the testing conditions of the actual MCAT
Day 77	• Thoroughly review AAMC MCAT Practice Exam Two • Make new flashcards for information that is absent from current preparation materials
Day 83	Take AAMC MCAT Practice Exam Three; closely mimic the testing conditions of the actual MCAT
Day 84	• Thoroughly review AAMC MCAT Practice Exam Three • Make new flashcards for information that is absent from current preparation materials
Days 85-89 Start: T minus 1 week; End: T minus 1 day	• Re-review AAMC Practice Exam One-Four or review flashcards made from AAMC Practice Exams One-Four • Review preparation materials that are not yet mastered • Complete practice questions that boost your confidence, such as the AAMC Question Pack questions
Day 90	• Rest • Prepare meals for MCAT test day • Try to get at least seven hours of sleep
Day 91	Destroy the MCAT

Critical Analysis and Reasoning Skills (CARS)

Critical analysis and reasoning skills (CARS) seem to be the most anxiety-provoking MCAT section for the greatest number of test-takers. Why is this? From what I have heard from students, their performance on CARS almost feels immutable. Either you were born a master of reading analysis, or you weren't. Adding to the anxiety, students do not know how to prepare for CARS. The other three sections - C/P, B/B, and P/S - come with clear study plans. We have spent our undergraduate careers dissecting the sciences – by now, we are more or less pros in STEM. Critical reasoning is the squishy skill set that all but the English majors have left untouched since taking the SAT or ACT.

These nerves surrounding reading comprehension are not foreign to me. As a high schooler taking the PSAT, I bombed reading comprehension. Our school counselor brought me and my parents in to discuss my lackluster performance. Part of the issue was embedded in my learning disability, which particularly affects reading. Not taking time accommodations on the PSAT meant I didn't finish reading any of the excerpts that we were tested on. However, my mindset was my most formidable obstacle. I was a member of the immutable club: I stunk at critical reasoning, and nothing could be done about it. This was my hymn. Boy, was I wrong.

Princeton Review's SAT preparatory course taught me reading comprehension skills as a high schooler. And to be clear, reading comprehension is, in fact, a skill that can be perfected. The Princeton Review course, specifically, showed me how to read critical reasoning passages efficiently and then answer the corresponding questions effectively. In some ways, critical reasoning is a test of the test-taking strategy itself rather than a test of superior reading skills. Oodles of practice later, I went from scoring in approximately the 40th percentile for reading on the PSAT to not missing a single question on the actual SAT – eighty critical reasoning questions. I didn't miss one of them. This transformation didn't happen overnight. It was during the course of several months spent making a strategy, perfecting reading and question-answering skills, and then completing plenty of sample passages that the perfect score was achieved. Reading analysis capabilities are not stagnant. In fact, **I believe CARS is one of the most easily improvable sections on the MCAT.** Compared to the effort that it takes to achieve top scores in C/P, B/B, and P/S, a top score in CARS can be earned with relative ease – no matter where you are starting from. For those who performed well on AP English Exams or the SAT Literature Subject Test, the same skill set with some modifications can get you a top CARS score. For those who didn't take those exams or did not perform well, you can improve to a 128 and above on CARS.

What skills do I need to kick CARS butt? CARS is one of those sections where you want to develop a plan to attack each passage. Multiple different strategies can work. I will share my own strategy, but please make whatever adjustments work best for you. Step one is to figure out the timing. The CARS section has nine total passages, with five to six questions per passage. Fifty-three questions total. We are given 90 minutes (according to normal time standards – no time extensions) to finish. Ideally, I like to leave 10 minutes for review. Quick math tells us that with 10 minutes for review, we must spend about 8.5 minutes per passage. This takes eight and a half minutes to both read and answer the corresponding questions (AAMC: Critical Analysis and Reasoning Section: Overview).

How do I read passages and answer questions in order to obtain the greatest number of correct responses within the time limit? First, here's a glimpse of what not to do. Unlike AP Exams and the SAT, you actually have to read the *entire* passage. Reading the two sentences above and below the target information won't work. Trust me, I tried. Reading is the most time-consuming aspect of CARS, so I was scheming for any way to cut down on reading time. If you managed to ace CARS by not reading the passages from beginning to end, please let us know your secrets. Also, with AP Exams and the SAT, I would read the questions first and then search for the answers within the passage. This technique didn't work for me on the MCAT. Many CARS questions focused on tone, attitude, potential beliefs of the author, and other larger, overarching ideas. To answer these correctly, I felt that it was critical to read the passage in its entirety. You may be tempted to peek at a few questions before reading the entire passage. This way, you can remember those questions while reading and get started with a few slam-dunk correct answers. I have tried this plan and would discourage it. Keeping specific questions in mind when reading made me focus too much on those questions and not pay attention to the big-picture ideas. I would also miss out on other key details that I would have otherwise picked up on. Ultimately, I found myself needing to re-read the passage rather than just have one pass-through and then move on to the questions.

On the MCAT, CARS was, admittedly, my lowest scoring section – I earned a 128 (90th percentile on my official exam version). Because I started out strong in CARS, since I had done the heavy lifting when learning critical reading for the SAT, my CARS score always fluctuated between 128-131 on practice exams. CARS was my rock from the beginning. Due to these consistently strong scores, I didn't do much practice for CARS. All of my work was maintenance-driven. Looking back, however, I would have drilled more practice passages in order to move my 128-131 range to the 130-132 range. This is absolutely a possible change to make. I happened to be too busy freaking out about C/P to focus more on CARS, but I am confident that my strategy works well for scoring consistently high, and additional practice can make for near-perfect on CARS.

Now, here's the strategy that worked best for me. Do not look at the questions when beginning a passage. Read the passage from beginning to end. While reading, you need to do several things: highlight dates and important names and underline strong emotive words (exceptional, decrepit, best, dull, etc.) in addition to words of similarity (likewise, additionally, furthermore, etc.) and words of contrast (although, however, but, etc.). As you complete each paragraph, make an outline of what you just read. Your outline should be a few keywords or a summary sentence of what was in each paragraph. What was the message? What topics were mentioned? This outline and your highlighting will serve as a map when searching for testable information within the passage. The underlined words give insight into the author's perspective. Once you finish reading all of the paragraphs, add to the bottom of your outline what the author's tone was as well as the main idea of the passage (why was the essay written?). Tone and main passage idea are two of the most common big-picture questions on the MCAT.

Reading is now complete. Time to turn to the questions. The AAMC divides the 53 CARS questions into three distinct types: 1) Foundations of Comprehension (30% of questions), 2) Reasoning Within the Text (30% of questions), and 3) Reasoning Beyond the Text (40% of questions) (AAMC: Critical Analysis and Reasoning Section: Overview). Kaplan did an outstanding job describing these three question types, which I have included below.

- Foundations of Comprehension questions determine whether you've understood the basic components of the text in the passage. These questions tend to focus on a single fact or idea, either on a broad scale or with a very narrow focus. You might be asked about the passage's main idea, whether or not a specific detail was mentioned, why the author included certain elements in the passage or the meaning of words or phrases in the context of the passage. These questions are closest to the traditional reading comprehension questions that you may be familiar with. However, the MCAT has ways of making them more difficult, such as asking which of the answer choices is NOT mentioned in the text or the meaning of a phrase that is very different in the passage from everyday usage.

- Reasoning Within the Text questions require a generally higher level of critical analysis of the MCAT CARS passage. These question types ask you to infer something from the passage or to bring together two disparate pieces of information and recognize their relationship. Reasoning Within the Text questions often focus on an argument made in the passage and ask about unstated assumptions or conclusions. They also ask you to identify evidence from the passage used to support or weaken an argument or, conversely, correctly identify the argument that a piece of evidence strengthens or undermines.

Reasoning Beyond the Text is often considered the most challenging of the MCAT CARS questions. This type of question will introduce new information and ask you to determine how it relates to the passage. You might be asked to extrapolate an inference from new evidence or to apply what the passage states in a new context. Alternatively, you might be required to understand how new facts might challenge or support an argument that the author discussed.

With practice, you will discover which of these three question types you are best at. After reading the passage, start by answering the type of questions you are best at to build confidence and quickly knock out several problems. Leave the toughest questions for last, as they will take the most time. The main idea and overall tone of the questions should be somewhat straightforward because of your outline. Your underlined words should help with Reasoning Within the Text and Reasoning Beyond the Text questions, as these problems focus a lot on the author's opinions and relationships between ideas. Highlighted words should be useful for Foundations of Comprehension questions because these often focus on specific details.

Beware of some of the detail-focused questions. A few of these are designed to waste your time. Let me give you an example. The first question on my official MCAT's CARS section was a list of vocabulary words, and the problem asked which of these words was *not* in the passage. This was such a dumb question, but it was used to test how I managed my time. I could have easily spent 10 minutes searching for whichever word was absent from the passage. This is the trap set by the test makers for you to fall into. As soon as I read the problem, I skipped it. It was the last question that I ended up answering on the test. With several minutes remaining, I decided to guess the question after I couldn't answer it with skimming. I used the remaining time to return to the problems that I was unsure of, but that also wouldn't take a lifetime to come to a correct answer. You will likely have a similar trap set for you in your official CARS section. Do not fall for it. Skip any super crazy detail-oriented questions, and come back to them at the end.

The most important piece of advice I was given in high school that helped me ascend from critical analysis flunker to dominatrix was understanding that there was only *one* correct answer to each question. What does this mean? Out of the four answer choices, three choices *have to be* wrong. What used to freak me out about reading comprehension – and I have a hunch others share this source of nerves – is that I thought the answer choices were subjective. I could narrow almost every question down to two choices but struggled to pick the best response from there. *Best* response? Who determines what is best? What is wrong with the second-best answer? I learned that there had to be something concrete that you could point to to show why one answer was correct, and the other was incorrect. The Princeton Review instructor from high school taught me to approach the critical reasoning section like an attorney. You can find hard evidence as to why one juicy, tempting response is wrong, and the other is right. This detective work is a skill that you will improve with more and more practice. More often than not, you can narrow down CARS questions to two possible answers. It is practicing that will allow you to master the job of the attorney: You will learn to reason why a tempting answer is incorrect and thus select the remaining choice as the correct response. How do you become a master attorney? With each question that you flag or get wrong, truly understand why the one answer was correct and why the others were incorrect. Fully understanding these subtle differences will sharpen your skills when distinguishing right from wrong answers. Over time, this ability will become second nature, and your critical analysis performance will improve drastically. If you struggle to determine why one answer choice is right and the other is wrong, do not skip the understanding part. Consult the internet, ask a friend, or find a tutor to explain the intricacies. Similar intricacies that separate right from wrong answers will show up on your official MCAT. The time to learn the difference is now – not on test day.

If you need practice, where are the best places to get it? During your initial practice, the AAMC CARS Question Pack and UWorld have outstanding CARS sample passages and questions. UWorld's ability to replicate the actual exam is astounding. Wink wink! Love you, UWorld! If you want an additional resource for practice, the Kaplan CARS passages are quite good as well. I took the Kaplan MCAT Practice Exams, and while the C/P and B/B sections were trash, CARS was pretty on point. Princeton Review, Examkrackers, and other outside companies may have good CARS practices, but I can't testify to them personally because I never used them. Once you are in the final four to five weeks before your test date, the AAMC Practice Exams are your main swig. Like all sections on the AAMC Practice Exams, the CARS sections are the best predictor of your CARS score on test day. I know CARS can be intimidating for many people, but you can ace this section! If I can ascend from being a critical reading disaster to a professional, so can you. For those who are shaky in CARS, do one new passage every day until exam day. Understand why certain answers are correct and incorrect, just like we discussed. Over the months of studying, your performance will become stronger and more consistent. Consistency in excellence is our aim. You can do this chipmunk.

Test Taking Strategy for CARS	
Minutes 1-80	• Working from least to most formidable, read nine passages and complete corresponding questions • Eliminate answer choices when stuck between two or more answers • Flag unanswered and wobbly questions • Note page numbers where passages begin, so it becomes easy to navigate the exam when returning to difficult passages
Minutes 80-90	• Review unanswered questions first; if taking too much time to arrive at the correct answer, eliminate as many choices as possible and select one answer choice; move on to reviewing other questions • Review questions when stuck between more than one answer choice • Review flagged questions • Make sure all questions are answered by the end of time

Chemistry and Physics (C/P)

Medusa is to Perseus what chemistry and physics are to me. Snake-like heads that grow back at twice the rate you chop them off. Chemistry and physics for a long time have been my toughest subjects to conquer. For me, the MCAT's C/P section was an opportunity to show medical schools that I understood this difficult material. Undergraduate courses left me with Bs in all my physics and chemistry courses (apart from biochemistry, where I clutched the A+). My goal was to earn at least a 128 in C/P to demonstrate to the admissions officers that I knew my stuff. Of the four MCAT sections, C/P was the segment I studied most for. Not only were these my most challenging subjects, but they were also the ones that I had taken at the beginning of college. The years between then and my senior summer meant that the information had faded to faint memories in the back of my mind.

To earn a 128+ on C/P, I first needed to internalize that this score was possible for me. My Bs in chemistry and physics courses made me insecure about my academic abilities in these domains. By reminding myself that my study habits had vastly improved from my underclassman years and that my undergraduate exams were much more difficult than what was found on the MCAT, I assured myself that a 128 score was possible so long as I put in the work. These were not one-time reminders but continuous lines of motivation throughout the summer. Concoct your own mantra to gain confidence in your toughest subject.

What work is needed to score well in C/P? To nail down the basics, the Kaplan MCAT Quicksheet and the AAMC Question Packs work wonders. The Quicksheet covers 101 physics, general chemistry, organic chemistry, and biochemistry. Biochemistry is technically concentrated in the B/B section, but a lot of biochem shows up in C/P. Turn the Quicksheet information into flashcards and study materials - like diagrams to learn basic organic chemistry reactions and charts to become fluent in glycolysis. Chemistry and physics are such difficult subjects to begin with that the good news is that they are not tested at an extraordinarily difficult level on the MCAT. The Quicksheet will give you the tools to nail down the high-yield C/P questions along with the AAMC Question Packs. The Question Packs provide easy and medium-difficulty problems to test that you know the basics. For tougher practice and to become proficient in low-yield C/P material, UWorld, and the AAMC Section Bank are your best resources. Genuinely comprehending the Quicksheet, UWorld, and the AAMC Section Bank is all you need to score a 130+ on C/P. These three resources range from easy to difficult material. They will prepare you for nearly anything that the AAMC will throw your way. As stated earlier, UWorld has phenomenal explanations for its questions. If you are struggling with a certain concept, UWorld's explanations will help you grasp the foundational material necessary to consistently discern correct answer choices.

When first using UWorld, don't time yourself on the questions. Give yourself time to practice critical thinking effectively. With more practice, your time will be cut down naturally. By the time you take the AAMC Practice Exams, take them under the same time conditions that are used on test day. That way, your practice exam score will most accurately predict your official MCAT score, which is the whole reason that the AAMC exams are beneficial. On the MCAT, there are 59 C/P questions. Forty-four of these are passage-based questions, and 15 are stand-alone. The passage-based questions correspond to ten total passages with four to seven problems per passage. Ninety-five minutes is given to complete C/P on test day. When you begin the AAMC Section Bank and have practice with UWorld, feel free to experiment with setting time limits. Consider starting by setting looser time limits and then working your way down to how you want to spend your time on test day. Give yourself 10 minutes to review wobbly questions (questions where you are not confident of your answer), and 85 minutes remain to tackle the 59 official questions. Plan to dedicate 15 minutes to the 15 stand-alone questions. The seventy minutes for the 44 passage-based questions are divided into seven minutes for each of the ten passages. Work toward this pace as you improve your accuracy with looser time limits in UWorld.

Unlike with CARS, do not read the C/P passages from beginning to end. Much of the information in the C/P passages is a distraction. Test takers are giving superfluous information in order to see if you know what details are needed to answer the corresponding questions correctly. This is cheesy, but, in medicine, there is a lot of background noise that will not contribute to a correct diagnosis. Because of the nature of medicine, perhaps that is why the test makers report excessive information in passages. Sharpen that scalpel and cut through the bull poop.

Arriving at a passage, your first job is to read the questions and highlight what the problem is asking for. Are you identifying an amino acid? Are you selecting the product of a particular acetal formation? Are you determining the angle of light refraction through a substance? Knowing what you are looking for will then permit you to skim the passage and find the necessary information. Start with the questions that are easiest and quickest for you to answer. Difficult questions can be saved until last, when you may need to check out the answer choices – particularly the units – to know what information is relevant. Especially challenging questions can be flagged and saved for your 10-minute review at the end of the C/P section. Don't be afraid to skip problems when you are totally stuck. This is a far better strategy than fumbling around for five minutes and squandering time to correct other questions. The super complicated questions are not worth any more points than the easy questions. The MCAT is a game of collecting the greatest number of points possible. Lastly, there are no penalties for incorrect answers. Finding yourself stumped should be handled by trying to eliminate any answer choices, as this will increase your odds of a correct guess. From the responses that remain, call upon cosmic energy to lead you to your best guess. Side note: according to Cristina Yang, "If you don't know the answer, choose B. It's always B!" Do with that advice what you will, Georgie!

Here is my test-taking advice on the AAMC Practice Exams and on the official MCAT: Start by knocking out the 15 stand-alone C/P questions before turning to the passage-based questions. With the stand-alones, you will either know it or you won't. If you don't know the answer, again consult the answer choice units if any are given, and then give it your best shot. Flag problems that you are unsure of to return to during the final 10-minute review. Begin your passage-based questions next. If there is a topic that you are uneasy about (this was organic chemistry for me), skip the passage and tackle it toward the end. I have a sneaky hunch that the test makers like to put the harder passages toward the front of the exam in order to slow you down. On my official MCAT, I literally answered the passage-based questions in reverse order. I began with passage 10 and worked my way backward to passage one - the sticky ochem passage. Gross!

The Kaplan Quicksheet, UWorld, and the AAMC materials should be enough to keep you busy while studying. I found that outside companies' materials, like the Kaplan practice exams, were way too challenging for C/P. The problems also did not mimic the MCAT well. I've heard similar scaries about Princeton Review. Be wary about what you invest your time into. The Kaplan question bank that I used was helpful in comprehending the high-yield C/P material, but it is redundant if you are using the AAMC Question Pack.

No matter what happens on test day, remember to breathe deeply and ace C/P. My goal was to earn a 128+ on the MCAT. I started out with a 122 on Kaplan's practice exams – literally, these exams are soul-crushing. Such a bad idea. But once I began AAMC's Practice

Exams, I was scoring 128 and 129 consistently. On the official MCAT, I scored a 129 and couldn't be happier to have overcome the beast. Snakeheads and all.

Biology and Biochemistry (B/B)

Preparing for biology and biochemistry is quite similar to preparing for chemistry and physics. Luckily, I needed fewer rhythmic mantras to build confidence for B/B since biology was my major, and I love the subject. B/B and I are tight, dawg!

Due to both majoring in biology and working as a teaching assistant for biochemistry and introduction to biology laboratory, the breadth of information covered in B/B was fresh in my mind. Working as a teaching assistant has the tremendous benefit of keeping knowledge up-to-date in your memory, which is one of the reasons that I recommend TAing jobs for undergraduate students.

Like C/P, lay your B/B foundation by making flashcards and study materials from the Kaplan Quicksheet. Some of my study materials included a fill-in chart to memorize the amino acids as well as diagrams of the different enzyme inhibitors. Along with studying the Quicksheet material, complete the AAMC Question Packs in order to lock in easy to medium-difficulty information into your long-term memory.

Moving into more advanced material, UWorld is your calling card. UWorld prepares you to ace the high-yield questions and handle most of the low-yield questions thrown your way. There were several low-yield B/B questions on my official exam that I was able to answer correctly because I had seen them on UWorld. Wrapping up with UWorld and the AAMC Section Bank will, again, fortify you against the most difficult questions on the MCAT. The Section Bank also gets you used to the AAMC format of asking questions and presenting background information in paragraphs.

As you study these resources, devise a strategy to answer B/B questions. Similar to C/P, it is unnecessary to read the entire passage corresponding to B/B problems. Much of the information is there to distract you and test if you know the relevant material to answer the questions given. Start by reading the problems and highlighting what the question is asking for. If you are stumped, any units given are a useful clue. Next, skim the passage and highlight details that will help you solve the questions. Move through the problems one by one, starting with the easiest for you to answer and ending with the most difficult. Give a shot at responding to each question. If you are completely stuck or unable to confidently choose one correct response, flag the problem and return to it at the end of the B/B section. With challenging questions, do your best to eliminate as many answer choices as possible in order to increase your odds of a favorable guess.

Untimed practice sessions with the AAMC Question Pack and UWorld are a perfect place to start. Focus on getting questions correct and becoming comfortable with your question-answer strategy. As you practice more, restrict your time until you match the pace at which you will answer problems on AAMC Practice Exams and the actual MCAT. For B/B, you will have 95 minutes to complete 59 questions. These 59 problems encompass 15 stand-alone and 44 passage-based questions. The 44 passage-based problems are divided over 10 passages, with 4-7 questions per passage.

When thinking about how to distribute your testing time, copy your formula for C/P. Spend the first 15 minutes addressing the stand-alone problems. Turn to the passage-based questions, and use 70 minutes to answer those. Reserve 10 minutes at the end of the B/B section for review. Review is your time to revisit flagged questions where you are unsure of your answer and to check over the entirety of your work to ensure that no silly mistakes were made. By starting with the stand-alone problems, you will kick-start building confidence and working speedily, as you will have knocked out a large number of questions in 15 minutes. Arriving at a challenging passage should be handled by skipping it entirely and returning to it toward the end of your 70-minute block. Finishing easier problems first allows you to shoo away any nerves while using your time most efficiently. As you know, the easy questions are worth the same number of points as the hardest questions – focus on collecting as many points as possible.

This is the game plan that I recommend using as you begin the AAMC Practice Exams. Tinker with your strategy as you complete UWorld and then execute the final version on the AAMC Practice Exams in order to get comfy for the real deal. As you work through AAMC's four Practice Exams, you will also be completing the AAMC Section Bank. The Section Bank contains 100 B/B problems that are more challenging in nature. Don't fret if your timing is tight on the Section Bank – the difficulty level of the problems will slow you down. The AAMC Practice Exams are the best resource to predict your B/B score. All of my B/B scores on the Practice Exams ranged from 128-131. On the official MCAT, I earned a 129. My actual B/B MCAT performance was not my best work, but I was still comfortable with the range that I scored in.

Looking for additional practice material beyond what we have discussed here? Get a hobby! How do you have that much time? I've found that Kaplan, Princeton Review, Examkrackers, etc., all have shaky student reviews. Kaplan's practice exams were never helpful to me with their B/B section. Save your money and do a second pass through UWorld. B/B is a very doable section to score well in so long as you put in the time. Luckily, there is heavy biochemistry overlap between C/P and B/B, so studying for one section will prepare you for the other. Just remember that the mitochondria are the powerhouse of the cell, and you'll do fine!

Psychology and Sociology (P/S)

Relieved – this is how I felt knowing that the rebooted MCAT included psychology and sociology as a new section. Seriously, we all must breathe a collective sigh of relief. Compared to the vast amounts of information that we need to cram into our heads for C/P and B/B, P/S is a walk in the park. Sure, there is a decent amount of information to know, but it is definitely less than what you need to nail down for the other two science sections. Another benefit is that it's harder for test takers to come up with challenging P/S questions. So long as you memorize what is needed, you should be gucci for a 130-132 on this section. The erreur fatale (fatal flaw) that test-takers make with P/S is not learning the necessary information. No, I don't speak a lick of French apart from "croissant mademoiselle?" Google Translate helped with the 'fatal flaw' translation.

My second major, psychological and brain sciences, may be skewing my perception of the P/S section. However, most of the psychology information that was relevant to the MCAT was covered in the Introduction to Psychology class. So long as you take that course, you're caught up to me in terms of preliminary MCAT psychology knowledge. My upper-division psychology courses didn't seem to give me much of an advantage – four years of college and not one sociology course for me. Funny enough, my sister was a sociology major. Sociology was a new subject for me to learn, and it did not take much effort.

Secure your basics with the Kaplan Quicksheet. You know the routine! For P/S, I stuck to flashcards, but diagrams of the brain or charts dividing the different information processing theories would be useful study material. Just as with C/P and B/B, complete the AAMC Question Packs alongside the Quicksheet to seep P/S details into long-term memory. UWorld is next. UWorld covers everything and anything P/S. The toughest questions will be yours to conquer on UWorld. Know it inside and out, and a 130-132 will be yours for the taking. Despite P/S being the newest section, I remember the AAMC Section Bank being the least helpful for P/S. Definitely aim to complete the 100 questions, but heads up that a number of them seemed almost outdated and not in line with the material that is tested. Still, put in the time to know what is on the Section Bank, as it may be your saving grace for a low-yield problem.

AAMC Practice Exams will be the best predictor of your score on test day. My Practice Exams scores ranged from 128-130. On the official MCAT, I exceeded my top score and earned a 131. My ability to jump a point on the actual MCAT was due to finishing more UWorld questions. Complete each of the four AAMC Practice Exams and review them thoroughly.

Same as with C/P and B/B, there are 95 minutes allotted to complete 59 P/S questions. Forty-four of the problems are passage-based, and the other 15 are stand-alone. You've been here before. Let's break down that time! Give 15 minutes to the 15 stand-alones. Seventy minutes are for the 44 passage-based questions: 10 passages total with 4-7 problems per passage. Ten minutes should be reserved for returning to challenging questions and checking for any mindless errors. One of the best parts about P/S is that most test-takers finish the 59 questions with far more than 10 minutes left for review. On my MCAT, I believe that I had 40 minutes remaining when I was done with everything (don't forget, though, that I had time extensions, so this number will likely be different for you). Make use of your extra time. First, with my extra 40 minutes, I addressed the difficult questions to choose an answer I felt confident in. Second, I double-checked all my responses to ensure that I had not selected the wrong answer or misread anything. I believe that I caught a silly mistake on my exam, which may have made the difference between a 130 and a 131– the final review really pays off.

Knock out the 15 stand-alone questions first when beginning the P/S section. The 44 passage-based questions should follow the stand-alones. Complete the easiest passages for you and work up to the most challenging ones. Approaching each passage, read the questions first and highlight what each problem is asking. Then, skim through the passage and highlight the information that will help you answer the questions. Unlike C/P and B/B, I found myself reading more of the P/S passages. Focusing on just a few sentences made it harder to extract the needed information. No worries, however, about taking more time to read because P/S is the quickest section for the vast majority of test-takers.

Perfect this blueprint as you make your way through UWorld and the AAMC Practice Exams. Although time is usually not an issue on P/S, ensure you complete all 59 questions with time left to review. Kaplan's practice exams were okay for P/S. Overall, there was relevant information on Kaplan's exams, but it wasn't worth the purchase, considering that everything and more is covered in UWorld. I'm unsure how Princeton Review's and Examkrackers' exams are with P/S, but I would wager that they're not worth the time and money. Treat yourself to a massage instead. Your neck will thank you!

Khan Academy's P/S review mega-document is well-known in the premed world. My version is 280 pages long and covers literally everything you need to know for P/S. Clearly, the Khan Academy document is extremely thorough. The biggest issue is, if you read the 280 pages all the way through, it is likely that you will forget many important details. Photographic memories excluded. Heroes who turn the Khan Academy P/S document into Anki cards will serve future MCAT testers tremendously. As I mentioned in the *How To Study* section, use the Khan Academy mega-document like so: study the Quicksheet, UWorld, and the AAMC materials. When you are done with those, skim the mega-document to see if there are any areas that weren't covered. Fill in any holes, and you will be set to score a 131-132.

Test Taking Strategy for C/P, B/B, and P/S	
Minutes 1-15	• Complete 15 stand-alone (a.k.a., not passage-based) questions • Eliminate answer choices when stuck between two or more answers • Flag unanswered and wobbly questions

Minutes 15-85	• Working from easiest to hardest, read ten passages and complete corresponding questions • Eliminate answer choices when stuck between two or more answers • Flag unanswered and wobbly questions • Note page numbers where passages begin, so it is easy to navigate the exam when returning to difficult passages
Minutes 85-95	• Review unanswered questions first; if taking too much time to arrive at the correct answer, eliminate as many choices as possible and select one answer choice; move on to reviewing other questions • Review questions when stuck between more than one answer choice • Review flagged questions • Make sure all questions are answered by the end of time

POST-MCAT BLUES

Blue is the month that follows the MCAT. Whether you felt that you aced it or totally choked, the weeks between completing the exam and waiting for your score are anxiety-ridden. Many minds comb over each of their uncertain questions, desperate to determine if they arrived at the correct answers. Days ago, you were on a roller-coaster of studying, reviewing, practicing exams, crying, waking up, and repeating. You faced the monster, and then... all is quiet.

For me, the worst part about post-MCAT blues was that I had no idea how I had performed on the exam. I think a lot of people have this same feeling. On the AAMC Practice Exams, I felt confident about a lot of my answers. Many of my mistakes were silly errors that could be cleaned up with careful reading and double-checking my responses. I enjoyed taking the Practice Exams. I saw my hard work pay off as I earned a 516 on Practice Exams One and Two and then a 518 on Practice Exam Three. The official MCAT held a different narrative.

Shock – that is how I felt walking away from my MCAT. My test version was much more difficult than the Practice Exams. Immediately, C/P had hit me with back-to-back organic chemistry passages, my weakest subject by far. Assured that I would only see a few organic chemistry questions on the MCAT, I had only skimmed the basics.

Big mistake, darlin'. No mercy was shown with B/B. The number of low-yield problems that I encountered was surprising. I had never seen so much low-yield information on a Practice Exam. Overall, I departed the testing center having no idea what my score would be.

Hastily, I scoured Reddit to listen in on what other test-takers thought of the exam. Most people had a rough ride. "At least it wasn't just me!" I thought to myself. My hope was that the curve on the exam would be lenient, considering the difficulty level. Yet, in truth, I could easily see a world where my Practice Exam scores were far higher than what I earned on the official test. I read post after post assuring other terrified test takers that the actual MCAT usually feels a lot harder and that the Practice Exams were still excellent predictors of their test day performance. I wanted to believe these words but couldn't fully accept them as truth. I was looking for certainty where there was none to find. Waiting out the next four weeks was the only path forward.

October 1st was my score release date. Months before I took the MCAT, I intentionally decided not to know when my score would be released. Knowing would only cause me to fixate on the date and get a terrible sleep the night before. Even with premeditated ignorance of the release date, my Spidey senses kicked in around four weeks post-exam. The time was nigh. On October 3rd, I finally built up the courage to look for my score. Distinctly, I remember biting on a kitchen towel as I opened the score report. Another towel covered the computer screen so I could slowly peel back my fate. After freaking out once the first cluster of mysterious numbers turned out to be my birthdate and AAMC ID number, I ripped the band-aid off. My eyes darted around the screen (I didn't know where I was supposed to look) until I found my results. 517. I DID IT! Immediately, my fingers whizzed around my phone as I called my parents to share the news. Unfortunately, not being a member of Delta Nu, my bouncy sorority sisters were not gathered around our spiral staircase with streamers at the ready. Phooey. Nevertheless, the relief that washed over me was spectacular.

To date, the MCAT is the hardest exam that I have taken. Cue USMLE waiting in the wings to blow the MCAT out of the water. I was thrilled that my AAMC Practice Exams had accurately predicted my MCAT performance. At the same time, I realized that setting 517 as my target score was risky, knowing that I would have been disappointed with anything lower. The rule of thumb is that your official

MCAT score will be within plus or minus two points of your average practice scores. For me, this range would put me between a 515 and 519. Since a 515 and 516 were below my target score, I should have made the low range of my potential outcomes a 517 and set a target score of at least 519. Looking back, preparing for a 520+ would have settled my nerves. Those additional study hours spent finishing my first pass at UWorld, mastering the basics of organic chemistry, and not resting on my laurels with CARS would have saved me from serious post-MCAT blues.

My advice throughout this section covers everything I did right, as well as missteps that I would correct if I had to suffer through another MCAT. All-in-all, the MCAT can be enjoyable if you prepare properly. I've heard the same words spoken about USMLE. **Dedicated, intentional preparation puts you in control of your MCAT outcome.** Don't surrender the driver's seat to fear and self-doubt. I was never a naturally gifted test-taker. The SAT gave me the confidence that I could conquer standardized exams, and the MCAT has reinforced this feeling. Again, I was never a gifted test-taker. I have *become* a talented student who commits herself to hard work and intensive preparation. These were choices that I made every day when studying for exams. There is nothing that separates you from the 520 scorers besides work ethic. With discipline and a touch of confidence, you can make the same choices to execute your study plan to completion. My challenge for you is to beat my score. Earn a 520+. We likely haven't met, but I know you have it in you. Godspeed, young grasshopper.

MCAT RETAKES

Avoiding Retakes

To paraphrase a line from Chuck Palahniuk's novel *Fight Club*, the first rule of MCAT retakes is "you do not retake the MCAT." Seriously, let's dig in to understand how to avoid a low MCAT score, which is the primary reason for a retake. There are five steps main steps –

First, set a target score that you will be happy with. Part of why I suggest that you set a target score of 520+ is because no one could be unhappy with a 520 (so long as you don't bomb one section and perform perfectly in the others). That score will open doors at every school in the country. Nothing will be off-limits due to your MCAT performance. While I did set a target score that I would be thrilled with (517), I played it too close. Had I earned a 515 or 516, I would have been disappointed. By setting my target at 520, a couple of points below that mark would still have been an amazing score for me. I've mentioned this before, but ***I'm a big believer that we study for the score that we set.*** If we set our goal at a 510, we will prepare for a 510. If we set our goal at a 520, we will prepare for a 520. It is hard work that separates the 510 scorer from the 520 scorer. Put in the hours with UWorld and the AAMC materials, and you will be unstoppable. The first step to avoiding a retake is to set a target score that will make you proud.

Second, make a study plan that will allow you to achieve your target score. Wanting to score a 520 won't work if you give yourself three weeks of preparation. Carve out the appropriate amount of time to prepare and follow the study plan etched out in the *How To Study* section.

Third, stick to your study plan. I can't tell you the number of students I know who craft well-thought-out study plans and then simply do not execute. Preparing for the MCAT can absolutely be boring. Yet, it is much better to condense that boredom into three or four months and walk away with an outstanding score rather than extend it with a retake. Make the game plan, stick to it, and a happy camper you will be.

Fourth, only take the MCAT when you are ready. If you have put in the day-to-day work (Kaplan Quicksheet, UWorld, AAMC materials) and are scoring well on your practice exams, then you are ready to sit for your exam. Get a good night's sleep, bring snacks and an empty bladder, and calm your nerves – you are prepared to excel on the MCAT. Do not – and I repeat – *do not* take the MCAT when you are unprepared. If you are not scoring within range on your AAMC Practice Exams, figure out what is going wrong. Did you not execute your study plan? Are you overwhelmed with anxiety? Are you not taking the Practice Exams in exam-like conditions? Is your study plan not working for your learning needs? Figure out the problem, and don't hesitate to bring in an advisor or a close friend for a consultation.

Fifth and final, if you take the MCAT and something goes terribly wrong on test day, then void your score. It is much better to void your score due to anomalous circumstances than to bomb the exam. These circumstances are legitimate and could include issues such as having a migraine, another test-takers' incessant pen tapping, facility power outage, or an unexpected and crippling panic attack (among others). Voiding means that your exam will not be graded, and it will be as if it never happened (a.k.a. the medical schools will not know that you took an official MCAT). Don't forget, though, that feeling like crap after the exam is not a reason to void. I felt horrible after my exam, but the curve worked its magic. From what I have seen, the number one reason for retakes is people sitting for the exam when they are unprepared. The silliest thing about this is that it is completely avoidable. Sitting for the MCAT unprepared surrenders your autonomy to fate. Put the outcome of your score into your own hands – don't let luck have anything to do with it. Few people get the miracle when they hope for a score they are unprepared to achieve.

If your study plan was supposed to be executed in three months, but it is taking longer to complete, push back your test date. If you are suffering from paralyzing anxiety, get that addressed before taking your exam. If you need accommodations, make sure those are met before taking the MCAT. Whatever reason is keeping you from your target score on the AAMC Practice Exams, deal with it, and you will likely avoid the retake trap. One of the most important reasons not to schedule your MCAT near the AAMC primary application submission date is that it takes away your ability to comfortably push back your exam. Build in a cushion (a few months, ideally) for you to push back your test date if necessary. Originally, I planned to take my MCAT near my primary application submission date. When I realized that I would not be adequately prepared to achieve my target score, I pushed back my test date by four months to give myself the summer to study. Changing my timeline meant that I needed to take an additional gap year. Sometimes I wish I had that year back, but overall, I wouldn't change the additional gap year. I am now at my dream medical school because I completed benchmarks on my own timeline. Friends made a bit of a fuss when I said I would be taking two gap years, not one gap year like everyone else. But many of them ended up doing the same later on or not matriculating to a medical school that they loved. I am happy with where my choices have taken me.

Speaking of how poor MCAT preparation can snowball into troubling outcomes, let's visit Nyra. Innocent Nyra sat for the MCAT exam after a hastened month of studying. She gave herself winter break to prepare for the exam and was unable to cover the necessary topics for her to succeed. Nyra's 508 on the MCAT was not what she had aimed for and was certainly not what she was capable of. The MCAT would have been an outstanding opportunity for Nyra to make up for her shaky undergraduate GPA, particularly her lower science GPA. Despite her MCAT performance, Nyra applied to medical schools only to receive zero interview invitations. This young woman who was planning to take one gap year is now taking three gap years to overhaul her application. She has invested the time to properly study for the MCAT and is now scoring above a 520 on every practice exam. Nyra was always capable of this superb performance. How different her application cycle could have been if she had put in the time to ace the MCAT on the first go-around. More on Nyra later.

What Score Should I Retake?

How do you know if you should retake the MCAT? Here are a few questions to ask yourself. Will your score keep you out of the schools you want to attend? Would a higher score open doors at a dream school? Why am I considering a retake? Why did I earn a lower score than I wanted? Will I be able to improve my score when I take the MCAT for a second time? Let's go through these questions one by one.

Questions one and two are connected. Will your score keep you out of the schools you want to attend? Would a higher score open doors at a dream school? Dr. Ryan Gray, Medical School Headquarters' founder, has said this about the MCAT score: The MCAT either opens or closes doors for you but does not move you through those doors. Two years ago, I would have rejected Dr. Gray's analysis. Having gone through the cycle, I now believe that Dr. Gray is spot on. Look at your school list and ask yourself where your score stands in comparison to a school's median and mean scores. There is nothing to worry about if you are a few points below their averages. For example, if a medical school has a median MCAT of 522 and you have a 517, it is not your MCAT score that will prevent you from gaining admission. You are good to go. I used to worry that my 517 could keep me out of schools like WashU, Mayo, NYU, and Vanderbilt because their averages were several points higher. I interviewed at all four schools and was accepted at two, waitlisted at one, and rejected from one. Boom boom! It was my scores that opened the door. My interview performances, essays, recommendations, and fit with the programs earned the three different outcomes. If an MCAT score opens and closes doors, when do doors become closed? Both fortunately and unfortunately, there are no hard cut-offs. Fortunately, because everyone can still reasonably apply to their dream schools. Unfortunately, because we are not working with clear, defined numbers. In my application year, one of the first students to be accepted to NYU had a 508 MCAT. For most people, a 508 would close the door at a school with an average MCAT of 522 (NYU Langone Health: MD Admissions Requirements, 2020 matriculate statistics). Clearly, there are exceptions for students with outstanding applications and personal stories. Overall, if you are reaching seven points below a school's average, you may be approaching closed-door territory. Every year, plenty of students with sub-510 MCATs gain admission to top research medical schools. However, these students are the exception and truly not the rule for admission into this tier of medical school. Look at the school's metric averages as well as the 25th and 75th percentiles. If you are nearing the seven points below your school's average MCAT, you may want to consider a retake. This advice goes for the top research institutions but also all other medical schools. If your prospective school's average MCAT is 510, and you scored 503, you may want to consider a retake.

Questions three and four also go hand-in-hand. Why am I considering a retake? Why did I earn a lower score than I wanted? Perhaps you are considering a retake because your school list changed. The average MCAT of your old school list may have been a 510. You prepared for a competitive score at those schools and earned a 509. Now, with more experiences under your belt, you may be considering a list of schools with an MCAT median of 519. While your 509 was sufficient for your old school list, you may want to pump up your performance for a new list of medical schools. Another scenario is realizing that you can perform better on the MCAT than you originally thought you could. Maybe you were stuck in a mental rut of believing that a 505 was your ceiling. With more information, you might be empowered to score a 515+. Something may have gone wrong on test day that caused you to underperform. Sudden illness, a panic attack, chaotic life circumstances, problems at the testing center. Hopefully, you decided to void your score if any of these issues happened. Yet, you may have decided not to void and ended up performing below your capabilities. Each of these reasons is sufficient to justify an MCAT retake.

Sometimes, a retake is considered because a student took the MCAT unprepared. Nyra, who we discussed above, was one of these students. To these individuals: absolutely retake the exam, but be sure first to understand why you were unprepared the first time and make a plan not to let the past repeat itself. Taking the MCAT for a second time is not without risk. Schools view each completed attempt, and there is no superscoring. Retaking the MCAT only to score marginally better (first attempt: 510; second attempt: 511) can hurt your application in addition to scoring equal to or below your previous score. Admissions committees will wonder how seriously you take the exam and if you understand the effort that it takes to prepare for a large standardized test. Since standardized testing is far from over with the MCAT (oh, hi there, USMLE), it is in medical schools' interest to select strong test-takers for their incoming class.

Question five: Will I be able to improve my score when I take the MCAT for a second time? This is the essential question to ask yourself before deciding to retake the exam. In the next section, let's address the answer to this inquiry on when and how to retake the MCAT.

Preparing for an MCAT Retake: When and How

There is no point in spending significant time and money for an MCAT retake when the results of the past are likely to be repeated. When and how, then, should you retake the exam? Through exploring question four in the section above (Why did I earn a lower score than I wanted?), you should have a strong grasp as to why your first MCAT score was lower than you wanted it to be. Based on an understanding of those factors, let's address the *how* of the retake.

Craft your new study plan. Maybe you did not budget enough time to study. Moving forward, give yourself the necessary preparation time. Maybe you were not using the right resources. This time, take advantage of the brilliance of UWorld and the AAMC materials. Maybe something wacky happened on test day that caused you to vastly underperform what you were capable of, and you had decided not to void. Double-check that you are truly ready for the exam, and schedule your retake sooner rather than later so that your studying doesn't go to waste. Whether it's needing beta-blockers, applying for testing accommodations, committing to a strict study schedule, or any other reason, be sure to execute fully on your revamped MCAT preparation plan. Take your AAMC Practice Exams following your necessary work, and if your scores are at or above your target score, then you are ready for the retake.

Something to note is that if you have taken the AAMC Practice Exams before, your score might be slightly higher than it would actually be since you've seen the questions previously. Personally, I think this "inflation of score" depends on the individual. If you took the AAMC Practice Exams over a year ago and aren't touting a photographic memory, I question how much you're actually remembering – even subconsciously – from the first time you took the Practice Exams. I don't think I would remember a hoot of AAMC material if I looked at it today (about a year and a half after my MCAT). It would be brand new to me. If you happen to be completing your retake within a shorter time frame (say within the same year as your first MCAT attempt), then you might remember more specifics about the Practice Exam questions.

Needing an accurate assessment of where you stand before your retake is important. Perhaps knock a couple of points off of the Practice Exams if you've taken them within the past few months. If you haven't done UWorld before, make a mock MCAT out of UWorld questions, as we discussed in the *How To Study* section. I still warn against using Kaplan, Princeton Review, and Examkrackers to gauge your scoring capabilities because I think that they generally deflate your score, damage your confidence, and are not representative of the real exam. Must you use an outside source – I've heard that Examkrackers is the best of the three for not tanking your score with heavy deflation. Kaplan CARS is actually pretty spot on for the actual MCAT, so you could use their practice exams to predict your CARS score specifically. Also, Kaplan's P/S isn't bad, so it could also be useful for predicting that subsection score. I can't comment on Princeton Review with any specificity, as I didn't use their materials for the MCAT. Overall, though, I heard that Princeton Review is a big score deflator similar to Kaplan. When it comes to retakes, the most important advice to follow is this: **only retake the MCAT when you are ready.** That is the *when* rule of retakes.

People have made miraculous improvements happen through MCAT retakes. There are many students whom I've read about who earned around a 505 on their first attempt and scored above a 520 on their retake. Nyra is one of these people whom I know personally. Putting in the time and effort can absolutely make you someone with an incredible MCAT retake story. As we move into the Essays chapter, think about how you may want to talk about your MCAT retake in your writing to the medical schools.

CHAPTER

09

TO GAP YEAR OR NOT TO GAP YEAR

That is the question!

GAP YEAR: THE PROS AND THE CONS

Gap years used to be the stuff of weirdos. Back in the day, students went straight from college into medical school. Ah, what a life! Those were the times when you only needed to apply to five medical schools. Your school list would be comprised of Harvard, UCSF, Yale, Hopkins, and Columbia. You would get into all five, and in order to piss off your parents, you'd choose UCSF over Harvard. All joking aside, getting into medical school used to be *so much easier!*

As medical school admissions have become more competitive, taking gap years between college and medical school has become more common (Premeds: Capitalize on Gap Years Before Applying to Medical School). Like, *much* more common. It is now the norm to take one year off before matriculating to medical school. Taking two gap years is skyrocketing in popularity. The once common breed of students moving straight to medical school from college is now rarer. Some speculate that gap years might become if they haven't already, a new soft requirement for admission. To help you decide whether a gap year is the right choice for you, let's investigate the pros and cons of the gap year.

The biggest pro of the gap year for many applicants is having time to improve your application. One can accomplish more in five or six years compared to three or four years. When I decided to take a gap year and then a second gap year later on, my choice was grounded in the logistics of not wanting to interview while in school and then wanting to study for the MCAT after college graduation rather than during the school year. Yet, two years before my expected matriculation, I found that my gap years gave me the flexibility to craft a more competitive application. Increased competitiveness was not my initial impetus to take time off, but my application was enriched due to my pursuit of additional research and volunteer work.

Personal circumstances are another reason for gap years. A loved one may be ill, you and your partner are planning a wedding, or maybe you want time to bond with your family after being away at college for four years. Numerous life events might cause you to take time off before medical school, and these are great reasons to take a year or more for yourself. Exploring a passion such as starting a business, serving in the military, caring for a group of people in need, or earning a master's degree may prompt you to pursue those interests. In fact, the time before medical school and before starting a family (if a family is part of your future) could be the only opportunity for you to pursue these passions to their fullest. Medical school is expensive. Medical school is also a time when you make little to no money to pay off mounting student loan debt. Choosing to work for several years before medical school is another popular reason for gap years. This money can help reduce the amount of loans needed to pay for your medical education or support your family while you are not actively earning income during training.

The cons of the gap year are important to consider. Delaying the start of medical school means delaying future income. These are numbers that I have run over in my head. My two gap years mean that rather than making marginal income as a resident at 27 years of age, I will be 29 years old when I begin residency. This two-year difference has prompted me to want to graduate from medical school in four years rather than take an additional year to earn another degree or conduct research. For women particularly, gap years stall the beginning of residency, which is a hectic period of post-graduate training. Residency and the years when women want to begin their families often overlap. Residency is a demanding three to seven years that absorbs the late twenties and early-to-mid thirties of a person's life. These are the same years when female fertility begins its decline. For many aspiring doctors, completing residency sooner rather than later can then free up these important years for them to dedicate to their own families. Not to mention, the pay during residency is abysmal for the work being done, and the level of training these young doctors have earned. This low income makes it difficult to support couples wanting to have their own children. As medical school is approaching, I have begun seriously favoring specialties with shorter lengths of residency training to free up my thirties for a family.

Lastly, according to data that Dr. Joan Downey at WashU shares with her students, too many gap years may be criticized by admissions committees (The Components of a Successful Applicant: Q&A Session). Now, I believe that this outlook on "too many" gap years is changing, but I will explain what the data indicated for those interested. The data showed acceptance rates to medical school based on the number of gap years an applicant has taken. Taking up to two gap years did not affect an applicant's ability to earn an acceptance. Acceptance rates began to decline once someone took three or more gap years. Dr. Downey, who sat on Harvard Medical School's admission board for ten years, explained that with three or more years off, some admissions committee members question an applicant's desire for a career in medicine. From my perspective, the interpretation of an applicant taking three or more gap years cannot be generalized. If an individual spent the last few years doing nothing related to the medical field or community service, then yes, I can see how committees may question their commitment to the profession. Yet, if the last several years have been spent immersed in research, volunteering, or patient engagement, I only see the gap years strengthening an application. More and more students who have taken significant time off before medical school (three or more years) seem to make compelling applicants whose differentiation of life experience is valued by admissions committees – not dismissed. While taking a larger number of gap years is something to think critically about, it should not be avoided if it is the right step forward for your circumstances.

Reflect on your own goals, current strength of candidacy for medical school, as well as your personal circumstances to determine if taking a gap year will benefit you. Gap years have transformed some applicants into candidates for top medical school programs. Other gap years have been unproductive. Whatever decision you make, be sure to make your time off an asset. We will get into how to spend your gap years in the upcoming sections.

HOW MANY GAPS

How many gap years you take depends on your application's current state and your ambitions for getting into medical school. We will discuss what kind of applicant might choose to take zero, one, two, or three or more years off between college and matriculation to medical school.

Zero gap years are for students with strong applications going into the summer following their junior year of college – the summer when applications will be submitted. An MCAT score, as well as both the cGPA and sGPA, should be competitive for admission. Recommendation letters need to ardently and enthusiastically advocate for the candidate's admission. These students must be prepared to interview during their senior year of college – a complicated task when balancing interviews with classes and extracurricular activities. Due to the mounting pre-matriculation requirements for students to meet, the zero gap year candidate is becoming less common. Using college summers intentionally can help to prepare someone for a successful application cycle at the start of their junior summer. Zero gap years may be risky for those aspiring to attend a top research medical school. It is true that each year, plenty of matriculants to the top programs haven't taken any time off between college and medical school. Yet, these students have top grades and MCAT scores, well-written essays, as well as compelling, meaningful involvement in their extracurricular pursuits. If you believe that your application could notably benefit from taking time to improve your grades or bolster your resume, taking a year off may be the move.

Applicants taking one gap year will submit their applications the summer following their senior year of university. These students will be able to submit all four years of undergraduate grades with their applications – a favorable option for students who stumbled academically during their first or second years. An additional summer and academic year of activities will strengthen the applicant's candidacy and is particularly useful for those lacking involvement in community service, research, leadership, or another core area prior to beginning senior year. One gap year allows people to avoid interviewing during college, which is an important consideration if interviews return to in-person over the upcoming years. The MCAT should have been taken before primary applications are submitted, and the applicant should be happy with her score.

Two gap years are attractive for a number of different reasons. Students wanting to improve their GPAs can take classes during their first gap year that will be seen by medical schools when applications are submitted. Post-baccalaureate programs for students who have not completed the premed course requirements or need to amend poor grades can be taken in one or two years. Those who did not take the MCAT during college or who performed poorly can take the summer following senior year to prepare for the exam without distraction to earn a top score. Two years is also the time it takes to complete many fellowship programs. Fulbright Scholars and Rhodes Scholars often take two years to complete their projects and education, respectively – thus, two gap years are necessary for people in these programs. For those needing to make more significant improvements to their applications, two gap years give the time to do so. Say you haven't completed any volunteering or your involvement in research is minimal; two gap years can transform a weaker applicant story into a gripping narrative.

Candidates taking three or more gap years are often called nontraditional applicants. Although nontraditional implies that few students fall into this category, in truth, this group of applicants has been growing at an alarmingly high rate. Earlier, we discussed the data that acceptance rates to medical school are lower among those taking three or more gap years. Although this data may be intimidating, I would speculate that the lower acceptance rate is because those being denied admission haven't explained how their time away from school has better prepared them for a career in medicine. That is to say that applicants should not feel pressured to spend their gap years focused on work and activities related to medicine. What you should spend your gap years doing depends on your individual application. Taking time before medical school to chase a passion that is not medically related is a fantastic decision. For those making this choice, be sure to keep a hand in part-time community service and be able to explain through essays and interviews how your pursued interest will still contribute to who you will be as a physician.

More often students pursuing post-baccalaureate programs take three or more gap years, particularly those who did not know that they wanted to go into medicine in college. This time is used not only to complete the prerequisite coursework and take the MCAT but also to engage in research, volunteering, and other health-related pursuits. Reapplicants to medical school may find themselves taking three or more years between college and medical school. Nyra is one example. After an unsuccessful 2019-2020 application cycle, Nyra decided to overhaul her application. She retook the MCAT to improve her 508 to a 520+, she joined a research laboratory where she was published on two papers – one as first-author – in leading research journals, she began volunteering at women's and children's shelters, and she enrolled in a master's program to help overcome her lower undergraduate GPA. Nyra's unwavering diligence has prepared her to have a successful application cycle for 2021-2022. I believe that the changes she has made to her candidacy will bring her much success as a reapplicant. What a babe!

Throughout the guidebook, I have mentioned my own two gap years between graduating from WashU and matriculating to Yale

School of Medicine. How did I come to the decision to take two gap years? Beginning college, I set out to join the zero gap year crew. I knew I wanted to study medicine, and what was the point of delaying such a long path to my eventual career? Delays would cause me to lose out on years of income and put further time constraints on when it was convenient to start a family. Early on at WashU, I realized that one gap year would be a necessity for my success as an applicant. My grades suffered during my freshman and sophomore years. Only Bs were earned in my science classes. The courses at WashU were challenging, and my senior year grades would suffer if I tried to interview while taking a full set of classes and participating in extracurricular activities. Thus, the choice to take one gap year was made.

Approaching the spring semester of my senior year, I had yet to take the MCAT. While I had prepared for the exam during the summer and fall leading up to my senior spring, the work I had put in was cursory. My efforts hadn't scratched the surface of what I would need to invest to earn a top MCAT score. Due to my respectable but meh grades (3.70 cGPA; 3.56 sGPA), I saw the MCAT as an opportunity to prove my academic prowess. My goal was to score in the top 5% of test takers, meaning I would need to earn a 517 or higher according to the 2019 exam curve. It became clear that with a full load of math and science classes for senior spring, I would be unable to effectively study for the MCAT during that semester. Delaying my application for the MCAT worried me, as the advice given to me by my advisors was to submit the application as soon as possible. Fortunately, I listened and decided that delaying my application would hinder my potential success as an applicant. Only one path became clear for me: I would spend the summer following college graduation studying for the MCAT and submit my application for the 2020-2021 cycle rather than the 2019-2020 cycle. Two gap years. Oh boy. I was in for the long haul.

Reflecting back, I am tremendously glad I took the time I needed to have a successful application cycle. Too many of my classmates rushed their applications and ended up with poor MCAT scores and grades, lackluster resumes, and sloppy essays. These students with tremendous potential ended up as reapplicants or matriculants to Caribbean medical schools. <u>Two gap years allowed me to do the following</u>:

1. Improve my cGPA to a 3.70 by taking a course at a Portland Community College following graduation,
2. Score in the top 5% on the MCAT,
3. Volunteer with older adults in memory care units and secure a generously supportive recommendation letter from the Life Enrichment and Wellness Director at Touchmark Senior Living,
4. Start my own online service for older adults and their caregivers through CaregiverZone (caregiverzone.com),
5. Earn significant savings through working in research and at my family's company,
6. Present at five additional regional and national research symposia,
7. Participate in the Harvard Chan School's Summer Research Program,
8. Write outstanding essays for my primary and secondary applications, and
9. Prepare thoroughly for interviews.

 I credit much of my success through the application cycles to taking the time necessary to become the best candidate I could be. Over the past two years, I have also decided that I will likely pursue a career in dermatology with a focus on geriatric dermatology. Dermatology is one of the most competitive specialties to match into. Thus, being able to attend a top medical school program through YSM, where the Yale System allows students the freedom to engage notably in research, has set me up with every opportunity to match into dermatology. I am especially grateful to attend YSM with Step 1 moving to pass/fail and the unknown effects of this change on match statistics into competitive specialties. When deciding how many gap years you should take before medical school, I urge you not to fall to peer pressure to take too few or too many gap years. Examine your application, know your weak points, and use the time to your best advantage. Would I have been accepted to Yale School of Medicine without my gap years? Possibly. But I felt a heck of a lot more confident applying on my own timeline, and after I pursued every advantage to become an excellent candidate for medical school.

WHAT TO DO DURING YOUR GAP YEAR

The last point to discuss around gap years is what to do during your gap year! We've brushed over different ideas for how to spend your time between college and medical school, but now we will hit each idea separately to ensure that all bases are covered.

Finding the weak points of your application is the first step to take in crafting gap year plans. Have you taken the MCAT and performed well? How are your grades? Have you presented at research conferences? Have you shadowed physicians? How are your volunteer hours? Poke at your resume from different angles to find which places are squishy and need fortification.

Your imagination is the only limit to what you can achieve during your gap year(s). For simplicity, below I will list the most common and, often, impactful gap year activities for medical school applicants. As you peruse the list of activities, see which ones speak to you and where you can improve your candidacy. Maybe another pursuit not listed will be your calling card. If so, like all that we invest ourselves into, pursue your ambition enthusiastically and with intention.

<u>List of potential gap year activities:</u>

- Complete a post-baccalaureate program
- Earn a Master or Ph.D. degree
- Take classes to improve your undergraduate GPA (does not need to be through a post-baccalaureate program if small-scale grade improvement is the goal)
- Take the MCAT
- Start your own business
- Work and build up your savings
- Volunteer with a population whom you are passionate to serve
- Conduct research surrounding a disease or community of interest
- Present research findings at symposia
- Apply for research or public health fellowships
- Spend time with your loved ones and tend to any difficult personal circumstances
- Write outstanding essays for your primary and secondary applications
- Prepare for your interviews
- Apply for medical school scholarships

CHAPTER 10

MAKING YOUR SCHOOL LIST

Yippie! Making your school list means you are getting ready to apply for medical school. How exciting! From GPA and MCAT to resume strength and from URM or ORM status to in-state or out-of-state positioning, many factors affect how to comprise a school list. As you consider these factors in regard to your own application, they can help guide how many schools you should apply to and which programs those should be.

HOW DO GPA AND MCAT AFFECT YOUR SCHOOL LIST?

GPA and MCAT open and close doors with regard to a candidate's competitiveness at a particular medical school. GPA and MCAT do not push someone through those doors (Dr. Ryan Gray, Medical School Headquarters). Determining which doors are open and which may be closed due to one's metrics is tricky business, as the numbers are not clean-cut. The rules are smudged.

Generally speaking, if your MCAT and GPA are above a school's 25th percentile marks, then you are good to apply from a scores perspective. What happens if one or both of these factors is not at the 25th percentile? In these cases, head to the medical school's website and look at their statistics for the last incoming class. Many schools share not just their matriculating students' GPA and MCAT averages but also the ranges of these two metrics. Feel free to submit your application if your scores are within their ranges or close to them. However, be aware that the students at the low ends of these ranges likely had superior achievements and remarkable personal narratives.

One factor to consider is that if your MCAT is above a school's 25th percentile, but your GPA is not, you likely have a better chance at admission compared to your GPA being above the school's 25th percentile and your MCAT not meeting that mark. Why is that? Since the MCAT is a standardized exam, admissions committees are able to put more faith in your academic readiness based on your MCAT score compared to your GPA, which can fluctuate wildly depending on your university and area of study.

Looking at the top research medical schools, these institutions have incredibly high MCAT and GPA averages. We know the 25th percentile rule, but let's look deeper into what scores make you competitive for the 20 leading research programs. ORM students with GPAs of 3.70 and above and MCAT scores of 517 and above are academically competitive for all top 20 institutions (even if these marks fall below a school's 25th percentile). URM students with GPAs of 3.60 and above and MCAT scores of 515 and above are contenders for all of the top 20 research schools (again, even if these marks fall below a school's 25th percentile) – more on this in the *URM and ORM Applicants* section.

STATE SCHOOLS VERSUS PRIVATE SCHOOLS

State schools (especially in-state versus out-of-state considerations) and private schools shape school lists. The die-hard rule is to always apply to your state school(s) if you have one. If you are a resident of a state with low numbers of in-state applicants relative to the number of medical schools, for example, West Virginia has three medical schools (two M.D. and one D.O.), you likely have a stronger shot of admission compared to applicants from California and New York where there are many more in-state applicants per seat. State schools are required to admit applicants with state residency, as these individuals are deemed more likely than out-of-state individuals to return to said state and serve the locals through medicine. Usually, there are specific percentages of in-state matriculants that state schools try to meet with each incoming class. Pretty nifty stuff. Because of this, many premed advisors discourage applicants from applying to state schools where the student does not hold residency. Let's examine this notion.

Generally, if you are from Florida and have no association with Utah, applying to the University of Utah School of Medicine makes little sense. It would be a waste of money. Having ties to the state of Utah (such as attending university there, working in the state during a summer or throughout your gap year, or having family who live in Utah) are compelling reasons to still apply to medical school without having residency. Many state schools have specific missions for the work they aspire to train their graduates to do. For example, serving communities in rural Oregon is a mission for Oregon Health and Science University (OHSU School of Medicine MD Program: Mission-Based Groups). Whatever the particular mission, if you have a connection to that work regardless of residency status, you have a strong reason to apply to that state school. Whether it is a personal tie to the state or a connection to the mission, you must be able to articulate through your writing and interviews *why* you are applying to a state school without residency status, *how* you connect with the mission of the school, and *in what ways* you will carry forth their mission through your work as a physician. These three points are necessary for you to hit to be offered an interview and then a seat in the incoming class.

There are graphs available that show how friendly schools are toward out-of-state applicants. Some state schools are more friendly (i.e., more likely to offer admission) to out-of-state applicants, while other programs are extremely unlikely to offer a spot to an out-of-state (OOS) student. In *Appendix D*, you'll find one of these tables for your reference based on 2022 *Accepted* data. This table is one of the best I've found in terms of how the data is presented in determining whether or not you should apply to an OOS program - check out *Accepted* for more details on their analysis.

Certain state schools have a network with other state schools, encouraging applicants living within this multi-state network to apply to each participating program. The most well-known network exists between Washington, Wyoming, Alaska, Montana, and Idaho (WWAMI). Through this network, residents of all five states are favored when applying to the University of Washington School of Medicine (WWAMI: A Five-State Medical Education Creating National Impact). Although Wyoming, Alaska, Montana, and Idaho do not have allopathic medical schools to participate in an exchange, the relationship with UW is greatly beneficial to students in these four states without allopathic medical schools. Similar networks are not as established and official as WWAMI, but generally speaking, applying to state schools that are adjacent to the state where you have residency may be your best shot at capitalizing on a more informal relationship between neighboring state schools.

If you particularly love certain state schools, you may want to consider moving to that state during your gap year and working to establish residency before applying to medical school. This strategy can be especially beneficial if you move to a state with fewer in-state applicants, such as West Virginia or New Mexico. Years ago, my dad's classmate moved to New Mexico to complete a post-bac and simultaneously establish residency before applying to and being admitted to the University of New Mexico School of Medicine. I know one young physician who established residency in order to attend medical school in California. She moved to San Francisco for her gap years, became a Californian, and was admitted to UCSF. UCSF was the only medical school to which this young woman (now a young physician) was admitted. Whew! What a close call! Another consideration comes with residency training. If you want to match into a certain state for residency, your chances increase if you attend medical school in that state. In love with Florida for residency? Consider applying to Florida state schools for medical school.

Private schools are fair game for all applicants. I do believe that many of these schools have a slight preference toward in-state applicants. The Out-of-State Applicant vs. In-State Applicant Friendliness Table above shows acceptance rates for in-state (IS) and out-of-state applicants at allopathic medical colleges in the United States. This table shows the slight IS preference for many private medical schools. The majority of medical schools you apply to should be private to avoid OOS limitations at many public schools. While the cost of private medical schools is typically higher than that of public medical schools (Kaplan, What's the Real Cost of Medical School?), these private programs often have robust financial aid resources, with many schools committing to meet 100% of a student's demonstrated financial need. Furthermore, private schools usually have more funding for merit scholarships than their public counterparts.

INTERNATIONAL APPLICANTS

Admittance to American and Canadian medical schools for international applicants is undoubtedly difficult. However, success in earning multiple acceptances to top programs is possible. Beware, though, that the bar of achievement is higher for international applicants (Medical Schools that Accept International Students: How to Get In). Top grades and MCAT scores are expected. Particularly for the CARS subsection of the MCAT, medical schools look for top scores to know that international students excel at understanding the English language. A large proportion of international applicants aim for a CARS score of 128+ to demonstrate proficiency in English. Beyond academic metrics, well-written and intriguing essays, phenomenal involvement in activities, and outstanding recommendation letters are critical for the triumph of international students in the application cycle.

The major hurdle for admission is that, as of 2021, only 64 allopathic medical schools in the U.S. and Canada accept international students into their incoming classes. A number of these schools either only accept international students with Canadian or U.S. citizenship or permanent residence or international students with a degree from a U.S. or Canadian college. Many programs require applicants to demonstrate that they are able to pay for all four years of medical school (tuition plus expenses) – some mandate that these students place the funds in an escrow account prior to enrollment. So basically, you better be hella rich. Calling all sugar daddies! Among the remaining programs, international applicants with financial need are able to apply. Below is a table with the names of the 64 medical schools that accept international students (source: Shemmassian Academic Consulting). I'm sure that the requirements to apply, as well as the school list, change frequently, so be sure to check the rules of each school you are interested in to ensure that you're working with updated information.

US and Canadian Medical Schools that Accept International Applicants	
Boston University School of Medicine	TCU and UNTHSC School of Medicine
Case Western Reserve School of Medicine	The Warren Alpert Medical School of Brown University
Columbia University Vagelos College of Physicians and Surgeons	Tufts University School of Medicine
Duke University School of Medicine	Tulane University School of Medicine
Emory University School of Medicine	Universidad Central del Caribe School of Medicine[†]
Faculty of Medicine Université Laval	Universite de Montreal Faculty of Medicine
Geisel School of Medicine at Dartmouth	Universite de Sherbrooke Faculty of Medicine
George Washington University School of Medicine and Health Sciences[*]	University of California, Davis, School of Medicine
Georgetown University School of Medicine	University of California, Los Angeles David Geffen School of Medicine
Harvard Medical School	University of Chicago Division of the Biological Sciences The Pritzker School of Medicine
Howard University College of Medicine	University of Colorado School of Medicine

Icahn School of Medicine at Mount Sinai	University of Connecticut School of Medicine
Johns Hopkins University School of Medicine	University of Hawaii, John A. Burns School of Medicine
Loma Linda University School of Medicine	University of Illinois College of Medicine
McGill University Faculty of Medicine	University of Kentucky College of Medicine§
McGovern Medical School^	University of Louisville School of Medicine^
McMaster University Michael G. DeGroote School of Medicine	University of Nebraska Medical Center College of Medicine§
Medical College of Wisconsin–Milwaukee	University of New Mexico School of Medicine§
Memorial University of Newfoundland Faculty of Medicine	University of North Carolina at Chapel Hill School of Medicine
Morehouse School of Medicine	University of Pittsburgh School of Medicine
New York Medical College*	University of Rochester School of Medicine and Dentistry§
Northwestern University The Feinberg School of Medicine	University of Southern California Keck School of Medicine
Perelman School of Medicine at the University of Pennsylvania	University of Toronto Faculty of Medicine
Queen's University Faculty of Health Sciences	University of Utah School of Medicine
Renaissance School of Medicine at Stony Brook University	University of Virginia School of Medicine
Rutgers New Jersey Medical School	Vanderbilt University School of Medicine
Rutgers Robert Wood Johnson Medical School†	Virginia Commonwealth University School of Medicine†
Saint Louis University School of Medicine	Washington University in St. Louis School of Medicine
San Juan Bautista School of Medicine	Wayne State University School of Medicine
Sidney Kimmel Medical College at Thomas Jefferson University	Weill Cornell Medicine

Stanford University School of Medicine	West Virginia University School of Medicine*
State University of New York Upstate Medical University	Yale School of Medicine

Notes:

* Denotes medical schools requiring international students to have completed all or the majority of a bachelor's degree at an accredited U.S. or Canadian college.
^ Denotes medical schools only accepting international students with pending U.S. citizenship or permanent resident status.
§ Denotes medical schools that only accept international students who hold a bachelor's degree from the same university or a university in the same system or who have specific geographic ties to the state.
† Denotes medical schools that accept international students on a case-by-case basis.

Although the metrics can feel daunting, each year, there are hundreds of international applicants who earn seats in the top medical school programs. One international student I interviewed at Yale School of Medicine (YSM) shared her story. Let's call her Inka. Inka is an international student from South America who completed her undergraduate degree at Swarthmore College and spent two gap years conducting research at YSM. She was anxious about entering the medical school application process as an international applicant who could not apply to schools requiring her to produce four years of tuition and other expenses at matriculation. Inka was limited to applying to schools that gave financial assistance to international students. She applied to twenty medical schools and was accepted to Yale, Stanford, and Duke, among many others. Having met Inka, I believe that some factors that played into her outstanding application cycle were her compelling personal story, dedication to research, strong recommendation letters, warmth during interviews, and impressive academic marks. Speaking to Inka, I learned she knew several international applicants who shared her success. While the competition is tougher for international students, acceptance to top medical school programs can absolutely be achieved with hard work. These 64 schools *want* international students to add to the diversity of their incoming classes. Market yourself thoughtfully in essays and interviews, and opportunities for admission will open themselves up.

Remember that if placement in a U.S. residency program is your goal, this ambition can still be achieved if you graduate from an international medical school. It is much easier to match into a U.S. residency from a U.S. medical school (especially now with Step 1 going pass/fail). However, this feat is still possible for international medical graduates (IMG) (BeMo Academic Consulting, International Medical Graduate: The 2021 Ultimate Guide). Study up to crush Step 2, obtain generous recommendation letters, and significantly engage in your community through research, community service, etc., and your chances of matching to the U.S. will skyrocket.

URM AND ORM APPLICANTS

Metrics are the most concrete data when examining differences between URM (under represented minority in medicine) and ORM (over represented minority in medicine) applicants. Because fewer URM candidates are applying to medical school compared to ORM candidates (AAMC, Table A-8: Applicants to U.S. Medical Schools by Selected Combinations of Race/Ethnicity and Sex, 2017-2018 through 2020-2021) and because many schools aim to fill at least 20% of their class with URM students, the GPAs and MCAT scores of URM matriculants are lower than that of ORM matriculants (AAMC, Table A-18: MCAT Scores and GPAs for Applicants and Matriculants to U.S. Medical Schools by Race/Ethnicity, 2020-2021).

Looking at the 2020-2021 data released by the AAMC regarding the MCAT scores and GPAs of matriculants based on race and ethnicity (inserted below), we see that Asian matriculants (ORM) had on average a 514 MCAT and 3.77 total GPA and white matriculants (ORM) had on average a 512 MCAT and 3.77 total GPA. The statistics for the groups of URM matriculants – American Indian or Alaskan Native, Black or African American, Hispanic, Latino, or of Spanish Origin, and Native Hawaiian or other Pacific Islander matriculants – are the following, respectively: 504 MCAT and 3.54 GPA (American Indian or Alaskan Native), 506 MCAT and 3.53 GPA (Black or African American), 507 MCAT and 3.62 GPA (Hispanic, Latino, or of Spanish Origin), and 507 MCAT and 3.62 GPA (Native Hawaiian or other Pacific Islander). The table of average (mean) MCAT and GPA of applicants by race and ethnicity is also found below.

URM and ORM Average MCAT and GPA - Applicants

Applicants	American Indian or Alaskan Native	Asian	Black or African American	Hispanic, Latino, or of Spanish Origin	Native Hawaiian or Other Pacific Islander	White	Other	Multiple Race/Ethnicity	Unknown Race/Ethnicity	Non-U.S. Citizen or Non-Permanent Resident	Total
Total MCAT	500	509	498	501	501	508	505	505	509	508	506
GPA Science	3.31	3.53	3.17	3.32	3.34	3.57	3.45	3.43	3.51	3.58	3.49
GPA Non-Science	3.64	3.76	3.58	3.66	3.68	3.77	3.72	3.70	3.73	3.75	3.74
GPA Total	3.44	3.63	3.35	3.46	3.49	3.66	3.57	3.55	3.61	3.65	3.60
Total Applicants	73	11,240	4,363	3,332	41	22,891	1,288	5,314	2,644	1,844	53,030

URM and ORM Average MCAT and GPA - Matriculants

	American Indian or Alaskan Native	Asian	Black or African American	Hispanic, Latino, or of Spanish Origin	Native Hawaiian or Other Pacific Islander	White	Other	Multiple Race/Ethnicity	Unknown Race/Ethnicity	Non-U.S. Citizen or Non-Permanent Resident	Total
Total MCAT	504	514	506	507	507	512	512	511	513	513	512
GPA Science	3.42	3.72	3.39	3.53	3.52	3.71	3.69	3.62	3.68	3.75	3.66
GPA Non-Science	3.69	3.84	3.69	3.75	3.72	3.84	3.84	3.79	3.82	3.84	3.82
GPA Total	3.54	3.77	3.53	3.62	3.62	3.77	3.75	3.70	3.75	3.79	3.73
Total Matriculants	36	4,803	1,767	1,524	14	9,944	470	2,311	1,094	276	22,239

How do these numbers translate into crafting school lists as a URM or ORM applicant? Recall the numbers cited from the *How Do GPA and MCAT Affect Your School List?* section. When looking at the top research programs, ORMs with 517+ MCATs and 3.70+ GPAs have the numbers to earn an acceptance. URMs with 515+ MCATs and 3.60+ GPAs are rocking the scores for the top 20 schools. Overall, students above the 25th percentile for MCAT and GPA are set to apply to said school. There is more leeway, however, for URM candidates. The numbers on this have not been analyzed. Use your best judgment, and always throw your hat in at your dream schools.

If you are an American Indian or Alaskan Native applicant, apply to schools where your MCAT and GPA are above the 25th percentile, but also feel free to apply anywhere you want. If you have a 500 MCAT but want to apply to Harvard Medical School, give it a shot. There were only 73 American Indian or Alaskan Native applicants during the 2021-2022 cycle. Schools are so excited to include students from diverse racial backgrounds in their cohort that being one of 73 applicants of your racial makeup makes you a compelling candidate by this demographic measure alone.

Activities are a critical component of the application. On the whole, both ORM and URM matriculants have impressive extracurricular involvement. Due to the slightly lowered GPA and MCAT bar for URM candidates, one could see how this trend may extend to the resumes of URM students. This conjecture may be true, but as far as I know, there is no hard evidence to support the claim that URMs have less robust achievements compared to their ORM counterparts. Personally, each URM matriculant whom I know has sterling leadership, research, and community service records. A greater percentage of ORM candidates may have distinguished resumes compared to the proportion of URM applicants with the same accomplishments. But, in total, the URM matriculants I have met are on par with ORM matriculants in terms of personal and professional accolades.

SAFETY SCHOOLS? FACT OR MYTH

Remember applying to colleges, and you could round out your school list with safety schools (a.k.a. schools where you had a very high chance of admission)? Yeah... safety schools don't exist for medical school. Verdict: Safety schools = myth!

Why is it that safety schools don't exist for medical school admission? One point to consider is that the average acceptance rate for the top 100 *U.S. News* ranked medical schools in the 2020-2021 application cycle was 6.3% (Accepted). This number will continue to decline as the number of applicants rises yearly. With nearly 94 students being denied a seat for every six students who earn acceptances, it is easy to see how no one can feel "safe" applying to medical school.

Many applicants often think that applying to schools with lower GPA and MCAT averages compared to their own scores can create a cushion of programs that will want to admit them for their academic prowess. Unfortunately, this rationality does not seem to pan out, and in fact, applicants who apply to programs with lower academic metric averages compared to their own scores are often at a *disadvantage* for admission. Let me explain.

Each medical school has a limited number of interview spots they can allot. Interviewing applicants is extremely costly in terms of resources – particularly when applicants interview in person. A large number of faculty, staff, and students give their time to conduct *multiple* 30-minute to hour-long conversations with each applicant. Multiple informational presentations are conducted about the medical school on each interview day. If on-campus interviewing returns, meals, and gifts are prepared, and sometimes housing and transportation are provided for low-income interviewees. Following months of interviews, the school selects which candidates are a strong fit for their program and who they believe will matriculate. As matriculation rates affect the ranking of medical schools in the *U.S. News and World Report* "Best Medical Schools: Research" and "Best Medical Schools: Primary Care" rankings, programs are further incentivized to admit students who will accept the offer of admission.

Let's look at George Washington University School of Medicine by putting these observations into a real-world example. For the 2020-2021 application cycle, George Washington University School of Medicine received more than 14,000 applications (MedEdits Medical Admissions). If GW interviewed 1141 applicants in the cycle prior (2019-2020) and accepted 349 of those interviewees (DataKing and Limeyguy, data pulled from *U.S. News and World Report*), then it is crucial that admissions officers interview candidates who are of high likelihood to matriculate to the program. GW could likely easily select 1,000 applicants to interview who far exceed their average MCAT and GPA metrics. However, GW knows that many of these students will likely earn admission to other outstanding programs – some of which hold greater "prestige" than their own program. While these candidates may have superb resumes and accomplishments, the school may struggle to fill their own class if only the top applicants are interviewed. Instead, excellent students who are more on par with the average GW statistics are more likely to be interviewed than the top-scoring students. This sort of gymnastics in deciding who to interview is often termed 'yield protection' because institutions are working to protect their yields by choosing applicants who are desirable *and* likely to enroll (The Admissions Strategist).

Anecdotal evidence is fun to look at with regard to yield protection. Shaman, from the MedBros YouTube Channel, described his difficulty receiving interviews at less "prestigious" medical school programs, while he more easily secured interviews at the top 20 research programs. In his video titled, "Why My 4.0 at UC Berkeley Actually Hurt Me," Shaman speculated that his higher GPA and MCAT score likely kept him from being seen as a likely matriculant to institutions whose metrics were far above their enrollee averages. Candidates with top academic marks but lack the exceptional experiences to earn admission to a top 20 research medical school often find themselves in a tough spot. Their resumes are not competitive enough for the top 20 schools, but their metrics are too high for the mid- and lower-tier programs. I really do use 'mid-tier' and 'lower-tier' loosely, as every U.S. medical school is phenomenal and very difficult to get into. Shaman conjectured that had he earned a lower GPA and MCAT that was still strong enough for top research schools, he would have more easily earned interviews to non-top 20 programs. You can see these occurrences play out in my own cycle.

My metrics of a 517 MCAT and 3.70 GPA were competitive for top research programs but put me below the averages for their typical matriculant. These numbers put me above the averages for mid-tier and lower-tier programs but still within range of their enrollee statistics. I applied to 23 of the top 25 research medical schools. Of these 23 schools, I earned interview invitations to 13 (56.5% interview rate). Looking at the other 11 schools that I applied to that were not ranked among the top 25 research institutions, I was offered six interviews (54.5% interview rate). Thus, my interview rates at top-tier and non-top-tier programs were nearly identical. Yes, I am an 'n of 1', yet, nevertheless, anecdotal evidence is interesting to think about.

From my own analysis, I believe that the combination of my great but not exceptionally superior numbers combined with outstanding essays and activities are what earned me interviews through all strata of medical school programs. It's quite funny to think how great but not near-perfect metrics may have advantaged some people like myself, while those 4.0/528 candidates could be passed over for interviews due to flawless academic performance. If you are a high-stat applicant who wants to earn interviews to mid-tier and lower-tier medical schools, your best bet is having a personal connection with the school or being able to clearly and specifically articulate why you want to attend a particular program.

While safety schools really are the things of college admission, not medical school admission, the best shot that you have at something resembling a safety school is your state school (if you have one). As we discussed earlier, state schools are required to admit certain proportions of in-state (IS) applicants, so as an in-state applicant, you are favored for a seat in the class. The degree of advantage you receive as an IS applicant depends on how many total IS candidates apply. The David Geffen School of Medicine at UCLA received 5703 IS applicants in 2019-2020 for 163 IS acceptances. Contrast those numbers with those of Oregon Health and Science University, which received 664 IS applications during the same cycle (2019-2020) for 185 IS acceptances (DataKing and Limeyguy, data pulled from *U.S. News and World Report*). Quite the difference in benefit of IS status depending on which state you live in.

HOW MANY SCHOOLS?

In today's competitive admissions market, apply to at least 20 medical schools. The average medical school had an acceptance rate of 6.3% during the 2020-2021 cycle, meaning more applications better your chances of admission (Accepted). While paying for the primary and secondary applications is costly, it is far less expensive than the cost of reapplying following an unfruitful cycle. Considering both the monetary and time costs of applications, around 40 programs should be the maximum you apply to. If your MCAT and GPA are above the 25th percentiles at most of your schools, you show dedicated, meaningful, and sustained involvement in your activities, and you produce well-written essays that thoughtfully and zealously articulate your personal narrative, a well-distributed list of 40 medical schools should be a large enough docket. Choosing to apply to more than 40 programs is understandable, given the low acceptance rates, but be sure that you are still able to produce high-quality writing for each school's essays (otherwise, you are throwing away your chance at an interview). The exception to the 40 max rule is an international medical school applicant. Because it is even more difficult for international candidates to earn a seat at a U.S. medical school, apply to as many programs as you are eligible for.

During my application cycle, I applied to 34 schools. Although 34 applications ended up being way more than necessary, I am happy that I cast a large net. The competitiveness of my candidacy was unknown to me going into the cycle. I know this may sound strange, considering that I had great research and leadership as well as a strong MCAT, but I really overestimated how much my good but not great GPA would hinder my success. I mistakenly believed that my 3.70 GPA would shut doors at a lot of the top research medical schools. Obviously, I failed to understand that GPAs only really open or close doors, and it's your writing, recommendations, and experiences that earn you an interview and then acceptance. Witnessing other WashU students have tremendous triumphs and devastations when they applied to medical school added to my anxiety. Doing the cycle over again, it's true that I could've saved a few hundred dollars in application fees by applying to fewer schools, but my wide net gave me peace of mind that I was more likely to secure an acceptance. In total, 34 applications were worth the stress relief.

WHICH SCHOOLS?

Part of knowing how many schools to apply to comes from understanding *which* schools to apply to. As we've gone over, all of your state schools are a must (if you have any). Did you attend an undergraduate institution associated with a medical school (e.g., Tufts, Boston University, Tulane, etc.)? Check those boxes, too. Are you associated with any other medical schools? In other words, did you complete a summer project at a medical school or college associated with a medical school? Did you take organic chemistry or another class or perhaps complete a post-bac at a program connected to a medical school? Do you have any loved ones who are alums or who teach at a medical school? Honey, apply to any and all of these schools! If you resonate strongly and specifically with a school's mission, submit an application and clearly articulate why you are a great fit for their program. Do you have any dream schools? You know what to do, babe! My philosophy is to always try for your dream schools, even if they seem out of reach. Each year, students with GPAs and MCATs far below your dream school's average are admitted. Take your shot because one of these incoming students may, in fact, be you.

What about the schools that don't fall into any of these categories? We've discussed throughout this chapter the rule of applying to schools where your GPA and MCAT are above the 25th percentile for a program. That's a good guideline for filling out your school list. Now, many programs may fall into your "above the 25th percentile mark." Research the schools and choose your favorites. Your total list should be twenty schools or more.

For candidates with lower MCATs and GPAs, ask yourself if you want to apply to M.D. as well as to D.O. programs. To me, M.D. and D.O. degrees are the same. The only difference between the degrees that may cause someone to concentrate on M.D. is if you want to match into a highly competitive specialty. Historically, competitive matches are more easily obtainable by those with M.D. degrees. The chance of matching to these specialties increases among those attending top medical schools – that's one of the big pluses of prestigious institutions. Unfortunately, with Step 1 going pass/fail, those with M.D. degrees may benefit in the match, while D.O. students and IMGs may suffer. The effects of the Step 1 change are unknown since the exam doesn't move to P/F until 2022. However, these disparate consequences for M.D., D.O., and IMG candidates are suspected among the current medical community (MedBros, USMLE STEP 1 is Now PASS/FAIL!? Why this is a HUGE DEAL!). Therefore, if ophthalmology, radiology, radiation oncology, plastic surgery, or another competitive specialty is your jam, you may want to concentrate on M.D. schools.

A note for those targeting the top 20 research medical schools: You have to apply broadly. Definitely apply to every top program you are interested in, but also target mid-tier and low-tier schools to round out your application. These are rough definitions, so bear with me. Typically, top-tier schools are denoted as the top 25 programs according to the *USNWR*'s 'Best Medical Schools: Research' list (these 25 are pretty consistent from year to year), mid-tier are the next 25-35 schools on the list (i.e., schools ranked from 26 to either 55 or 65), and the remaining schools are low-tier. To be clear, I think that getting into medical school itself is a tremendous accomplishment, and the tiers are silly. I still talk about tiers because they allow us to clearly communicate about which specific programs to apply to based on competitiveness (competitiveness not in terms of the number of competing applications, but rather in terms of average academic metrics of incoming students). It is an operable term more than anything, but regardless, I know that it still frustrates people to break an extraordinary accomplishment down into finer and finer ranks of perceived excellence. When I was researching how most people parse medical schools into tiers, I came across a source that said the top-tier was the top 10 research programs, schools ranked from 10-20 were mid-tier, and low-tier was everything else. By this person's standard, Vanderbilt is a mid-tier school. Now that's just bonkers! Before coming after me for sharing my tier list, go after this person first!

Before we move on, here is my school list and an explanation of why I applied to each school to guide your thinking as you craft your own list.

Medical School	Reason(s) for Applying
Baylor	top-tier
Brown	middle-tier; aunt is professor
Case Western	top-tier; regional
Chicago	top-tier; regional
Cincinnati	middle-tier; regional
Columbia	top-tier
Cornell	top-tier
Duke	top-tier
Dartmouth	middle-tier
George Washington	middle-tier
Harvard	top-tier; research fellowship; o-chem course
Johns Hopkins	top-tier
Loyola – Chicago	lower-tier; regional
Mayo	top-tier; regional
Michigan	top-tier; regional
Mount Sinai	top-tier
North Carolina	top-tier
NYU	top-tier

Northwestern	top-tier; regional
OHSU	middle-tier; in-state school
Penn	top-tier
Pittsburgh (Pitt)	top-tier
Southern Cal	mid-tier
St Louis U (SLU)	lower-tier; regional
Stanford	top-tier
Tuffs	middle-tier
UCLA	top-tier
UCSD	top-tier
UCSF	top-tier
Vanderbilt	top-tier
Virginia	middle-tier; regional
Wake Forest	middle-tier
WashU	top-tier; undergraduate school; research
Yale	top-tier

Q: What changes to my list would I make if I were to apply again?
A: I would swap out the University of Cincinnati College of Medicine for the University of Missouri School of Medicine. That way, I would apply to a state school where I attended college (Missouri) versus a state school where I have no connection besides geographic region (Ohio). Besides that, I would keep everything the same! Considering my scores, essays, experiences, and recommendation letters, it felt like I had a good range of schools. Whatever you end up deciding for your own list, be sure to run it past your advisor for some feedback. And no matter what anyone tells you, apply to those dream schools!

CHAPTER 11

EARLY DECISION

E*arly decision is weird waters.* Weird waters is a term coined by one of my friend's flings who texted her post-fling, "I don't know if I can see you again. Everything with my ex is kind of weird waters. You know?" No. I don't know, Todd.

This sterling young man was never heard from again.

In its own way, early decision is weird waters. General advice about early decision for medical school: don't do it! I will explain. The early decision for medical school is very unlike the early decision for college. For college admissions, early decision does not limit the number of schools you can apply to in the regular decision pool and does not affect when you can apply to those institutions. For medical school admissions, applying early to one school means you *cannot* apply to any other programs until you hear back from your early decision program (EDP) by October 1st (AAMC, Early Decision Program). You must accept your place if offered admission (AAMC, Early Decision Program), which cripples any power you have in negotiating scholarships and financial aid. Let's just be frank. If you are not given a spot in the incoming class through EDP, your odds of being interviewed and admitted at another medical school through the regular admissions cycle are severely limited (The Princeton Review, Should You Apply Early Decision to Medical School?). October is extremely late to submit primary and secondary applications. Even if you hear back from EDP in September, you are still super late in the cycle (*U.S. News*, What Late Medical School Applicants Need to Know). Stacks of thousands of other applications likely loom before readers at the admissions offices, with your profile near the bottom of the pile. By the time medical schools reach candidates' applications that were submitted in September and October, few interview slots, if any, are left, meaning that you have to be a top candidate to get one of those coveted spots (Shemmassian Academic Consulting, Applying Early Decision to Medical School: The Ultimate Guide). Save yourself from the bloodbath and the likelihood of becoming a reapplicant and just apply for the regular decision like everyone else. Do not get seduced by the increase in the percentage of people accepted through early decisions compared to regular decisions. The candidates admitted are superbly high quality and have strong reasons for applying via EDP. Those who aren't admitted are essentially screwed for the cycle.

Who are these minxes getting in through early decision? There are exceptions where an applicant should consider EDP, but these exceptions are specific and rare. Let's discuss while you think about if any of these exceptions apply to you. Exception one is if you have an extremely sick family member or another critical reason why you cannot leave a specific geographic region. In these cases, focusing on the program closest to you makes sense. To be clear, these crucial circumstances do not include people who want to stay close to their partner or spouse. Students are dragged around the country for medical school and residency. This is a sacrifice we all make for our careers. Trying to control that is risky business. Ultimately, you and your honey need to either be committed to moving wherever medicine takes you or feel comfortable with long-distance travel. Homesickness is also not a reason to apply for EDP. I love my family bunches, and attending school on the other side of the country (I'm in Connecticut, and they are in Oregon) is the biggest bummer of YSM. Still, I suck it up and Zoom with my mom, dad, and sister. Learn to do the same – I know it's tough, but once you're a doctor, you can literally live wherever you want in the U.S., and you will have a high-paying, extraordinarily stable job. Your time away from loved ones is temporary. The second reason to apply to EDP is if you have remarkably close ties to a medical school. For example, if you have worked at the medical school during your gap years and are well-acquainted with the admissions committee, applying to EDP is much more likely to work in your favor. If your immediate family member or very close mentor is on the admissions board and you are heavily involved with the medical school, EDP could work out well for you. None of these circumstances, however, are guarantees of admission. Tread carefully.

No matter your personal affairs, before you apply for EDP, several things must be done to protect yourself, your time, and your money as you apply during this risky process. First, ensure that the school where you want to apply to EDP is somewhere you want to go. If you are admitted, you are locked in. Second, research the requirements for applying early to the program and make sure that you satisfy every requirement. Third, speak with an advisor or trusted mentor about the circumstances leading you to apply early to ensure that no alternative options would allow you to apply during the regular cycle. The regular cycle carries much less risk than the early cycle. Fourth, if you need financial aid, make sure that applying early will still allow you to be considered for aid and scholarships. Fifth, you absolutely must reach out to the admissions team at the medical school and discuss whether you should apply early. A conversation with the admissions team is required before applying to a number of medical schools that participate in EDP. Admissions officers understand what a blow it is not to be accepted early. Hence, the admissions committee wants to be sure that they are not wasting your potential success during the regular cycle. When speaking with admissions officers at the school, ask if you are competitive and what you can do to improve your application. The program should give you clear, honest answers to those questions. If they are skirting around their answers, you may want to speak with someone else at the school or consider applying elsewhere. I know that it sounds weird waters to reach out to an admissions team and ask about the competitiveness of your candidacy for early admission, but you must ask. These inquiries are the norm among applicants applying early. You may also want to schedule a phone call or Zoom meeting with one of the admissions committee members to introduce yourself more formally and put a face to your name.

If you are applying early, I wish you the best of luck! People do get accepted through EDP every year. Think through the decision, take the steps outlined above, and hopefully, all will go in your favor. For a few months, I was kicking myself for not applying to Yale through EDP, but once I reflected on it, I'm not certain that I would have even been accepted early even though I got in through the regular cycle. I would hope that the result would have been the same, but I had no connections to YSM to warrant applying early, and maybe my interviews would have been a flop. Who knows! Regular decision may work out. Good luck to you and any EDP endeavors!

CHAPTER 12

ESSAYS

HOW IMPORTANT ARE MY ESSAYS?

Next to personal overarching narrative, essays are the most overlooked and underappreciated yet vital component of the best medical school applications. Essays are misunderstood by most applicants, which is why so many people write mediocre statements. Because most applicants don't use their writing to give their application a sharp advantage over others, crafting strong written work is an efficient strategy to make yourself truly stand out among the competition. I am convinced that my personal statement and secondary essays landed me such a large number of interviews, especially those with top medical schools - including two California state schools (UCLA and UCSD) as an OOS applicant.

Because I was confident in my writing ability, I knew I could describe myself, my ambitions, and my experiences through essays, unlike all other applicants. The dirty secret is that I was not always a good writer. From this guidebook, you're probably thinking: "Umm... sorry to break it to you sweet cheeks, but you're no writing savant." And you would be correct. My writing for my medical school essays was some of my better work. This book is a casual conversation. But seriously, throughout middle school and high school, I earned one A on one essay over six years of English classes. *One A*. And I think it was an A-. My writing throughout middle and high school was no good. Once I got to college, I invested in improving my writing to get the best grades in my classes. The work paid off. I earned high marks on essays, allowing my confidence to grow. You, too, can produce introspective, gripping statements for admissions committees to read. It takes time, but the work will be worth it.

Your essays are very important. Do not underestimate them. From everything I have seen from my own application cycle and the application cycles of my classmates, essays can separate those who land interviews and those who do not (Medical School Headquarters: Why is the Med School Personal Statement So Important?). Admissions officers want to talk to people who interest them. When pouring over thousands of generic, bland statements about why someone's curiosity in some scientific topic sparked their undying love for medicine or how grandma's cancer drove them toward becoming a physician, essays that break the mold are sweet relief. Readers love stumbling across the rare, fresh, and honest piece of writing that allows them to see into the author. To be fair, you can talk about generic topics but still write an outstanding essay. I myself wrote about my grandfather's dementia, which is an extraordinarily common topic. **What made my writing stand out was how I told the story.**

You may be wondering how I know that I wrote tremendous essays. Why should you trust that my writing was any good? Here is the evidence that I can cite. Numerous mentors and one of my advisors told me that my essays were top-notch. Several of my interviewers at top medical schools told me my personal statement was the best that they had read. One interviewer said that she knew I would become a writer in addition to a doctor (does this guidebook count?). Another person said that medical school essays are broken down into the following categories: 10% are horrible, 80% are boring, and 10% are superb. You know where this person put your girl in that ranking!

No one is born a great writer. Indeed, some are naturally gifted in articulating their thoughts. Yet, writing is a skill that can be grown and developed. If you take time with your primary and secondary applications, there is no reason why you cannot end up in the 10% superb essay category. The secret to the superb essays is that few people put in the work to earn such merit. Through the next couple of sections, we will go into when and how to write your essays to maximize the chances of impressing your readers.

WHEN TO WRITE

One word: pre-writing. Pre-writing essays is the name of the game. When should you write your primary and secondary applications? The answer is simple: *before* you receive the applications. Don't you dare wait to have the primary and secondary essays pile up in your inbox before you start writing. Frankly, I don't think that your essays should be partially done when you receive your primary and secondary applications. They should be done, done! Like copy, paste, and submit kind of done! There may be some adjustments needed for character count, and occasionally a medical school will change a question prompt, but overall, you better be gucci for that smoochie.

The personal statement is the centerpiece of your application. The prompt does not change from year to year, meaning that you have every opportunity to produce outstanding work. Simple and open-ended: "Use the space provided to explain why you want to go to medical school." Fifty-three hundred characters (Kaplan, Medical School Personal Statement FAQs).

While the AMCAS primary application opens during the first week of May and is not able to be submitted until a month later, you should not try to write your personal statement in those four weeks. Your personal statement should be polished, within the character count, and ready to submit before the primary application opens in May. Start writing your personal statement by January of the year when you apply at the latest. Honestly, you should be thinking about your personal comments throughout college and any gap year(s), as the prompt is simple and unchanging. Even if a wave of inspiration hits you sophomore year, or perhaps you are sick of studying for an exam and want to write creatively, take a shot at a draft of your personal statement.

It was in WashU's Law Library during the summer following my junior year that inspiration washed over me. I was quietly reading the Kaplan MCAT books when the first few lines of my personal comments popped into my head. I went with it and kept writing. Soon, what would end up as the first half of my personal statement was laid out on the page before me. I didn't wake up that summer morning thinking that I would work on my application, which I was two years away from submitting. At that point, I hadn't even read the personal statement prompt. What I did know and was finally able to articulate was why I wanted to become a physician.

About one year later, when I met with my mentor, I wrote the second half of my personal statement. Meetings with my incredible mentor, Patti, always inspired me to work my booty off to get into medical school. After showing Patti the first half of my personal comments, she said that she loved what I had written but needed to finish what I had started. Coming home from our meeting, I set out to do just that. Planted at my desk, I fueled myself on Patti's encouraging and warm energy to complete my personal statement. This was about a year before I applied to medical school. From there, Patti and I made minimal word choice and paragraph order changes.

Next, I handed off my personal statement to my bench mentor and good friend, Zosia, to review. They both gave great insights. My bench mentor, Phat, pointed out where I had used a complex research term in a setting meant to be understood by any reader. Zosia explained that the paragraph where I specified what I wanted to do as a physician read more like an MD-Ph.D.'s aspirations than an M.D.'s ambitions. She was right. I reworded a few of my sentences. Both Phat's and Zosia's edits made a huge difference in how my comments came across. I am going into the details of my writing and editing timeline to show that it can take some time to write and then perfect such a critical piece of writing. You do not, by any means, have to carve out two years pre-submission to begin writing your personal statement. My early writing start date happened unexpectedly. Please give yourself several months to really think about why you want to become a physician and how you want to communicate your past experiences and future goals in your writing. Your comments will then need to be reviewed by others and edited, so leave time for that as well. I want you to be as confident about the cornerstone of your application as I was. Give yourself the time to craft something that you're proud of. When receiving feedback, be gracious in accepting input, but don't be shy about deciding not to implement these suggestions. Confidence in your narrative and preserving your voice should be the lens through which you make edits to your writing.

While writing your personal statement, begin to work on the activities section of the primary application. Like the personal statement, the activities section does not change from year to year. A maximum of 15 activities can be entered, and three of these can be designated as most meaningful (AAMC, Section 5 of the AMCAS Application: Work and Activities). <u>The AAMC categorizes activities as the following</u>: Artistic Endeavors; Community Service/Volunteer - Medical/Clinical; Community Service/Volunteer - Not Medical/Clinical; Conferences Attended; Extracurricular Activities; Hobbies; Honors/Awards/Recognitions; Intercollegiate Athletics; Leadership - Not Listed Elsewhere; Military Service; Other; Paid Employment - Medical/Clinical; Paid Employment - Not Medical/Clinical; Physician Shadowing/Clinical Observation; Presentations/Posters; Publications; Research/Lab; and Teaching/Tutoring/Teaching Assistant (Shemmassian Academic Consulting, 2021 AMCAS Work and Activities Ultimate Guide [Examples Included]).

Seven hundred characters (including spaces) are given to describe each activity. The three activities designated as 'most meaningful' are given an additional 1,325 characters (including spaces) of writing space (Shemmassian). While the short character count may make it seem like the activities section of the primary application can be knocked out quickly, do not be deceived. It is difficult to write comprehensively and clearly about experiences that you have been involved in over months and years. There is so much information to compact into a few sentences. Don't take my word for the difficulty of compact writing. In the words of Mark Twain, addressing a friend, "If I had more time, I would have written a shorter letter." The best writers know better than anyone that brevity is the raging battle of penned expression. To be brief, yet complete - that is the challenge.

It will take time to decide what activities to include within the 15 allotted by the primary application. Some people will struggle to contort their many experiences into 15 distinct points of involvement. Others will not use all 15 slots. No matter where you are on that continuum, organizing your activities, writing about them, and editing takes at least several weeks.

Secondary applications are a beast. Typically, there are two to four secondary essays for each school where you apply. Some places like Duke will hit you with ten secondary questions to test if you want them. Then, after pouring out your heart and soul and contracting a mild case of carpal tunnel, the Duke adcoms will leave you on read. Not that I'm speaking from personal experience or anything... Not that I'm still salty...

Like the primary application, secondary essays need to be prewritten. These very often do not change from year to year. Shemmassian Academic Consulting keeps a record of each year's secondary prompts, which can be found under their post titled "Medical School Secondary Essay Prompts." Take advantage of this resource to prewrite your secondaries. Each year, there are thousands of students exhaustively writing their responses once the floodgates of secondary applications are opened. And it is a *floodgate* that opens. Schools largely send supplemental essays at the same time since most programs do not have cutoffs for receiving a supplemental application. Personally, I believe that programs should follow Vanderbilt's lead and make cuts before the supplemental applications, but that is a discussion for another time.

Let's do some quick math. Say you apply to 20 medical schools, which have three secondary essays on average. Three times 20 equals 60 essay responses in total. Keep your panties on, math majors - I know that was impressive. SIXTY ESSAYS! That is a lot, mama! You are asking for a world of hurt if you try to write 60 high-quality essays in a matter of weeks. Note that it is critical to submit supplemental applications as soon as possible. There are two reasons necessitating early submission. One: Often, there is a clock on secondary applications - they need to be submitted within ~two weeks of receipt. Two: The quicker your turnaround of supplementals, the faster the admissions officers can decide whether to invite you for an interview. Since interview slots are plentiful at the beginning of the cycle and wane thereafter, being evaluated for an interview earlier rather than later increases the odds of being invited to speak with the program, thus advancing in the selection process.

Here's some good news. The supplemental essays for each medical school heavily overlap. This means that you do not have to write sixty unique essays for 20 medical schools. You will likely write five or six core essays that will be submitted to most schools with minor tweaks. Then, there will be some oddball questions that will require deviation from the core essays. The standard questions asked by most schools are 1) How will you contribute to the diversity of the class?, 2) If you took a gap year, what did you do?, 3) What is a challenge that you overcame, and what did you learn about yourself in surmounting this obstacle?, 4) Why do you want to attend this school?, 5) Write an autobiography, and 6) Is there anything else that you would like to share with us?

I recommend not skipping the "Is there anything else that you would like to share with us?" prompt - write a short response that gives the committee a little more insight into who you are. I will share my answer to this prompt, as well as other secondary questions, below.

Lastly, when it comes to supplemental applications, don't get sloppy. Too many students think, "I wrote a great personal statement. No need to go all out for my secondaries." This line of thinking is a fatal flaw. Personally, I believe that admissions officers use supplemental essays to tease out who is genuinely interested in their program versus who is uninterested. Investing your time to produce intentional, engaging responses to secondary essays may be what allows you to be selected for an interview over other applicants. One of the reasons that I believe that I earned 19 interview invites was because my supplemental responses were strong. Many of my interviewers shared that they enjoyed my diversity essay - what I think was a standout of my application. Avoiding sloppiness, again, underscores the importance of prewriting. Beginning to write secondaries right after submitting your primary application should give you sufficient time to draft and then polish all supplemental applications. If you are a slower writer, then consider beginning secondary essays before the primary is submitted. The goal is to submit your secondaries within hours of receiving the supplemental application invitation. One exception to the lightning-fast turnaround: if there is a new prompt, take time to perfect a new essay and submit your responses within a few days of receiving the secondary invite rather than speeding through the new question.

It is rumored that some schools look at secondary turnaround time as a metric for the enthusiasm and engagement of an applicant. Generally, I don't believe medical schools would have the capacity to consider secondary turnaround as a factor even if they wanted to. They are swamped with information to consider for each applicant. The only place where secondary turnaround time might come into consideration is if you submit the supplemental application after a given deadline. For example, if a school asks you to turn in your secondary within 14 days, and then they don't receive your response on day 21, it is reasonable that your passion for the program would be called into question. If chaos happens that prevents you from turning your application in within the deadline, I would note that with either an email to the school or a few sentences before jumping into the meat of your secondary response.

Below, I am sharing ~exclusive~ Caroline content. Here are my primary application essay, three activities section responses, in addition to four of my secondary essays. Feast my munchkins!

Primary essay:

We have the same eyebrows. Bushy, black. Mine are lightly tweezed, hinting at my obedience to modern beauty rituals. Their shape, however, I have faithfully preserved. You gaze off to a cage of chirping birds in a distant corner, and I steal another glance in your direction. There they are: my eyebrows stitched onto your face, your eyebrows stamped onto mine.

These defining rows of thick, dark hair tie us together – back to the torrid village in Puerto Rico where you are from and where I have never been. These eyebrows brand us with Caribbean origin, a constant reminder of our kinship. But you don't notice that.

Your warm eyes flash over to me and grab hold of my presence. A smile broadens across your face, chiming with politeness yet void of recognition.

You were robbed of me. You were robbed of my mother, her three sisters, and her one brother. We were robbed of you.

Did you know you were losing us as dementia steadily overtook you? Our faces, our voices sinking into the thick, hazy curtain that now stifles your memory from the clarity of the present.

Years ago, you and I sat twenty feet from where we sit now. We faced each other seated in soft, cushioned armchairs. I fought against gravity for an erect posture. Gravity won.

Slouched in comfort, I told you about my life. I had started work at an Alzheimer's research laboratory. In your honor, I had chosen to study the disease that was suffocating our family in fear and anguish. I was going to disarm it of biological mystery. Pinpoint the cascade of molecular nuances that led to neurodegeneration and, ultimately, to your functional decline. Once exposed, I would strike back. Gluttonously assemble a brigade of researchers to contrive a drug that will prevent the onset of this disease or halt its effects, perhaps both.

A rough hand claps down on mine, yanking me back to the present. "Hi," you hesitate, your brow furrowing in bewilderment. "Who are you?" And I want to tell you everything.

I want to tell you about my twelve-hour days spent hunched over ELISA plates. How my mentor's eyes roll as I make cooing sounds to each new mouse born into our colony. I want to share my mentor's and my discovery with you: We reduced amyloid plaque levels – the same culprit devastating your brain – using a novel designer drug.

I want to tell you about my time spent with the residents of the memory care units at Touchmark and Stonecrest. Meg solves any and all math equations. Stooped over, shoveling soil into planter boxes, Russell taught me that the primrose thrives in the shade. Celeste recalled that peaches are the state fruit of Georgia. It took five minutes while her daughter and I dropped clues, but then she remembered. Kurt gets nervous when his wife, Deborah, forgets to call. We distract him with board games until she arrives. Each is remarkable, but the disease has forever disrupted their lives, and their memories are fading.

I want to tell you I didn't give up on treating dementia. I want to tell you I never will.

While Alzheimer's strips one's reality of coherence, it has brought my career sharply into focus. I am pursuing a career as a physician that will allow me to treat geriatric patients, all while continuing to stretch our understanding of Alzheimer's so that I may help unravel dementia's enigma.

Like that of many others who came before me, my ambition is to move arm-in-arm with older adults as we, together, face age-related illness and injury. I know the loneliness that too often accompanies neurodegenerative disease. I know the overwhelming questions that older adults and their caregivers confront as they navigate eldercare. Using biostatistics research to allow persons living with dementia and their caregivers to make informed and individualized choices surrounding eldercare is where my vocation lies. I choose to dedicate my life to Caring for the spirits and the bodies of older adults, always reminding them that they are not alone in facing illness and injury.

Alzheimer's is extraordinary in how it devastates. I am taken back to one of our visits and my sudden realization that you and I are not unalike. We, both, have had our lives torn into disparate worlds. Yours is a fading past, a confused present, and an unrealized future. Mine is years of knowing you and loving you, and now speaking to a man whose mind dementia has molded into a hardly recognized form. And here we both stand – overwhelmed by the chasm between then and now. The familiar now made foreign.

Dementia tears. It tore you from us and us from you. It fragmented our worlds into two: You and I, once family; you and I, now strangers. Our lives exist in pieces – marred by the devastation brought by disease. We seek solace in the ephemeral cosmos of memories. Yet, memories are stagnant by design. Together, we will never again move forward.

Because, to you, my eyebrows are just that – dusky and fuzzy and trivial, not warranting hesitation, much less a second thought. To me, they are all I think about when I see you – the man who lived an extraordinary life.

I remember the look on your face when you knew me, and I knew you, and you understood what I had chosen as my life's work. I remember you were proud.

I finally respond, "I'm Caroline. I'm your granddaughter."

Activities response 1:

As a volunteer in the memory care units of Stonecrest and Touchmark, I engage with residents living with memory disorders in order to promote life enrichment and wellness. Life enrichment activities often include exercise, self-care, current events, gardening, and brain games. While I could not visit with residents during the coronavirus outbreak, I made and delivered over 600 masks to Touchmark to help protect one of our most vulnerable populations from viral exposure. I look forward to continuing in-person visits once it is safe to do so! Overall, interacting with individuals living with dementia and other neurodegenerative diseases has been paramount to bringing my work as an Alzheimer's researcher full circle. As an aspiring geriatrician, I aim not only to treat the symptoms of disease but also to continually connect my work as a clinician and researcher to the community in need of care. Above all, the moments I have shared with my adopted grandparents have enriched my life beyond measure, as I have found kindred souls abundant in warmth, vitality, and spirit.

Activities response 2:

During my sophomore year of college, I began work investigating Alzheimer's disease (AD) at Washington University School of Medicine under Dr. David Holtzman's mentorship—the neurology department's chairman. As a research assistant during my undergraduate summers and during my sophomore, junior, and senior academic years, I focused on studying the relationship between the apolipoprotein E gene (the greatest genetic risk factor for late-onset AD) and amyloid-beta – one of the foremost biological hallmarks of AD. During the summer prior to my junior year, I was awarded Washington University's Biology Summer Undergraduate Research Fellowship to fund my research. Following graduation, I rejoined the Holtzman lab as a research technician, where I worked full-time in the lab investigating the relationship between the apolipoprotein E gene and microgliosis and neuritic dystrophy as well as the effects of tau – the other foremost biological hallmark of AD – on cellular senescence. My time with the Holtzman lab not only allowed me to contribute to furthering our knowledge of a devastating and widespread progressive neurodegenerative disorder but also formalized my desire to incorporate research into my career as a physician.

Activities response 3:

I was the teaching assistant (TA) for two courses at Washington University in St. Louis. As the laboratory TA for Principles of Biology II, I assisted students in their laboratory experiments, held weekly office hours to address student questions, proctored weekly quizzes, and graded weekly quizzes and laboratory reports. As the TA for Introduction to Biochemistry, I assisted students with their problem sets at weekly help sessions, held exam review sessions, proofread problem sets, quizzes and exams, proctored exams, and graded quizzes and exams. My most rewarding role as a TA was forming strong bonds with students by supporting them in achieving academic success.

Secondary essay - diversity:

It walked the line between tangible and intangible. Something in her eyes had changed. My religion. It didn't fit into her world, and suddenly, no longer did I.

She had carved a line splitting people into two. Within moments, I fell into the abyss where she cast me and all those like me as we stood silenced, condemned by the rejection.

My firsthand experience of religious discrimination has forever altered how I see the world and how I behave. I know now what it is to be seen in fragments. To be disassembled and then sifted through grates until only pieces of myself remain. It seemed that the entirety of my personhood hinged on the God I worship. But, above all, how does this experience relate to my potential as a physician?

I know that the time I spend with my patients, however critical, will be relatively brief. The sum of moments in their lives that led up to the time we now share is unknown to me.

Strangers are seen in pieces: color, gender, appearance, and polite introductions. Yet, physicians see even further: drug tests, alcohol levels, and sexual histories. The private lives of those whom I may hardly know will lie quietly in a tidy printed chart in my lap. Patients are a particularly vulnerable type of stranger. They sit defenseless to a cheerless fault of our human condition: unconscious judgment. Unconscious judgment is automatic and misguided and affects how we view and treat one another.

As a physician, unconscious judgment would alter my patient interactions, corrode the trust that is foundational to our relationship, and ultimately undermine the care that I am able to give.

There was grief through my experience with discrimination, but I also found tremendous gratitude. I was taught the significance of seeing people for their sum and not their parts. I was taught the gravity of bigotry. I was made more conscious of my own potential to unconsciously judge others. Because of my personal encounter with discrimination, I believe that I will be a better physician and a better caretaker of my patients, to whom I pledge never to become lost in the minutiae but rather to steadfastly honor each person as a whole.

Secondary essay - overcoming challenges:

Two years ago, I was notorious for failed public speaking performances. Words stumbled out of my mouth, shaking rocked my voice, flashes of heat marked my cheeks red, and at times, tears threatened to flood my eyes. I would, without fail, stand close to the nearest door in case panic drove me to flee. My embarrassment became my audience's as my symptoms of dread were uncontained. Inherited discomfort would settle upon the crowd.

The trembling and shaking, however, did not reflect my feelings toward my coursework or research. I desperately wanted to share my findings with peers, colleagues, and faculty. Presentations were, to me, a celebration of intellectual discovery. A well-articulated, enthusiastic delivery had the power to insight into conversation and discussion among the audience and introduce novel discoveries or insight to a field with excitement.

It wasn't until the spring of my junior year that I thought public speaking would be my lifelong handicap and limit my ability to present my research as a student and one day as a physician. That spring, I was given an opportunity to deliver the opening address at my university's undergraduate research symposium and share my mentor's and my research, which had recently been published in Neuron, with an audience of classmates and instructors. I was incredibly proud of our work and yearned to confidently and passionately communicate our findings. I knew that if I allowed fear to rob me of this uncommon opportunity, I would be filled with unshakable regret.

Leading up to the symposium, my professor helped me master fear management techniques, and both my mentor and the symposium director critiqued my presentation. I received loving support from my family and friends as I grappled with angst and doubts in overcoming my phobia.

The credit for my achievement lies with guidance and unflappable encouragement from each of these individuals. With all acclaim belonging to those who supported me, I delivered my address with enthusiasm and clarity, free of stuttering speech and quaking hands. Beyond the symposium address, independence from my phobia allowed me to, for the first time, actively pursue other public speaking opportunities. Notably, I have since been able to present my mentor and my work at five national research conferences. I cannot express enough gratitude to the people who helped me overcome my fear and taught me how to speak effectively.

My mother was not educated beyond high school and worked simultaneously as both a maid and waitress before launching her own company and eventually helping thousands of people find employment. She taught me never to let my circumstances define my outcome. She would tell me that although I was not in control of the result, I was in complete control of my own effort. My mother anchored my upbringing in these values – it is through such values that my mother transcended her circumstances, and I dared greatly to break my silence.

Secondary essay - gap year:

Pink is my favorite color. Eighteen years ago, this was considered a critical piece of personal information. Today, not so much. If favorite colors informed one's medical specialty, pink would possibly suggest my future in gynecology and obstetrics or perhaps neonatology. Surgeons would be clad in red. And the unfortunate gastroenterologist would strut sporting hues of brown. Luckily for us, no such connection exists. Otherwise, my rose sweaters and blush blouses would be replaced with the notorious groutfit (gray + outfit). Why? Because I am passionate about serving our aging population.

When graduating from Washington University in St. Louis in May 2019, I was determined to immerse myself in gerontology prior to matriculating to medical school. The U.S. is undergoing a marked demographic shift in the age of our population. By 2030, one in five Americans will be aged 65 years and older (AARP). By 2034, older adults will outnumber children (US Census). These changes mark a turning point for our country, and with it comes new challenges we will face in healthcare.

I began exploring these challenges through the lens of disease. As a sophomore, I started researching Alzheimer's disease (AD) – the third leading cause of death among older adults (NIH) – under the mentorship of Dr. David Holtzman, chairman of the neurology department at Washington University School of Medicine. This research continued into my gap year as I completed several projects investigating the relationship between tau (one of the foremost biological hallmarks of AD) and cellular senescence. During my gap year, I was selected to present our findings at five national research conferences. To me, advancing our understanding of dementia through basic science is critical, as the necessity for breakthroughs in treating and preventing dementia will continue to grow as more individuals live to confront the age-related disease.

To connect my research to the community most impacted by the disease, I began engaging with residents of memory care units as an undergraduate and have continued this work during my gap year. Currently, my primary roles revolve around promoting life enrichment and wellness by involving residents in physical exercise and self-care.

My time spent with the residents of memory care units illuminated the problems faced by both older adults and their caregivers – namely, the lack of resources and guidance to aid in decision-making regarding eldercare. In response, this year, I co-founded CaregiverZone, an online service that uses biostatistics research to provide data-driven resources grounded in helping older adults and their caregivers make confident, informed, and personalized choices surrounding eldercare (caregiverzone.com).

As a novice biostatistician, I was thrilled to be awarded a research fellowship at the Harvard T.H. Chan School of Public Health for Summer 2020. The biostatistics courses that I am taking, as well as the research project that I am competing alongside Chan School graduate students and faculty, will bolster my abilities to impact eldercare via biostatistics research – work I *would be enthusiastic to continue as an NYU medical student and one day as a physician-researcher.*

Pursuing a joint M.D. and M.S. in Translational Research at NYU School of Medicine would be an empowering next step toward my career as a geriatrician. Working with faculty whose research helps individuals make informed choices regarding care will allow me to learn from experts how I can accomplish the same objective with regard to eldercare. Moreover, the training offered by the Medical Students in Aging Research (MSTAR) program would anchor my research in the direct needs of the geriatric population. Learning patient-centered care through NYU's Geriatric Medicine Elective will provide me and my peers with a strong background in the numerous and diverse systems of eldercare: palliative care, outpatient geriatric clinics, assisted living and care facilities, and in-home care. By engaging with fellow students as we prepare for a vocation grounded in service, we will, together, realize our common devotion to providing exceptional patient care and advancing healthcare for many future generations.

Secondary essay - anything else:

I treasure the letters I have received from students I have mentored as a peer mentor, orientation counselor, and teaching assistant. To me, providing academic and emotional support and career guidance can have a tremendous impact on the lives of others. I have been remarkably fortunate to have been supported by my own caring mentors as I pursue a career in medicine and research, and I cherish the relationships I share with my own students.

As a medical school student, I would work to support my fellow students as they prepare to become physicians, researchers, and innovators in healthcare. I believe that by working together, communities are only made stronger. In this spirit, I would especially strive to guide and support fellow Hispanic students who, like myself, are the first in their families to pursue medicine and research. This work I would continue throughout my student tenure and maintain as a Tufts Medical School alumna.

HOW TO WRITE

It is challenging to tell someone how to write. It is more difficult to competently share how to write *well*. Each person has their own style of writing. I am by no means a writing expert, yet when I put my mind toward producing a thoughtful, provoking essay, many times, these efforts seem successful. I was not one of those kids who buried herself in books. In fact, it's been one of my ambitions to become a better reader because there are so many important literary works to read that provide insight into world history, economic and political philosophy, our shared human experience, and religion. The kids who grow up as reading friends tend to be great writers. So when asked, "how do I learn to write well?" one step forward is learning through reading great writers. Ayn Rand, Fyodor Dostoevsky, Louisa May Alcott, Friedrich Nietzsche, Mary Shelley. You will learn to write better from reading the greats.

Now, let's say that you're a college student or a working professional with limited time to read (which you probably are). Or maybe you have a month before you begin writing medical school essays and don't have time to basque in the Great American Novel. Fair enough. This was me, too. When writing the personal statement -the cornerstone of one's application - I would refrain from reading other people's personal statements before writing your own. Why is this? Didn't you just tell me to read great writers? Why not read the personal statements of successful applicants?

To answer these questions, from my experience, many personal statements - even the best ones - follow a cookie-cutter style of writing. The storytelling seems to be more academic. These essays may be well-written and stirring, but many follow a similar pattern of writing. I won't attempt to fully dissect what this pattern is, but if you eventually read a handful of personal statements, you will pick up on what I mean.

I wrote my personal statement without ever reading another person's medical school essay. Because of this, my writing was not affected by expectations of what I was "supposed to write" or "supposed to sound like." This hits upon the other big risk of reading other people's essays before writing: it is easy to become too focused on sounding like Colby, who got into Harvard Medical School, instead of just telling your story. The personal statement is where admissions committee members want you to reveal who you are.

It is supposed to be formal but not formulaic. Since I wrote my personal statement blind, I had no expectations of what I was supposed to write. My one job was to explain why I wanted to become a physician. I did just that, but in my own way. The style of my personal statement turned out quite different than most – this is what admissions officers seemed to love. My essay was highly praised throughout the admissions cycle by my interviewers and letter writers. The only person not so thrilled with my out-of-the-box writing was my premedical advisor at WashU, who worried that my style was too different and risky. My advisor encouraged me to re-write my essay and mold it to fit within the common formula. No way, José! The personal statement was an opportunity for my application to stand out from the hundreds of others it was sandwiched between. As my reader's eyes were drooping shut from reviewing the fiftieth bland description of my competitors' love of science and helping people, my essay would swoop in, and BAM, wake them up! Jolt your reader with your writing. Be appropriate. Be professional. But step out of the box with your writing and take a calculated risk or two.

To take risks with your writing, take your time. Don't rush the writing process, and don't force yourself to write when not in the creative headspace. If you're never in the creative headspace for writing, see what ideas strike you in the shower or bath. For some reason, many of my best essays strike me when in the tub. If the water doesn't work, then you may need to force yourself to do some brainstorming sessions.

Get feedback on your writing. You are going to want someone to review your personal statement before submitting it. This person should be well-credentialed in understanding what good writing looks like. They needn't be a professor or advisor. It is chiefly important to find someone who writes well, recognizes strong storytelling, can catch red flags in your essay, and will preserve your own voice. My premed advisor was clearly not this person for me. I received much more helpful feedback from my bench mentor, my close friend who was a current medical student at the time, and one of my dearest mentors and admissions consultants.

There's a saying that speaks to female beauty: "You don't have to be pretty like her. You can be pretty like you." I don't know who first said this, but I believe the same idea extends to writing. You don't have to write like Mark Twain to be a great writer. You can be an exceptional storyteller using your own voice. This same concept was shown in lines from Greta Gerwig's 2019 adaptation of *Little Women*. Jo turns to Friedrich, exclaiming, "I'm no Shakespeare." Friedrich responds, "Thank goodness, we already have him."

A final hint to share about strong writing: You've heard it before. *Show, don't tell*. The idea behind *show, don't tell*, is that our actions speak louder than our work. You may identify as a caring person, but what have you done to warrant this descriptor? When writing, it is much more effective to tell a story that shows your ability to think creatively, for example, rather than simply state, "I am a creative thinker! (Pick me for medical school!)." I will point to my own diversity essay (found at the end of the *When to Write* section above) as an example. In my diversity essay, I did not state that I would treat people who are different with respect and an open heart and then walk away. I described a painful personal experience of religious discrimination and then explained how this encounter changed how I thought about myself, other people, and the world around me. This was a *show, don't tell* moment.

Dr. Ryan Gray, founder of Medical School Headquarters, has a video series called "Application Renovation," where he works to improve the applications of students who will be reapplying to medical school. In nearly all "Application Renovation" segments, Dr. Gray shares with students that they need to show through storytelling why they will be good physicians rather than stating, "I am curious. I am a hard worker. I am passionate about caring for the sick and injured." One strategy effectively convinces admissions officers that you will be a great doctor. The other strategy is less convincing.

Best of luck to you, my angel, as you work to reveal the "self" through writing. Meditate, go to church, enjoy a hike, submerge yourself in a sensory deprivation tank. Do what you have to do to get in touch with your inner self. Then, let the inner self do your writing. Clearly, I am not an expert in instructing people how to write well. But I hope that some of what I have shared has been helpful.

CHAPTER 13

CASPER

For those who are unfamiliar with CASPer, ignorance is bliss, my friend. CASPer stands for Computer-based Assessment for Sampling Personal Characteristics (Shemmassian Academic Consulting, How to Prepare for the Casper Test to Get into Medical School). It is an online assessment lasting about 90 minutes that asks questions to evaluate ethics and behavior (Casper, About CASPer). The exam was first used among Canadian medical schools before reaching its greedy, toxic fingers into the wallets of medical school applicants in the United States. Can you tell that I'm not a fan of CASPer? To be clear, it isn't the fact that medical schools want to assess candidates based on ethics and behavior that bothers me. I know several sleaze balls in medicine, and it would've been great if there was some way to screen them out of becoming physicians. The issue with CASPer is that its effectiveness in screening out unethical candidates has not been thoroughly tested among medical school applicants since this tool has only recently become widely used. Medical schools don't even know if the tool works! And instead of telling CASPer to screw off and run studies to produce hard data regarding how the exam can select more ethical physicians, medical schools sold us out to be their guinea pigs. It gets better! You have the pleasure of PAYING to be a guinea pig. WTF?!?!?!?! It's incredulous to me that these medical schools claim to want to reduce the hoops that candidates need to climb through and then actively choose to throw new hoops in front of us. Bitch, please! All talk and no action. Consider this rant my official call for medical schools to stop allowing companies like the CASPer to enrich themselves on desperate and poor young students who have no choice but to take the exam or not be considered for a particular medical school. Do you know why applying to medical school is so expensive? Because there is no competition in the market. The AAMC, CASPer, and other organizations can simply charge whatever they want because we, as applicants, have nowhere else to turn if we want to become physicians. We are sitting ducks whom these executives choose as their prey to engorge themselves on. It sickens me.

My argument is not that applying to medical school should be free. I don't necessarily think that should be the case. However, allowing companies like CASPer to prey on us and allowing there to be no competition in the marketplace (a total monopoly by the AAMC, CASPer, etc.) has not served the premedical community well. These self-interested actors work with their own wallets at the forefront of their minds. For example, CASPer, during my application cycle

(2020-2021), raised the cost of their exam from $10 (*U.S. News*, What to Know About the CASPer Test for Med School) to $12 per school to send your result to (Shemmassian Academic Consulting, How to Prepare for the Casper Test to Get Into Medical School). Excuse me?! Why is this company charging to send an *electronic* score report to *each* medical school? It is because they are feasting on our sitting duck status. Why did they raise the price of the exam? Because they know that you either foot the bill or do not apply to the medical schools that have bought into this dirty scheme. Well, guess what, CASPer. I am coming for you. I may be a little medical student now, but mark my words: I am going to launch a blitzkrieg campaign to get your filthy hands out of the medical school admissions process. I have an army of tens of thousands of pissed-off students who will be eager to support this plan. To the medical school admissions directors who are using CASPer: stop. It's not as much about the money as it is about the principle of the thing. You say that you want to take hoops out of the process. Show us. Don't tell us. You say that you want more students from low-income backgrounds in medicine. Guess what? These standardized exams hinder those who cannot pay for them. The playing field has become more uneven because of CASPer. People pay for tutors and practice questions to raise their scores. The performance of students on this exam can be bought. CASPer is an artificial assessment of behavior and ethics because students' responses can be practiced and perfected. Can't you see this? I suppose that this is an open letter to all medical schools to tell CASPer to go to hell. Make them eat crow.

HOW IMPORTANT IS CASPER?

Okay! Now that my delightful outburst is over, let's discuss the importance of CASPer in the medical school admissions process. As I mentioned in the above tirade, the effects of the CASPer on accurately predicting performance in medical school and the ethics of incoming students seem not to have been shown. To do this, CASPer would need to perform a longitudinal study stretching years over a medical student's and then a doctor's career. So far as I know, no such studies have been conducted. The rumor as to why medical schools began using this unproven, shady measure is to test whether your score helps predict performance in medical school, particularly during clerkships.

Since medical schools have yet to determine the score's effectiveness, it is widely understood that your CASPer performance holds little sway over your ability to secure an interview and then be admitted to an M.D. program. Some people believe that a particularly low CASPer score could be a red flag for medical schools (maybe below the 25th percentile), but none of us know how each school views a poor CASPer performance. The cherry on top? There are no CASPer retakes within the same application cycle. What you earn is what you get. One exception to the no retake policy is if there is a technology malfunction. Another cherry? You do not get to see your CASPer results. I do not know how it is legal to have someone pay for a test - mandatory for certain programs - and then not release their score! How is it okay to have a literal black box in the application cycle? I never knew my CASPer score. I could've scored at the first percentile or the 100th percentile. I'll never know. How is this black box not extremely alarming to ethics boards who may note that a school can simply reject a candidate for any reason and then blame it on this mysterious score that the applicant has never seen? Are there even ethics committees overseeing the medical school application process? If such committees exist, are they bought and paid for, too? I can literally feel my blood pressure rising again, so I'll smoothly transition back to my point. Those bastards. ~Smooth transition.~

CASPer showed signs throughout 2020 that they are considering giving people information about their scores. Some candidates this past cycle were selected by CASPer to learn what quartile they scored within the $0 - 25^{th}$ percentile, $26^{th} - 50^{th}$ percentile, $51^{st} - 75^{th}$ percentile, or $76^{th} - 100^{th}$ percentile (Casper, FAQ: Quartiles. Maybe by the time you fall victim to this grimy conspiracy, CASPer will give applicants some knowledge about their scores. Any lawyers want to take on a class action lawsuit against CASPer? I'm all for testifying.

To wrap up, it is doubtful that CASPer has any notable effect on your admissions decision. Still, make sure to study up and do your best on the exam in order to protect yourself from any cuts that could be made to applicants who scored extremely poorly on the assessment. Uhhh! I hate CASPer and everything it stands for. Let's now talk about how to prepare for this dance with the devil.

HOW TO PREPARE

Back then, one could easily avoid applying to schools that opted to use CASPer. This maneuvering is becoming increasingly difficult each year as more medical programs dip their hairy toes into the cesspool that is the CASPer exam. My original plan was to cut the schools that decided to use CASPer. But once my state school (looking at you, OHSU) decided to hop on the bandwagon of corruption, I knew that I would have to suck it up and take the phony exam. It was too risky for me not to apply to my one and only state school. While I don't know and will likely never know my CASPer score (again, how is that legal?), I think that I did pretty well on CASPer. I don't have much hard evidence to back this claim, but here's what I've got. One – I did a LOT of practice for the CASPer and worked for my answers to closely match the recommended answers given by different consulting services, like BeMo Academic Consulting. Two – I applied to five schools (Baylor, Wake Forest, Case Western, OHSU, and UMich) that required CASPer, received interview invitations from four of those schools (Baylor, Case Western, OHSU, and UMich), and was admitted to two of the programs (Case Western and UMich). Baylor waitlisted me (oddly after I thought that I had withdrawn), and I successfully withdrew from OHSU before receiving an admissions decision.

Step one to doing well on CASPer is to apply for exam accommodations if you need them. Exam accommodations are important because CASPer is a timed exam. The minutes given to respond to a prompt go quickly. To apply for CASPer accommodations, a medical professional fills out part of your accommodations request form, and then you submit supporting documentation. The good thing is that since you likely already need a professional evaluation for the MCAT, the same professional can fill out the paperwork for CASPer.

Step two for acing CASPer is to do practice questions! People say that you can't prepare for CASPer. I disagree with them. People are correct in that you will not receive the same prompts you practiced for the actual exam, but your formula to answer the prompts should be finetuned even with different questions. Research CASPer answering strategies and practice questions to begin preparing for the exam. Overall, some consistent points to keep in mind for all CASPer prompts are to 1) remain non-judgmental at all times, 2) consider all parties affected by a situation (patient, physician, patient's co-workers, and family, reputation of hospital, reputation of physician, etc.),

3) acknowledge that there is missing information from the prompt and address the unknowns with if-then statements in your answer, and 4) discuss the pros and cons of each suggested response given by your if-then statements. These four markers are a good rule of thumb for responding to any prompt on CASPer.

Your research will find many practice questions and sample answers for the exam. Anywhere from one to three weeks of preparation time is needed before CASPer to nail down your response strategy. Complete a few sample questions each day (perhaps 25+ practice prompts total), and you will be ready for test day. I went a bit crazy with CASPer prep and typed out 30 pages of practice responses on a Word document before my exam. Yikes! I definitely could've done with less practice, but I was determined not to let the icky CASPer be my downfall in getting into medical school.

CHAPTER 14

INTERVIEWS

Now, let's move on to something positive and exciting: interviews! **Getting invited to a medical school interview is a big deal.** Congratulations if you have an upcoming interview! Anxiety is certain to come along with these huge opportunities, but be sure to celebrate your accomplishments.

We've discussed the average 6.3% acceptance rate to medical schools (Accepted) before. Well, here is the good news. Once you are invited to interview, your chances of acceptance skyrocket. Here is some data from 2019 to support this point (DataKing and Limeyguy, data pulled from *U.S. News and World Report*). In 2019, Emory School of Medicine had an acceptance rate of 3.99%. Pretty dismal, right? Yet, once you were invited to an interview, your acceptance rate became 46.6%. One in two odds of acceptance is a massive improvement from 4 in 100 or 1 in 25. Let's look at Georgetown School of Medicine. Pre-interview Georgetown's 2019 acceptance rate was 2.85%. Post-interview, this number rose to 36.4%. I could go through dozens of more examples, but you get the point. The citation listed for this information will take you to a chart that catalogs details of pre-interview and post-interview acceptance rates at all U.S. M.D. schools.

HOW IMPORTANT ARE INTERVIEWS?

One of the first questions that applicants find themselves asking after being invited to a medical school interview is, "How important is this interview in earning an acceptance?" In short, the interview is very important. However, the dimensions of *very* in "very important" can change depending on the applicant. To understand what I mean, let's first discuss why medical schools interview candidates.

Accomplishments, academic metrics, recommendation letters, and essays are all critical components of a medical school application that give admissions committees insight into what kind of doctor you will be. Accomplishments and academic metrics usually speak more to hard skills, while essays and recommendations focus on soft skills. While academic skills and grit are certainly important for physicians to possess, soft skills are equally important given that physicians deal in life and death matters for a living. Essays are an insight into soft skills. Yet, they are self-serving accounts of one's own empathy, compassion, etc. Recommendations also give a glimpse into someone's soft skills, but the applicant hand-selected these recommenders to give their perspectives to the committee. ***The interview is the sole chance for medical schools to independently evaluate a candidate's character***, communication abilities, motivations, and other personal characteristics. Only a small percentage of applicants are invited to interview. From there, the admissions committee must select the top students for a seat in the incoming class. The fact that medical schools invest notable resources into selecting who to interview, hosting selected candidates (usually on campus), recruiting an interview team, and evaluating interview results speaks to the importance that these conversations will have on an individual's chance of acceptance.

There is a component of the interview where candidates are screened for inappropriate, disengaged, and pompous behavior, among other undesirable characteristics. Few candidates are screened out for these types of character traits, but it's worth noting that applicants are evaluated on these dimensions. One of the more well-known examples of a competitive applicant reportedly having issues with their interview behavior is documented on the Student Doctor Network (SDN) website. During the 2019-2020 application cycle, a user of SDN with the handle u_raptor reported securing interview invitations to an inordinately large number of the nation's top medical schools. It was clear that u_raptor has an incredibly impressive written application. As final decisions began coming in, u_raptor was rejected or waitlisted from the vast majority of the programs where he interviewed. (I'm assuming u_raptor is a "he," but I could be wrong). This news shocked u_raptor, and I also believe many other candidates on the SDN forum. Some students who claimed to have met the real-life u_raptor on interview day did not have positive comments about his character. Personally, I believe that u_raptor was an extraordinarily compelling applicant who was screened out of many schools during his interview for poor interpersonal skills. Eventually, u_raptor reported that he was admitted off of the waitlist at Vanderbilt, which is apparently where he attends medical school today. Hopefully, he is not wreaking havoc on Vanderbilt's Class of 2024 and the people of Nashville!

Coming back to the various dimensions of *very* in the phrase "very important interview." What I mean by this is that the interview may be more important for some applicants than it is for others. Another famous SDN user with the handle *LizzyM* explains this idea using what she has termed the staircase analogy. LizzyM is reported to be an admissions officer at a top medical school and is given much credibility among the users of SDN. I'm going to insert her staircase analogy here, explained in her own words.

Question from SDN user Syialb: "Hi LizzyM, The answer to my question may vary from school to school, but here it is: Once you're at the interview stage, do med schools use just the interview to make their decision, or do they go back and look at the entire application, including GPA, MCAT, etc.? I've heard that once you get an interview, it's your acceptance to lose. But I can't help but think GPA/MCAT can still hold you back. Thanks in advance!"

Answer from LizzyM: "I've answered this before but here goes: It does vary by school. Imagine that people are standing on a huge staircase with those with the highest stats and the most remarkable experiences at the top stair and downward to the least among those interviewed. After the interview, the applicants can keep their place on their original stairs, go up a step or two or go down a step or many steps. In most cases, the people with the highest stats are still at the top, but some are sent to the bottom step, and some people move up or down according to their performance" (Student Doctor Network, Ask LizzyM (Almost) Anything 2012 edition.

To put LizzyM's staircase analogy into my own words, she says that before the interview, some applicants are closer to acceptance than others based on scores, experiences, and other factors. The best applicants are at the top of the staircase, with the door to an acceptance opening to those who are on a high enough step to move through the door. As the staircase descends, interviewed applicants are less competitive as deemed by the admissions committee. People interviewing at the top of the staircase have to perform well, but not as well as someone standing on a lower step to reach the threshold for moving through the acceptance door. Those with particularly poor interview performances can fall down so many stairs post-interview that they lose a chance at acceptance. I believe that this is what happened to u_raptor. Someone standing toward the bottom of the staircase will have to perform much better than someone at the middle or top to ascend across the threshold for acceptance. To me, LizzyM's analogy is quite useful for understanding the relationship between interviews and acceptance. That being said, I don't think the analogy would fit the admissions procedures for every medical school. But for the most part, the imagery is useful to keep in mind.

WHAT TO EXPECT FROM INTERVIEW DAY

Before jumping into interview preparation, let's go over what to expect from interview day. I will share what to expect for both virtual and in-person interviews, but please note that I was only exposed to virtual interviews, so some of my in-person interview knowledge may be lacking!

Both virtual and in-person M.D. interviews are usually scheduled for one interview day. There were two medical schools that I interviewed virtually who hosted their information sessions on one day, and then their interviews were scheduled for a separate day (Mayo and OHSU), but besides those programs, the other schools conducted information sessions and interviews on the same day. MD-Ph.D. applicants will often have two interview days, especially in-person interviews (this time may have been limited to one day during the 2020-2021 virtual application season). Two days are often necessary for MD-Ph.D. applicants because they are being wined and dined like no other, and the research interviews with faculty can take longer than the more general interviews for M.D. applicants.

The number of interviews that applicants will have will vary from school to school. Some programs like Baylor give applicants one interview. Other programs, like UCSD, have eight mini-interviews. The number of interviews given will depend on the type of interviews offered. Among the two-day timeline for MD-Ph.D. applicants, I am unsure how many interviews are given - consult another resource for their expertise.

The two most common types of medical school interviews are traditional one-on-ones and multiple mini interviews (MMI). Traditional one-on-ones are where you will sit with a faculty member or student and discuss topics such as your drive to enter the medical field, your interest in and fit with the program, details of your application, how you would handle challenging scenarios, and many other related topics. MMIs are set up as 6-10 mini interviews where an applicant rotates among different stations to either speak with someone on admissions or perform an activity. Speaking with a faculty or student on admissions can range from asking how you would handle an ethical scenario to asking what your greatest challenge as a medical student will be - basically a short version of the traditional one-on-one interview. Performing a task at a station includes activities such as solving a puzzle with a fellow applicant or acting alongside a trained actor to see how you respond to an ethical dilemma.

While the vast range of questions that can be asked of you on interview day may sound daunting, the following sections will prepare you to arrive ready for nearly anything thrown your way. Even the acting stations or puzzle solving, which can sound out-of-the-box, became some of my favorite interviews because all you had to focus on was communicating well, and the rest was just fun!

Presenting yourself professionally is another point we will hit on during this chapter. Some quick tips are to pack (in-person) or layout (virtual) a few outfit choices so you can choose the clothes you feel most confident in that day. Sometimes, even our favorite shirts can betray us on an off morning! Iron your clothes the night before the interview. Some students carry their suits onto planes to avoid wrinkles. Try to get as much sleep as possible by going to bed early the night before. Wake up early to have sufficient time to get dressed, eat a light snack to avoid nausea, arrive early at your destination, and have a buffer for any mishaps. When prepared for, interviews can become the most enjoyable part of the admissions cycle. Put in the work, and you will shine on interview day!

HOW TO PREPARE FOR ONE-ON-ONES

Preparing for your interviews is essential for success. If you dare wing it for your medical school interviews, you will get a personal spanking from me. A spanking, I tell you!

To prepare, be sure to schedule your first interview so that you have approximately two weeks to prepare. As you have more interviews, this time can be reduced to a couple of days of preparation or whatever timeline you are comfortable with.

There are three main things to prepare for medical school interviews: 1) prepare for the common questions interviewers ask, 2) make flash cards about your research, and 3) type out a list of questions to ask your interviewers. Let me provide some more detail on each area.

First, prepare for the common questions interviewers ask at the particular medical school. This can be achieved by searching "[Insert name of medical school] interview questions SDN." SDN houses a forum where past medical school interviewees post the questions that they were asked. Yes, these people are likely breaking a confidentiality agreement they signed with the program. However, medical schools know that these questions are leaked, and many still choose not to change their questions from year to year. Since this information is publicly available, other interviewees are taking advantage, and medical schools are not changing their questions, I would advise you to go on SDN and make flashcards out of the questions you will be asked at each school. Use Quizlet or Anki to put each question on the front of a flashcard, then bullet point your response on the back. Practice answering each question with flashcards until you are comfortable and confident in your responses. Be sure to run some of your responses by advisors, family, or friends to ensure your answers are clear, comprehensive, and engaging.

Second, make flashcards about your research. One common way students bomb interviews is by completely fumbling the questions about their research. Did you mention that you worked on a project? Did you complete a senior thesis? Did you report publications or presentations on your application? Medical schools have noted and want to test if you are actually knowledgeable and passionate about your research or if your accolades are simply the result of mindless, robotic work in the lab. These flashcards should cover why your study was done (i.e., what was the pretext), the question(s) under investigation, the methodology used, the results, the interpretation of the results, and future applications of the study's findings. Know it all. Especially if you're interviewing for MD-Ph.D. programs, you have to know your research backward and forward. I was asked about my research at almost every medical school interview. Several of my interviewers asked in-depth questions about the papers I was published in. One conversation about research lasted over thirty minutes. If you know your research, you will perform better than most interviewing applicants. Too many candidates enter the interview with rusty knowledge of their projects - they end up coming off as unprepared at best and unknowledgeable and dispassionate at worst. Plus, preparing for the research questions will give you room to make mistakes if someone asks you about a future application or method or another topic that you don't recall or don't know. This happened to me during my Vanderbilt interview. My interviewer asked me a methods question that was really quite basic (the background of the mice used for the experiment), and I realized that I had not reviewed this information. Although I thought that I remembered the mice's background accurately, I told my interviewer that I was not completely certain of my response. Because I could assuredly answer all of her other questions, this error did not feel like a big deal, and she was understanding of my one point of uncertainty. Do yourself a favor and know your research so that you have room for forgivable errors. Remember that your interviewers can ask about any research project you mentioned on your application. Make flashcards for all of them.

Third, type out a list of questions to ask your interviewer. By and large, these questions can be reused or tweaked for each interview. You don't have to come up with a unique set of questions for each school. Some of my favorite questions to ask faculty, staff, and current students were: From what you have seen, what makes for the most successful medical students at [insert name of school]? What are the mentorship relationships like between [insert name of school] students and faculty? What things surprised you about coming to [insert name of school]? How do students balance their involvement in clinical exposure, research, and studying? These are four of my most-asked questions, but for each interview, I brought a list of about 15 questions for faculty and staff and 20 questions for current students. Again, these really didn't change from school to school. I wanted a large list of questions so that I could tailor what I asked to the conversation. Whatever you do, do not tell an interviewer that you have *no* questions to ask. Think of something, even if it is totally made up. It is a put-off interviewing someone for a job – or, in this case, a seat in a selective program – and then hearing that they have no questions to ask. A deficit of questions shows that this person has either not put any thought into coming up with questions, is uninterested in the school, or is not a curious person. I had my share of interviews where I already had a ton of questions answered by panels and casually speaking with students. But I still ponied up and either repeated questions to get another point of view or asked about something spontaneously that my interviewer and I had discussed during our conversation. Also, it is okay to bring a sheet of questions with you on a piece of paper and read off of the sheet when you ask your questions. Of course, do not read off of anything when you are being asked questions. However, when it is your turn to ask the questions, tell your interviewer that you brought a list to make sure that you didn't miss anything that you were excited to ask them. Most people will find your list endearing, especially if it is hand-written. Bringing a list is also great because you won't feel pressured to think of questions on the spot or worry about forgetting questions that you had set aside for your interviewer. I told my interviewers that I wrote my questions down in every single one of my interviews, and no one had a problem with it. I'm still convinced that my dorky list helped me stand out on the cuteness factor.

HOW TO PREPARE FOR THE MMI

Preparing for MMIs (Multiple Mini Interviews) is much like preparing for the CASPer. If you feel good about your CASPer preparation, you will feel good about preparing for the MMI. First, the basics. In an MMI, you will move between six and ten interview stations, where you will spend around eight minutes at each station. Each station has its own interview, but usually, these interviews are unlike the traditional one-on-one interview. Typical MMI stations have interviewees respond to ethical and behavior-based scenarios, perform teamwork and problem-solving activities often involving multiple interviewees, and respond to predetermined scenarios by interacting with a trained actor (again, often an ethical or behavior-based situation).

Apart from the teamwork/problem-solving stations, which require a bit more finesse, preparing for the MMI will mimic how you prepared for the CASPer. The same ethical and behavior-based questions that you responded to for the CASPer will be very similar to what you are responding to in the MMI. Remember the four principles for ideally responding to these types of prompts: 1) remain non-judgmental at all times, 2) consider all parties affected by a situation (patient, physician, patient's co-workers and family, reputation of hospital, reputation of physician, etc.), 3) acknowledge that there is missing information from the prompt and address the unknowns with if-then statements in your answer, and 4) discuss the pros and cons of each suggested response given by your if-then statements.

In the MMI, you will be going through all of these same four steps, but instead of typing your answer like in CASPer, you will share your response verbally to the interviewer or the trained actor. Since most of us don't have experience acting, it's easy to feel awkward playing pretend with a total stranger. Definitely practice acting out some ethical scenarios with a friend, family member, classmate, or advisor before the real deal. This way, you can avoid grappling with the novel discomfort and embarrassment of being a green "actor" in the actual interview. One of my MMI stations was acting-based, and although it was unexpected, I enjoyed playing along with the interviewer. She did a great job staying in character, and I found the whole thing to be pretty entertaining. Mind you, I took a beta-blocker, which helped keep my anxiety at bay. Overall, prepare for these stations as you did for CASPer, except speak your responses rather than type them. Get into a rhythm and formula for answering each question (literally every prompt that is thrown at you can be answered with a practiced method), and you will rock it on interview day!

The teamwork/problem-solving stations require a bit more thought beyond what you prepared for in CASPer. The trap that too many students fall into is that they think the goal of the exercise is solving the puzzle in front of them accurately and quickly. Trust me. The interviewers do not care if you make zero progress or solve the problem in record time. They are not measuring your critical thinking abilities here – that is what the MCAT and your GPA are for. Again, the interviewers are assessing your soft skills. Frankly, I think it's quite smart to test soft skills with these teamwork stations because it seems harder for applicants to conceal major character flaws when working with a fellow interviewee to solve a puzzle rather than schmoozing faculty in the one-on-ones. The key to acing these teamwork/problem-solving stations is all in *how* you communicate with the other participants. Ask for their input. Complement what they're doing correctly. Acknowledge any criticism that you receive and take it with grace. Openly admit your own mistakes when you make one (and you will likely make an error). Ask your teammates for feedback and offer constructive feedback to others. Taking these steps with other participants, as well as sharing and receiving information in a respectful manner, is how you ace these stations. At one of my MMIs, my partner and I were botching the puzzle that we were working on. However, we both had excellent communication. We complimented each other's strengths, didn't get frustrated, openly acknowledged our deficits in solving the problem, and gently delivered constructive feedback to the other person. Even though other groups taught us to solve the puzzle faster, I believe my partner and I both scored high on the station. I was admitted to the school (UMich), and I would be surprised if my fellow interviewee wasn't admitted as well. I have heard of so many other interviewees who have botched the problem-solving but aced the communication at these types of stations and then who went on to receive an acceptance at the school. Let the fact that you are *not* being evaluated for on-the-spot problem-solving calm your nerves. Just communicate kindly and clearly, and you will receive high marks. **Medical schools need to select students willing to learn from one another and want to work together.** That is what they are measuring with these exercises.

ANSWERING THE MOST COMMON AND IMPORTANT QUESTIONS

Fun Fact

Being asked your fun fact is not always an interview question per se, but it is often asked during group activities on interview day. Since there are usually admissions officers present at these activities, it's understandable that people get nervous about what to share as their fun fact.

In my experience, the best fun facts have to do with your hobbies and unique interests and skills rather than your accomplishments. During the course of my nineteen interviews during the admissions cycle, I shared my fun facts numerous times and listened to many other applicants share their own fun facts. Students who excitedly told the group about their recent experience making their own popcorn or learning to ride a skateboard seemed to have their fun facts go over well with the group. Students who talked about being a published playwright or speaking four languages did technically share a fun fact, but their choice of fun fact came off as more boastful. It is very impressive when people can speak multiple languages or have their writing published. However, I don't think this should be the first thing you tell a group of strangers about yourself. It comes off as a bit icky to me.

Additionally, please do not share anything political as a fun fact. One prospective student discussed working on a political campaign in a heated election that had just been called - he directly stated to the group that he knew that his work would "piss some of us off" – his words. He was a particularly unappealing character to me. The whole shebang was really off-putting. Not only did he share his political stances in a setting where no one could freely respond, but he also came off as cocky, knowing and openly stating that people would be offended by who he worked for and that he didn't care. For interview day, for the love of all that is holy, just tuck your politics aside and be an apolitical person. You can do it for one day.

For my fun fact, I had multiple that I rotated between. One was that my favorite beverage is hot chocolate, and I would drink it with any meal, including salads. Another was that I love learning about aliens and UFO sightings. Specifically, I called myself an 'alien enthusiast.' These fun facts shared unique information about me with the group while not touting my accolades. Many people seemed to like my fun facts and would comment or laugh in response. If you can think of a niche topic you enjoy learning about (i.e., growing orchids, Reddit theories on the hit TV series Lost, etc.) or some odd food combination you enjoy (i.e., popcorn and watermelon, maple syrup, and cucumber), I would recommend sharing these with the group.

Tell Me About Yourself

Ah, the dreaded "tell me about yourself" question! This one really bugs people out. And I get it – the question is super vague. The "tell me about yourself" question is one that you want to be prepared for because you are virtually guaranteed to be asked this by your interviewers as the first question. Here is the formula that I recommend. Introduce yourself again and state where you are from and the members of your family. Then, I would add about three fun facts and end your answer. Here is a sample:

"Hi, my name is Caroline, and I am from Portland, Oregon! My family consists of my mom and dad, my younger sister, Claire, as well as our two cats, Hazel and Holly, and our dog, Max. One of my favorite pastimes is cooking, and I recently attempted to make an orange olive oil cake, which turned out a bit funky. In addition to cooking, I love hiking with my family, although my sister usually rushes up the mountains near us, while my parents and I struggle to keep up! I'm so excited to be here with you today!"

The key to this answer is not to touch on medicine and why you want to become a doctor. The interviewer is just wanting to know a few interesting things about you. I think talking about your family – if you are close to them – is a nice touch because it shows that you understand yourself through familial relationships. When choosing which fun facts to share with your interviewer, choose lighthearted ones, and you can even reuse the fun facts that you shared with the larger group during the pre-interview activities. I shared my alien enthusiast fun fact with many interviewers who loved it!

Like always, keep the fun facts apolitical and don't select information that is too boastful, and you will be fine. Also, you do not need to think of unique, fun facts for each interviewer you speak with at a school. I often reused my fun facts with interviewers at the same school and said, "I just told Dr. X this, but I have been learning to care for an orchid and have successfully kept it alive for three months!" Follow these guidelines and keep your response between 30 and 60 seconds, and you will be golden.

Why Do You Want To Be a Doctor?

Next to the "tell me about yourself" question, the "why do you want to be a physician" question is intimidating for many applicants. Numerous factors fold into why we are drawn to medical careers, and condensing these points down to a 60-second answer is a daunting task. The good news is that once you figure out what to say and how to say it, your response flows out of your mouth on interview day.

The "why do you want to be a doctor?" question is important to master pre-interview, as you are nearly certain to be asked this by an interviewer. Many people joke about the notorious "love of science and helping people" response that we are told to avoid. It's too bad that we can't talk about our desire to combine our passions for science and caring for people, as I think this is a perfectly appropriate reason to go into medicine. Alas, I am outvoted by admissions committee members who have grown weary from decades worth of variations of this reply. So, without our humdrum, go-to answer, how do we tackle the "why do you want to be a physician" question?

Honestly, this was the question that was hardest for me to come up with a comfortable, authentic answer to, and that could be condensed into a minute or less of talking. What I found to work for me was a summary of my personal statement. I started by saying when I was first interested in medicine and then transitioned to when my interest became more serious. I recapped how I explored this interest in medicine during my undergraduate years and gap years and then led into how this exploration has now fueled my passion for solving X problems and working with Y community. Here is what my exact response to the "why do you want to be a physician" question looked like:

"I'm one of those who wanted to become a physician since I was a little kid. However, my interest in medicine really sparked when I witnessed my grandfather's cognitive decline due to Alzheimer's disease. Through his illness, I watched a man who loved physical activity become unable to walk and someone who loved history and storytelling become unable to share his own life story and recognize his family. My grandfather's experience with Alzheimer's prompted me to work in an Alzheimer's research laboratory during my undergraduate years as well as engage with older adults in memory care units who were experiencing cognitive decline. The cumulation of these experiences has made me incredibly passionate about working with our aging population. Specifically, I am hoping to become a geriatrician who can help guide aging adults and their loved ones toward making personalized, informed and confident decisions surrounding eldercare."

I know this isn't a particularly zesty answer, but it gets the job done while being clear and honest. Most importantly, the answer is very specific to me and what prompted me to become a doctor. You couldn't just choose a random prospective student and have us share the same reasons that led us to medicine. From my answer alone, I think people familiar with my file would have known that these were Caroline's words.

When crafting your reply to the "why do you want to become a physician?" question, follow my formula and be sure that your answer is specific to your story. The narrative that ties your application in a pretty bow and is featured in your personal statement (i.e., working with older adults, caring for rural populations, expanding our understanding of pediatric oncology, etc.) should be the framework of your response. After building out your answer, practice, practice, practice! You will be set for interview day.

One last point: your narrative may no longer be a close fit for your current leading interest in medicine. Perhaps your narrative surrounds your passion for global health, but you've now leaned toward a private practice career in plastic surgery. Or maybe your narrative concentrates on your love of psychiatry, but recently, you've thought surgery would be a better fit. Changing your mind about the specialty you desire to pursue and which population you strive to work with is totally okay. This was the case for me. My narrative focused on geriatric health, but throughout my gap years, I began feeling like I wanted to become a dermatologist. The good news is that we can usually find ways to tie multiple interests into one career. For example, I now want to become a dermatologist, but I want to specialize in aging skin and treating older adults. While I may no longer want to solely be a geriatrician, I have found a way to include my love of older adults in the world of dermatology. You will likely be able to do the same if your specialty of choice changes. I brought this up because it is probably best not to mention this change of interest in your "why do you want to be a doctor?" response. Including your shifted favorite specialty is a strong departure from the narrative that you've built your application around. For example, if I said that I've done all this work with older adults, but now I'm thinking about dermatology, my interviewer would probably be confused. My interviewer would be perplexed as to why my application centered on eldercare, but now I'm saying that I want to become a dermatologist. Do yourself a favor and just stick to your narrative. Keep it simple. You are not being dishonest in not sharing every thought and interest that you have in medicine. Your job on interview day is to present yourself as a great candidate for a future career as a doctor. Of course, be truthful in your responses. But being too transparent can hurt you. No one is going to pin you to a fence and interrogate you as to why you said you wanted a career in pediatrics but now are trying to match into orthopedics. So many people change their trajectories in medical school just as they change their college majors. Your narrative is your anchor. Stick to it.

Why Do You Want To Go to Medical School Here?

The "why us" question is one that I think is most overlooked by applicants preparing for their interviews. Do not underestimate the "why us" question. Your answer is extremely important, as interviewers use your reply to help determine your authentic or fabricated interest in their program. Oh, yes. It's a doozy.

The good news is that this question is not hard to answer well if you do a little research. As with everything, your reply to the "why us" question returns to your narrative. Let me explain. My narrative surrounded my passion for working with aging adults. Because of this, I focused my research for each medical school on opportunities to connect with geriatric patients. Was there a center focused on healthy aging? Was there a longitudinal program where students could care for a senior citizen? If so, these points were included in my answer. Since my family comes from a Hispanic background and it has been a long-term goal of mine to care for Spanish-speaking patients, I also researched opportunities related to helping the Hispanic community. Does the medical school have a Spanish-speaking clinic? Is the school located in an area with a large Latino population? If so, you bet I mentioned these in my answer.

Based on your interests, research how each medical school connects to your narrative and will further your passions in medicine. If you are driven to provide health to Native American communities, does the medical school partner with Native American health centers? If you want to perfect transplant surgery, is the medical school a leader in transplants (looking at you, Pitt)? By framing the "why us" response through how a program fits with your narrative, your words will reinforce how you presented on paper and will show genuine, individualized interest in the school's offerings that other interviewees cannot replicate. Here is my "why us" response for UCLA.

"UCLA offers incredible opportunities for research that closely align with my drive and aspiration to care for older adults. Specifically, UCLA's Longevity Center - which is dedicated to improving the quality of life of older adults through the alleviation of age-related memory loss - ties into my desire to help older adults achieve happy, healthy aging. UCLA is one of a few sites that is home to the MSTAR program (Medical Students Training in Aging Research). The program is a summer fellowship dedicated to aging research, which is where I want to focus my research efforts in medical school. Lastly, within Los Angeles, I will be exposed to a diverse set of older adults where 48% of the population is Hispanic. Since I am dedicated to caring for Spanish-speaking older adults, engaging with Spanish-speaking patients as a medical student will help me learn to provide better care for the Hispanic community throughout my career."

Tell Me About a Time When... You Received Criticism, You Gave Criticism, You Failed, etc.

"Tell me about a time when..." prompts are a type of behavioral interview question. There are endless endings to the "tell me about a time when. . ." stem, but your job is not to prepare for every possible behavior question. Instead, focus your efforts on crafting solid responses to the most common behavioral questions asked by medical schools. Three of the most asked behavioral questions are: 1) Tell me about a time when you received criticism, 2) Tell me about a time when you gave criticism, and 3) Tell me about a time when you failed.

Behavior questions are the most fragile of all the question types I have encountered. In other words, responses to behavior questions can easily go off the rails. Where does this fragility come from? These questions are delicate because you are usually asked to share an honest experience from real life that does not touch upon your or someone else's most flattering moments. These unflattering memories can often be emotionally charged and hard to handle in the moment. Most people prefer to shove these memories to the back of their minds and leave them untouched - to be forgotten amongst the cobwebs that cover your eighth-grade geometry lesson on parabolas. Therefore, when these memories are suddenly yanked to the forefront of our minds in a behavioral interview, our recollection of how we handled these difficult situations can come off awkward and not present us in the best light.

Hold onto your Swiffers because to effectively prepare for behavioral interviews, you must analyze and package past difficult encounters into neat, clean stories that showcase your best attributes. The attributes that interviewers will specifically look for are: 1) being able to recall a difficult experience without denigrating anyone involved, 2) an ability to take personal responsibility for your role in the challenge, and 3) evidence that you have reflected upon and grown from the encounter. To demonstrate these attributes, I will share my response to the following behavioral interview question: "Tell me about a time when you disappointed your team."

"As an undergraduate, I was a writer and editor for AcStart - a student-written guide to WashU's first-year courses. Our team of writers and executive board members consisted of 38 students, and our president decided that we should use Slack to communicate amongst our smaller and larger subgroups. I was a new user of the Slack platform and became a bit overwhelmed with the hundreds of messages that were exchanged by our team every day on various channels. Many of the messages seemed more casual in nature, so I didn't check Slack often, but unfortunately this led to me missing an important meeting announcement. Our team had been planning to meet with the student government to request funding for AcStart. I was very much looking forward to the meeting but ended up missing the meeting notification date on Slack because I wasn't regularly checking the platform. I was so disappointed when I was at work and received a text from AcStart's president asking where I was for the meeting. Unable to leave work to attend the meeting, I ended up letting my teammates down by being unable to represent AcStart's interest to the student government. After this difficult day, I was dedicated to checking Slack multiple times per day to stay up-to-date on meeting announcements. We also began sending email reminders about meetings so that everyone was aware of important group events."

Tell Me About Your Research

The iconic "tell me about your research" question can either go very wrong or very right. The good news is that you are in complete control of which way this question swings. Our game plan for acing "tell me about your research" is simple. Step one: take note of what research you mentioned in your application. Step two: know this research inside and out. To know your research inside and out, review your studies in detail and make flashcards that cover the details of each study. Background, methods, results, conclusions, and future directions. Make sure to master these concepts for each project. All research mentioned on your application is fair game for interviewers to ask about. If you are only familiar with your main project, you leave yourself vulnerable to the possibility of an interviewer asking about a minor project. It will look bad if you aren't able to speak clearly and intelligently about minor projects. Know your stuff for the interview.

You may think that only MD-Ph.D. interviewees are grilled about research, but this is incorrect. MD interviewees are fair game for research grilling. My Vanderbilt interviewer and I spent 30-40 minutes of our time together speaking about one of my research projects. The interviewer asked one tough question after another, and the only reason that I could confidently answer her was because I prepared with flashcards. The best part about coming prepared was that my anxiety was tempered when the research questions began. Moreover, it was no big deal when I was unsure of a methods question because I had already enthusiastically responded to all other inquiries about the study. That is how to be a research boss in your medical school interview.

Many students show up to interview day unprepared to answer questions about their research. This line of questioning is a smart strategy for admissions officers to distinguish between those who know their work and come prepared for the interview and those who were asleep at the wheel. Because research questions blindside many students, fully comprehending your projects is a winning strategy to easily allow you to stand out from other applicants on interview day.

During my Vanderbilt interview, the faculty member shared with me the admission committee's apprehension about my early undergraduate grades in science courses (during my freshman and sophomore years, I earned only Bs in the core sciences). Although I returned with a vengeance during my junior and senior years, I understood their concerns. Personally, I believe that my ability to kick butt in the research interview helped give the committee confidence that I was proficient in the sciences. Your baby clutched that A at Vandy.

Explain X Activity on Your Application

Similar to "tell me about your research," the "explain X activity" questions all come down to knowing your application. So long as something is listed on the primary or secondary applications, it is fair game for interviewers to ask about. Preparing for "explain X activity" questions is simple. Re-read your primary application prior to interview day, as well as your secondary responses for the school. By preparing for behavioral interviews that we discussed with "tell me about a time when…" questions, you should have a strong grasp on your activities because many should be used as examples of times when you faced a challenge or had to give someone difficult feedback.

For each activity listed, know what you contributed and identify your favorite aspect of participating. Stating your favorite part of each activity is a nice way to wrap up discussing a particular activity with your interviewer. Here's an example using my involvement as a peer mentor (known as a Washington University Student Associate or WUSA for short). "Tell me about your experience as a Washington University Student Associate."

"I absolutely loved serving as a peer mentor! I pursued becoming a WUSA because I initially struggled to acclimate to college during my first year and wanted to help the incoming students successfully transition to being university students. Me and my co-WUSA, Xavier, provided academic mentorship and personal support to 70 first-year students living in Lien House. It was incredibly rewarding to help our students develop effective study schedules and testing strategies, help students cope with homesickness, and help resolve any roommate issues. We also took our students on trips off-campus each semester like going to the Missouri Botanical Gardens and the Saint Louis Zoo. My favorite part of being a WUSA was witnessing so many of our students thrive during their first-year and overcome obstacles that initially challenged them as new college students. I feel very humbled to have formed strong relationships with our students and have played, hopefully, a positive role during their first-year at WashU."

Now, that is how you butter up your interviewer. Pull on those heartstrings, maestro. In all seriousness, speaking coherently about your extracurricular activities is critical. Medical schools are looking for people who are passionately involved in what they dedicate their time to. Applicants who fumble when speaking about extracurriculars by being unable to describe what they were involved in and what impact they left on their team could come off as resume padders. Not a good look. But one that is easily avoidable. As a current alumni interviewer for WashU Undergraduate Admissions, I recall an interview where the student I spoke with gave little detail about her activities. I inquired further into her extracurriculars to learn more about her and her interests, but she consistently responded with cursory information. At the end of the interview, it was difficult to say that I had a strong grasp of the applicant and how she had contributed to her high school because there was a lack of detail and interest conveyed. As much as I enjoyed our conversation, it seemed the applicant was either unprepared for our interview or not deeply involved in her activities. Again - this is all avoidable. Review your application, have a few points to hit with each activity, and your interviewer will be buttered like a Thanksgiving biscuit.

PRESENTING YOURSELF: VIRTUAL AND IN-PERSON

First impressions really do matter. First impressions during a medical school interview matter a lot. In this section, we are exploring how to present yourself at your interviews, whether they are virtual or in-person.

Appearance is what we will discuss first. The appearance guidelines are pretty much the same for both virtual and in-person interviews. Wear clean, wrinkle-free clothes. Men should wear a shirt and tie with pants. A jacket can be added if the boys want to step it up. Women should wear a top with a high neckline (save that cleavage for your English professor) and pair it with either pants or a knee-length skirt. Jackets are also an option for women. Particularly for in-person interviews, I highly suggest wearing boots or flats and not heels. There are too many young women each year who are wobbling around because they're not used to heels (this would be me), wincing in pain from their shoes (also me), or falling when walking around the medical school campus (me, again). Now, the rules of what to wear change a bit if your interview is virtual. Everything from the waist up should be the same, except certain patterns can mess with computer cameras, so you might want to stay away from pinstripes for virtual interviews. From the waist down, you have more flexibility with a virtual interview. While I would discourage wearing just your undies or going cheek to cheek with your seat (a.k.a. bare bottom), it's up to you, so long as the camera doesn't show your lack of clothing. In one of my interviews, I had to get up from my chair and close the blinds because the sun was streaming in and having a weird effect on my Zoom background. Things would've gotten pretty awkward if I had been wearing undies or going commando. Wearing sweatpants or leggings is a preferable alternative. I wore leggings for all of my interviews, and it was fantastic! Highly recommend. One thing to consider, however, is that studies are showing that dressing more formally increases your performance on a task (*The Daily Universe*, Students Respond to 'Dressing for Test Success'). I'm not sure how much of the formal outfit needs to be worn to benefit from this improved performance effect, but it's something to think about. Personally, because all of my interviews were virtual, I showed up in a button-up Jackie cardigan, leggings, and a jacket (although I began leaving the jacket on the back of my chair because I was too hot). I was comfortable during my interviews and felt my outfit looked fine on camera. With an in-person interview, I definitely would've stepped up my game by wearing pants or a skirt. For the sake of comfort and expense, I hope all of your interviews are virtual like mine were!

    Any ladies out there? We need to chat about makeup. Most people in medicine don't seem to be makeup fanatics. I don't fit in with this generality – I love makeup! False eyelashes, bright lipsticks, blended eyeshadow. I adore it all. If you are a makeup person like me, you will likely have to tone down your everyday makeup routine for interviews – especially in-person interviews. Try wearing a neutral lip color rather than something bold and bright. Choose a shorter, more understated pair if your false lashes are voluminous. Men appear more uniform in appearance, on average. Because of makeup and women's clothing, it's easier for women to stand out from the crowd based on appearance. This self-expression is a great thing, but it can be tricky when it comes to interviews. Women tend to be judged more for their appearance than men (Science in Poland, Sociologist:

Women Judged More by Their Looks in Various Spheres of Life). Makeup is one of the facets by which women can be judged and stereotyped. Women who wear more makeup are sometimes viewed as less intelligent. That is why, on interview day, it's best to be critiqued for your responses to an interviewer's questions rather than a personal presentation. I was not looking forward to toning down my everyday look for interviews, so I simply hid my own Zoom video from my screen and wasn't thinking about my appearance all day.

Speaking of hiding your Zoom video, I highly recommend this if you are prone to getting distracted by your image and if it keeps you from concentrating on the medical school's presentations and the interviews. There's nothing worse than speaking to someone and feeling like they're not paying attention – that's an easy way to put off an interviewer. The two pluses of keeping your personal video visible to you are that you can catch yourself making weird faces or getting too close to the camera. If you position your own video right beneath your computer's camera, it will give the appearance that you are looking at the interviewer, even if your eyes drift slightly down to look at yourself. For each of my interviews, my personal video was either hidden or right beneath the computer camera so that I was making constant eye contact with the interviewer.

Interviewers notice where your eyes drift to on your computer screen - this extends to reading off of a script. Some "genius" applicants from the 2020-2021 cycle typed their answers to interview questions and decided to read these responses off of their computer screens during their interviews. Suffice it to say that this strategy did not go over well. I wouldn't be surprised if each of these candidates was cut from consideration for dishonesty. If you have glasses especially, do not look at any other screen besides the Zoom screen. Too many stories have come out about interviewers saying that they could see the reflection of another screen (not the Zoom stream) off of their candidate's glasses and what a put-off that was. Just do the work and practice your responses to questions, and you'll do fine. It is so much better to fumble through a question than to be caught cheating in your interview. The last quick point is to position your camera so that your background is clean and simple. It's too easy to get distracted by someone's stray laundry or shirtless posters of Justin Bieber. Keep your background boring, and your interviewers will more easily concentrate on what you're saying.

Just as your appearance and eye contact are important, so are the hellos and farewells with your interviewers. I like to say hello and goodbye for virtual interviews by smiling and waving with both hands. It's a bit dorky, but it comes off as endearing and friendly. Besides a smile and a wave, I would also recommend saying, "Hi! How are you [insert name]? It's so wonderful to meet you!" as your introduction. These words show the interviewer that you are warm, approachable, and excited to speak with them. To end the conversation, I would say, "It's been incredible speaking with you [insert name]! Thank you so much for your time today!" before bringing back the smile and waving goodbye. This will end the interview on a positive note and show that you are grateful for the interviewer's time. I would recommend the same strategy for in-person interviews with a few adjustments. Be sure to give a hardy handshake at the beginning of the interview, either in addition to or instead of the wave – play the wave by ear. Also, prepare to have small conversation topics at the ready in case your interviewer and you need to walk to their office or a private room for your conversation. At the end of the interview, your interviewer may go in for another handshake, which is perfectly fine, but I would highly recommend smiling and waving goodbye once you leave their office or once they drop you off at the admissions office. I swear the smile makes a big difference, and the wave is an added bonus.

NAVIGATING VIRTUAL INTERVIEW BLUNDERS

Virtual interview blunders have become the ruling memes of 2020 and 2021. Expect blunders to happen on your interview day (if it is, in fact, virtual), so any glitches do not take you aback. Setting yourself up for success online starts with kicking family, roommates, friends, and noisy pets out of the house. Ask in your sweetest voice to have the house empty for your interview blocks. Too many people or barking puppies are not only a distraction, but people in the other room can also make you self-conscious about being overheard in the interview. Kick everyone out. Bake them cookies as a thank you. Put a note on your door for delivery people so they don't ring the doorbell. Leave them a cookie too!

Medical schools during the 2020-2021 cycle were great about letting candidates know that we would not be penalized for any technology glitches. Nevertheless, I believe that students can be judged on how they respond to virtual mishaps. For example, if two people start speaking at the same time, which happens often, I recommend you allow the other person to speak first. Say something like, "You go ahead [insert name]!" with a warm smile on your face. This gracious gesture will come off well to admissions committee members who might be on the call. If your video is freezing, try to put your video on speaker view rather than cluster view (the cluster setting – the setting where you can see a bunch of people at once – slowed down my connection) or leave and rejoin the call if you have to. If your interviewer's video is freezing, it's better to tell them than to say nothing. I made the mistake of saying nothing during my OHSU interview, and it was so hard to speak to the physician when the audio and video were always freezing. I really should have said something to him. Besides NYU, OHSU was my worst interview by far because of the streaming issues. During two of my other interviews with audio problems, my interviewer and I talked on the phone instead of on video. It was a perfect solution. Sometimes, my interviewer suggested that we talk on the phone, and at least once, I was the one to suggest calling one another. Don't be nervous to suggest a phone call as a solution if Zoom isn't working. Also, if your camera faces a window, watch out for bright light that can seep in and blind your interviewer! You may want to reposition the camera or shut the blinds. The final comment about virtual interview issues: make sure to check whether you're on mute or not. Double-checking the mute button will save you from the slight embarrassment of launching into a monologue without anyone hearing you. On the other side, make sure that you are muted when you're not speaking. One young man let slip a few curse words at a WashU current student meet-and-greet event. Luckily, the medical students weren't perturbed, but if that had happened with faculty on the call, things might have become sticky for the boisterous candidate.

WHAT TO DO IF AN INTERVIEW BOMBS

Did someone make a stinky? The first question to ask is, "Was it you or was it them?" Sometimes, we make a mess of an interview, but other times, we have a terrible interviewer. I have experienced both myself. Neither is fun.

We'll begin by talking about what to do if you are the cause of the bad interview. An interview can go sour for many reasons. Some of the most common are anxiety attacks, unstated audio glitches if the interview is virtual, forgetting your response to an important question, and not giving the best response to difficult, unexpected questions. If one of these issues happens, here is how I recommend trying to resolve the situation. First, if you realize that things are going downhill while still in the interview, ask if you can take a sip of water and a few deep breaths to collect yourself. People completely understand that you are nervous. Interviewers much prefer that you catch your breath rather than not perform your best. Not for medical school but for a UCSF research program, I bombed an interview because I had a panic attack. I literally couldn't think straight, and the fact that my interviewer was a bit cold and stiff only made me more anxious. After the interview, I did what I recommend you do if you cause an interview blunder: email your interviewer. In your message, state that you weren't at your best and didn't articulate yourself the way that you had hoped. You can then transition into quickly stating a few points that you wish had come across clearly during your conversation. Your note may or may not change anything, but I think it's better to try and fail with an email follow-up than to wonder, "what if." For my UCSF interview, I didn't move on to the last interview round, which I definitely expected. However, my contact information was passed along to other faculty with research openings who offered to meet about working on their projects. By that time, I was accepted to the Harvard Chan School research program, so I didn't take the UCSF faculty up on those offers. You never know what can come from trying to save a poor interview performance. Maybe they would've reached out regardless of my Hail Mary email. Who knows!

A whole new can of worms is opened if an interview goes wrong because of the interviewer. Trust me, this happens all the time. Even in medical school interviews. The three most common reasons an interviewer causes issues are having a bad attitude or being disinterested, cutting the conversation short, or making inappropriate comments. I have personal experience with the latter two scenarios. Don't worry, Gossip Girl – I will spill the tea!

Ultimately, poor interviewers don't give you a chance to succeed, which is why it's important to take care of yourself if this happens. The bad attitude or disinterested interviewer is the trickiest territory to navigate for medical school interviews. Some schools ask faculty, staff, and students not to show emotion or be antagonistic to see how they respond under pressure. These tactics are idiotic, especially considering that candidates do not know they are in a stressful interview. This type of interview also confuses students who don't know if they are being subject to a stress test or if their interviewer is not fit to evaluate people for medical school. If you are subject to these tactics, consult your advisor, close friends, or family members. They may see signs that you were subject to a stress interview, or they may tell you that the interviewer was simply acting strangely. I would say the best move forward in these cases is to send an email to the admissions office. In your message, the key is to use neutral language and to ask whether the interview was meant to be a stress test. By doing this, you are not accusing anyone of anything but, at the same time, are making your concerns known. Here is a sample email.

Sample poor interview performance follow-up email:

Dear [insert name of school] Admissions Team,

Thank you so much for the opportunity to interview on [insert month and day]! It was wonderful speaking with faculty, staff, and current students. I especially enjoyed learning more about student involvement in the [insert name of clinic] Free Clinic and the [insert name of research program] summer research program.

I had a quick question about whether one of my interviews was supposed to be a stress test. I didn't see anything about having a stress test interview on my invitation and welcome packet, which is why I wanted to double-check with your team. I was so excited to speak with [insert name of interviewer], but I am concerned that our conversation didn't go as I had hoped. I'm more than happy to give further details if requested, and again, I appreciate the opportunity to interview with [insert name of school].

I'm incredibly enthusiastic about the possibility of joining [insert name of school]'s Class of [insert graduating year], and I send my best wishes to your team!

With gratitude,

[insert your full name and AAMC ID]

What I like about this message is that you've given enough information here to let a school know that something may have been awry during your interview without pointing fingers. You simply ask a question about the possibility of a stress test and then state your wishes that the interview had gone better. If the interview was, in fact, a stress test, they will either let you know or say that they can't disclose that information (which will likely mean that, yes, it was a stress test). If it was not a stress interview, they will reach out for further information and very often will grant you a rescheduled interview with a new faculty member. Medical schools want you to have a great interview experience and will work hard to correct any mishaps on their part.

Another possibility of a wayward interview is if your conversation is cut too short. By 'too short,' I mean a conversation that was truncated because the interviewer was late or had to leave early. If this happens, reflect on how the discussion went. Was your interviewer distracted by other things? Was your interviewer excited to speak with you? Did the discussion go well? Did you get to communicate the bulk of what you wanted? If the conversation was short but you felt good about it, I would err on the side of letting the sleeping dog lie. Don't roll the dice with a potentially worse interview if you felt that the first one went well but was just short. If you did not feel great about the interview, and even if you felt lukewarm, I would consider reaching out to the admissions team. My second interview with UCLA was cut short because my interviewer was 10 or 15 minutes late, which left about 10 minutes for our conversation. He seemed quite busy, and while our discussion was fine, I didn't leave feeling that we had made a strong connection. Instead of asking for a redo, which UCLA even offered because they knew that my interview was super short, I decided to stick with what had happened. Going back, I would definitely change this decision. I was nervous that my replacement interview would be a disaster and thought it was better to take a meh interview rather than risk a disaster. UCLA was my first medical school interview, so I didn't yet understand that very few conversations would totally implode. I ended up getting waitlisted at UCLA. I have no idea if a redo interview would have caused a better outcome, but I encourage you to take the replacement if the discussion wasn't ideal. Here's a sample email to ask for a redo interview if it is not offered to you.

Sample interview redo request email:

Dear [insert name of school] Admissions Team,

Thank you so much for the opportunity to interview today! I very much enjoyed connecting with current students, faculty, and staff and learning more about the program, especially the [insert name of program] global health efforts.

I'm unsure if [insert name of interviewer] reached out to you, but unfortunately, our conversation was cut short. We only had [insert number] minutes speaking with one another, and I wanted to reach out and ask if your team recommends scheduling another interview. It was wonderful speaking with [insert name of interviewer], but we didn't get to cover a few points that I was excited to share with [him/her]. Let me know what your team recommends connecting with another faculty or staff member. Thank you so much for your thoughts on this!

With gratitude,

[insert your full name and AAMC ID]

The final scenario of a bad interview isn't a fun one. Sadly, some people have interviewers who ask inappropriate questions or make distasteful comments. Inappropriate questions can include those touching on politics, religion, sexuality, socioeconomic status, marital status, and family planning, among many other topics. Something to be aware of is if you mention one of these off-limits topics in an essay, they become fair game for your interviewer to ask about (within reason). For example, if you talk about your experience as a gay man, your interviewer could ask if your experiences have affected how you will care for patients. Your interviewer should not ask whether you have come out to your family if that is not something you spoke about in your writing or brought up in the conversation. My experience with an inappropriate question was from my one-on-one interview at NYU. My interviewer, who I really liked, by the way, asked my opinion on whether a fertilized plant seed should be considered life. This question is slightly altered to ask whether a fertilized human egg or zygote should be considered life. Because this question directly asks into one's religious beliefs and also often informs their political leanings, it is an out-of-bounds question for an interview. I have a strong hunch that someone's views of a plant seed as life closely aligns with their views of a zygote as life. In other words, my interviewer used a plant seed as a backdoor to ask into my religious and possibly my political beliefs. I was stunned when I was asked this in the interview. Again, I made a mistake in not reporting the question to the admissions committee. Although I do not think that I performed particularly well in NYU's MMI interview (it was my worst interview performance by far), when the interview day ended, I had a strong feeling that it was the plant seed question that wouldn't work in my favor. Of course, I'll never know if it was my own poor MMI performance, the plant seed question, or a combination of the two that caused me to bomb the NYU interview. About two weeks post-interview, I received my rejection. NYU was the only program that rejected me post-interview.

If you are the subject of an inappropriate interview question, report it. I will give a sample email once we discuss interviewers who make distasteful comments. Distasteful comments are objectively offensive statements. Remarks on a candidate being physically attractive or unattractive, comments of a sexual nature, statements that disrespect someone's military service, or opinions on why someone shouldn't go into medicine because they're disabled, a woman, or of a certain religious background are a few examples. Although these scenarios are disturbing, they unfortunately do happen. My own experience with inappropriate and blatantly sexual remarks during an interview occurred when I met with a neurologist in Oregon about Alzheimer's research that he was conducting. This doctor, who was likely in his 70s or 80s, explicitly referenced masturbation in our conversation. Our discussion had nothing to do with that topic. I remember sitting in the room alone with him and feeling absolutely mortified. I never expected these words to come out of someone's mouth. I thought about walking out of the interview right then. I wish that I could go back and leave him to his filth. Instead, I remembered his personal relationship with my former boss, Dr. Holtzman. I was terrified that if I walked out of the interview, he would call Dr. Holtzman or perhaps medical school admissions officers and speak poorly about me even though he didn't even know me. I should've had faith that Dr. Holtzman wouldn't listen to this colleague. If this physician had revealed his depravity to me – a total stranger – so quickly, other neurologists in the field probably knew what he was like. Instead of walking out, I sat in the room, counting down the seconds until the interview was over. When it finally ended, this doctor asked me to email him with critiques on some blog or journal article that he had produced. I can't even remember because I was so focused on getting back to the safety of my car. Needless to say, I left that room and never contacted the monster again. Until that day in January 2020, I never thought something like that could happen to me. All of my male colleagues, bosses, and professors had been nothing but professional and kind. Please take it from me that if anyone makes repugnant comments to you in an interview, the best thing you can do is stand up and leave the room. You do not have to say anything.

These people are testing what you will put up with, and if you end up working for them or associated with them in any way, they will take advantage again. If this happens in a medical school interview, this is how you reach out to the admissions committee (use the same communication for inappropriate questions like politics, religion, etc. that we discussed above).

Sample inappropriate interviewer email:

Dear [insert name of school] Admissions Team,

Thank you so much for the opportunity to interview today! I very much enjoyed connecting with current students, faculty, and staff and learning more about the program, especially the [insert name of program] global health efforts.

I wanted to ask if it would be possible to schedule a call with someone on your admissions team about my interview with [insert name of interviewer]. I was very excited to speak with [him/her,] but I am concerned about some of the comments that [insert name of interviewer] made during our conversation. Please let me know if a phone call would be possible – I would much appreciate the time to speak with someone on your team.

With gratitude,

[insert your full name and AAMC ID]

From this message, the admissions committee should absolutely schedule a time to speak with you. If, for some reason, they don't, that will speak volumes about the school's culture, and you could report what happened and how the program handled it to the AAMC. From your email, the admissions team will know that something was off during the interview, and I think it's best to discuss the details over the phone. When you take the phone call with admissions, state what happened with as little frustration as possible, even though frustration is a normal response to what happened. I was frustrated and angry at the neurologist in Portland after our interview. It's okay to become emotional, especially if something notably bad happened. The admissions committee will probably be very apologetic, offer you a makeup interview, and inform you that they will reach out to your interviewer. If those steps aren't taken, again, the school may not have a healthy culture. Be sure to schedule your makeup interview whenever you have had sufficient time to recover from the debacle. Admissions committees should be very understanding when something goes sideways. Rest assured that an interviewer's poor behavior will not reflect negatively on you in any way. Handle the situation professionally and respectfully and protect yourself from any shenanigans on the interviewer's part.

THANK YOU NOTES

I don't care what people say. Even if you say thank you to your interviewer once the interview concludes, you still need to send them a thank you note. This note can be sent either by email or mail. In either case, pony up and send the dang thank you. One activity I've done during my gap year is interviewing students for WashU's undergraduate program. Although I submit my evaluation before anyone sends a thank you note, receiving a thank you or a lack of a thank you definitely affects how I think of the student. I learn a lot about people by the way they communicate. Those who are kind, respectful of your time, and get back to you in a timely manner are my cup of tea.

Although your interviewer will likely not receive your thank you before they evaluate you, I believe that receiving one will heighten their positive feelings toward you. If you end up on the waitlist of the school, a thank you letter may increase the chances that your interviewer will advocate for you to be admitted. Perhaps your interviewer is on the scholarship committee, and your note can influence whether you are given a merit award. Beyond the ways in which a thank you can serve you, the most important reason to share your gratitude with an interviewer is because it's the right thing to do. Someone took time out of their day to meet with you and then advocate on behalf of your candidacy. A thank you note is an important gesture of appreciation. Below is a sample thank you note for those in need of inspiration.

Sample thank you note:

Dear [insert name of interviewer],

Thank you so much for taking the time to interview me for [insert name of medical school]! It was wonderful speaking with you about [name two or three specific points you discussed]. I very much enjoyed our conversation and will reach out to you when [insert name of medical school] sends an admissions decision. Wishing you an incredible rest of your week!

With appreciation and gratitude,
[insert first and last name]

LETTERS OF INTEREST AND LETTERS OF INTENT

What's the Difference?

Letters of interest and letters of intent are two types of post-interview communications used to convey interest in a medical school. What is the difference between these two forms of communication? Letters of interest are used to tell a program that you are incredibly enthusiastic about the possibility of joining the incoming class and to eagerly state your strong fit for the program. Some people state that letters of interest should only be sent to three schools at most. I disagree with this advice. Medical schools have every advantage in the admissions process. For you to state your interest in more than three schools post-interview is not an act of dishonesty. Clearly, you are excited about each program that you applied to since you submitted an application and accepted the invitation to interview. Frankly, I recommend that you submit a letter of interest to every school you interview at. From there, it is up to the committee to accept, waitlist, or decline you – do everything in your power to earn an acceptance.

Letters of intent carry more weight for both you and the program. These letters are declarations that you will attend a school if admitted. The consensus is that only one letter of intent should be sent, as one cannot honestly state that one would commit to attending more than one school if admitted. This advice I agree with. I believe sending more than one letter of intent would be dishonest. As an applicant, I recommend sending a letter of intent to your first-choice program and letters of interest to the rest. I think this is the best way to bolster your admission chances of admission maintaining your integrity.

When To Send a Letter of Interest?

Since some committees meet to discuss your candidacy soon after your interview, I would aim to send a letter of interest within a week of when you are interviewed. Some medical schools specify that they only want a letter of interest or a letter of intent if you are waitlisted. If that is the case, follow the program's guidelines. If waitlisted at a school that you would prefer to attend over any programs where you are admitted, send a letter of interest or intent within a week of the waitlist notification. Timely messages show keen enthusiasm for joining the incoming class.

How To Write a Letter of Interest?

Four ingredients are needed to write a good letter of interest. Ingredient one is to thank the medical school for the interview. Two is to state a few things you enjoyed learning about on interview day (faculty-student mentorship opportunities, leadership in medicine electives, affiliation with local high school science programs, etc.). The third ingredient is not sugar, but it's a little sweet, and that is to state that you would love to join the incoming class. Fourth is a sprinkle of showing why you are an excellent fit for the program. These four points are a bit abstract, so to put them in concrete terms, I will share below the letter of interest that I sent to medical schools. This letter is, I think, a great model for communicating your passion for a medical school program.

Letter of interest:

> *Dear Vanderbilt Admissions Team,*
>
> *I greatly enjoyed my interview day at Vanderbilt and am writing to convey my continued interest in joining Vanderbilt's Medical School Class of 2025. As I am devoted to caring for older adults and Spanish-speaking individuals, one of my goals on interview day was to learn about opportunities for engaging with these two groups at Vandy.*
>
> *Through my conversation with Dr. Deborah Lannigan, we discussed the extensive clinical experiences for gaining exposure to our aging population as well as the studies being conducted at the Center for Quality Aging. Dr. Mario Davidson, as well as current students, shared that Shade Tree Clinic was an excellent way to gain experience working with Spanish-speaking individuals throughout Nashville. The panel of current students noted that medical Spanish classes can be taken that will teach important, useful vocabulary when communicating with patients.*
>
> *These conversations confirmed that Vanderbilt will shape me into the passionate geriatrician-biostatistician I am committed to becoming. I can see myself using my new Spanish medical vocabulary to speak with patients at Shade Tree Clinic. I can see myself investigating how older adults can make informed, confident eldercare decisions at the Center for Quality Aging. The Center's*

mission is to "foster multidisciplinary aging research to improve quality of care and quality of life for older adults" – this aim precisely fits my aspirations as a biostatistician. I am confident that the curriculum, which "develops outstanding physicians, who are also leaders in health care," will instill in me a clinician who will deliver exceptional patient-centered care for decades to come.

Lastly, throughout interview day, students and faculty members alike referred to a theme of kindness in Vanderbilt's culture. Kindness has long been a trait that I have cherished in others and fostered in myself. Yet, the value of kind people and kind interactions can too easily be forgotten or overlooked. Hearing that kindness rests at the heart of Vanderbilt's community spoke volumes to me about the quality of education for students and the quality of care given to patients.

Each of these conversations on interview day gave me steadfast confidence that Vanderbilt is an exceptional fit for my career goals and personal values. It would be an honor to join the Vandy family as a member of the Class of 2025.

Yours sincerely,

Caroline Echeandia-Francis

When To Send a Letter of Intent?

Sending a letter of intent is a bit more complicated than sending a letter of interest. There are two strategies if you interview at a school and absolutely fall in love. Option one is to send a letter of intent soon after the interview. Option two is to start by sending a letter of interest and then send a letter of intent after all your interviews are complete. Option two is also appropriate if you have several front-runners and need to complete all interviews before knowing which school is your top choice.

Similar to letters of interest, some medical schools may specify when they will receive letters of intent. For some programs, letters may be sent throughout the entire interview cycle, and others will only consider them if a candidate is waitlisted. If waitlisted at your first-choice school, send a letter of intent within a week of receiving your decision notification to show your passion for the program.

My personal experience with prematurely sending a letter of intent is when I sent one to Mayo soon after my interview. I was absolutely and unexpectedly blown away by Mayo during my interview. I left the experience certain that I wanted to attend medical school there above all other choices. Because of these feelings, I was eager to convey my intentions to Mayo to matriculate to their program if admitted. While I sent this letter with total resolve to attend the program, several months later, I began worrying that I sent the letter too soon. Over the months, I conducted more research on the schools where I interviewed. I learned more about the Yale System of Medical Education and how it fostered student collaboration. I was drawn to the flexibility of the curriculum and thus extra time for research and volunteering, no class rank, no shelf exams, and extremely high honors rates during clerkships. Listening to current Mayo students, I learned that the curriculum was more stress-inducing. Earning honors in clerkships could be quite difficult, and there seemed to be a ranking system denoted in letters to residency directors. Shelf exams consumed the lives of those on rotation, and mandatory classes meant that there was less flexibility for research and volunteering. After gaining a better picture of what my four years would be like at Yale and Mayo, I began to think that Yale might be the better fit. With this feeling came guilt. I did not want to go back on my word to Mayo and decided to let the admissions decisions come in before letting the trepidation overwhelm me. Ultimately, starting by sending Mayo a letter of interest and then waiting until all interviews concluded before selecting a program to send a letter of intent to would have been a better plan for me. Consider your options before choosing where and when to send a letter of intent. In the end, I believe everything worked out for the best. I was waitlisted at Mayo in mid-February 2021, and a week later, I was admitted to Yale.

How To Write a Letter of Intent?

Writing a letter of intent is much like writing a letter of interest. All four ingredients still apply, but with one exception: ingredient three must be tweaked. The recipe is as follows: first, thank the committee for the interview; second, outline several things that you loved learning about the program on interview day; third, state both your enthusiasm to join the incoming class *and* your intention to matriculate if accepted, and fourth, explain why you are an outstanding fit for the school. Below is the letter of intent I sent to Mayo after my interview for you to review and inspire your writing. Notice that it is very similar to my letter of interest. No need to reinvent the wheel for each medical school!

Letter of intent:

Dear Mayo Admissions Team,

I greatly enjoyed my interview day with Mayo, and if admitted, I am writing to convey my enthusiastic intent to join Mayo's Medical School Class of 2025. Before this week, I never anticipated being able to write a letter of intent for any medical school. I did not think my choice as to where to train for my future career as a physician would be so clear. Yet, the people I have met this week – from the Sunday student panel to my virtual host, Cecile, and from the admissions team at the Monday Welcome Session to my two interviewers, Hannah and Johnny – have made me resolute in stating my intentions. I would be honored for each of these individuals to become my peers, teachers, and mentors.

As I am devoted to caring for older adults and Spanish-speaking individuals, one of my goals on interview day was to learn about opportunities for engaging with these two groups at Mayo. Through my conversation with Johnny Dominguez, we discussed how Mayo's national medical school allows students to learn from the rich diversity that exists within Scottsdale's and Jacksonville's large and growing Hispanic and geriatric populations. Hannah Case shared that the Senior Sages Program allows students to immerse themselves in longitudinal geriatric care through a four-year mentorship with their Senior Sage. The panel of current students noted that medical Spanish classes can be taken that will teach important, useful vocabulary when communicating with patients. Cecile Riviere-Cazaux expressed how the 2+2 program – via both the Rochester-Jacksonville and Scottsdale-Jacksonville paths – is unmatched in training students through personalized instruction and mentorship to provide remarkably effective patient-centered care.

Together, these conversations confirmed that Mayo will shape me into the passionate physician leader, geriatrician, and biostatistician that I am committed to becoming. I can see myself using my new Spanish medical vocabulary to speak with patients throughout Rochester, Scottsdale, and Jacksonville. I can see myself investigating how older adults can make informed, confident eldercare decisions at the Center on Aging's Healthy Aging and Independent Living Program. The Program's mission is "to develop scalable and readily implementable solutions to improve the health and well-being of older adults" – this aim precisely fits my aspirations as a biostatistician. I am confident that Mayo Clinic's primary value of "putting the needs of the patient first" will instill in me a clinician who will deliver exceptional patient-centered care for decades to come.

Lastly, throughout interview day, students and faculty members referred to a family theme in Mayo's culture. The kindness and care that define families have long been traits that I have cherished in others and fostered in myself. Yet, the value of kind and caring people can too easily be forgotten or overlooked. Hearing that the traits of family rest at the heart of Mayo's community spoke volumes to me about the quality of education for students and the quality of care given to patients. Moreover, Mayo's students struck me as truly down-to-earth, humble individuals who continue to stand out as the happiest medical school students I have met.

Each of these conversations throughout the interview week gave me steadfast confidence that Mayo is an exceptional fit for my career goals and personal values. If admitted, I can say with enthusiasm and without hesitation that I fully intend to choose Mayo for my medical education. It would be a privilege to join the Mayo family as a member of the Class of 2025.

Yours sincerely,

Caroline Echeandia-Francis

CHAPTER

15

POST-INTERVIEW BLUES

COPING WITH THE BLUES

Blues often set in after interview season has concluded. Before decisions are released, we become trapped in a purgatory of juggling our potential futures. We could end up on one side of the country or another. In warm weather or under blankets of snow. Meeting one group of unknown friends or another. So much is uncertain in a process that we have little control over.

It is easy to take these feelings and become wrapped up in over-analyzing every word and gesture in each interview. Did I talk too much or too little? I forgot to mention my work as a teaching assistant – will that affect my prospects? My interviewer didn't smile much. Did he not like me? It becomes all too easy to talk oneself into a state of anxiety.

I have two remedies for dealing with post-interview blues. The first is to avoid Reddit's premed forum as well as the Student Doctor Network (SDN). The second is to distract yourself with productive activities. We will get into these distractions in the next few sections. For now, I want to say a few words about Reddit and SDN.

While these two websites are helpful for learning when secondaries and interviews are being distributed and can give insights to those filling out their applications (e.g., submit your transcripts to AMCAS as soon as possible), I have found that the post-interview negatives of Reddit and SDN vastly outweigh the positives. Once interviews have concluded, you will only find students neurotically fretting about the upcoming final decision and people posting their decisions, as these come out in waves at most schools. Specifically, seeing other students earn acceptances while you wait to hear of your fate can be quite devastating. I remember how down I felt when Vanderbilt sent out their first round of acceptances, and I was not a part of the group. I began questioning my interview performance and wondered what I could have done better to be one of the first people admitted to their class. As it turns out, there was nothing much to worry about. I was accepted several months later in their second wave of decisions. The other issue with watching for updates on SDN was that I focused too much on the schools that I hadn't heard from rather than celebrating my current acceptances. I was fortunate enough to be accepted to Northwestern Feinberg in their first round of acceptances. I was thrilled when I received the notification in late November. However, the excitement at the long-awaited decision to one of my first-choice programs was soon washed away by the anxiety that I felt about my upcoming results for the other medical schools. Do yourself a favor and block Reddit and SDN (especially SDN) after your interview. You will be much happier and better able to celebrate each acceptance when you hear back from your schools. Now, let's talk about distractions.

SENDING UPDATES

Sending updates to medical schools is a strategic distraction that can help push your application into the accepted pile. I recommend sending an update to each school where you interviewed. Updates can also be sent before an interview invitation is extended, but I've found them to be most effective post-interview. Some applicants choose to combine their letter of interest or intent with an update letter, but I recommend sending updates separately. Two post-interview communications will make you more memorable than just one communication to the committee. Furthermore, sending two notes post-interview conveys a stronger interest in the program than sending only one note.

Updates to medical schools can include the following: recent publications or presentations, completion of a notable course or certification (e.g., becoming a certified interpreter), continued volunteering hours or additional experiences, personal achievements (e.g., publishing a novel), earning a scholarship or honor, or beginning a new job. There are many other notable accomplishments that you can update medical schools about. In addition to your updates, be sure to reaffirm your interest in the school in addition to discussing how your updates are meaningful to you or how they will make you a better physician. All post-interview communications – including updates and letters of interest or intent – should be sent at least a month and a half before decisions are released or before the interview season concludes. As medical schools wind down interviews, the admissions teams will meet frequently to shape the incoming class. Some candidates wait too long to send updates or letters of interest or intent, which then aren't considered when evaluating their application for the final time. If you are wondering whether you should save updates for getting off of a waitlist and not send them before decisions are released, I would not encourage this. Getting into a medical school right off the bat is much easier and less hectic than trying to maneuver one's way off the waitlist. You can send an additional update letter if you are waitlisted. You may not think that you will accomplish anything of note between a first update letter and being placed on a waitlist, but you will. Perhaps you will begin taking an online Spanish course or have an impactful article published in your school's newspaper – these are accomplishments that medical schools would love to hear. Below are the two update letters that I sent to medical schools. The first was sent before interview invitations went out. I don't think this letter made a difference as to which schools interviewed me. They seemed to interview whomever they wanted. The second update letter was sent post-interview, which I think made the difference for some of my acceptances and waitlists.

Pre-interview update letter:

I am excited to share that on Friday, September 11, 2020, I was awarded a registration

scholarship to fund my participation in the 2020 SACNAS – The National Diversity in STEM

Conference. As a first-time participant, SACNAS will provide an excellent platform to introduce my mentor's and my Alzheimer's research to others in the neuroscience field, as well as an invaluable opportunity to incite discussion and build professional connections with experienced researchers in all stages of their careers. This conference will also grant me further experience in sharing complex scientific concepts with a range of audiences – a skill that will be critical to my future work as a clinician and researcher.

Screenshot of award notification:

> **Congratulations!**
>
> Dear Caroline,
>
> Congratulations! SACNAS is pleased to inform you that you have been awarded a registration scholarship for 2020 SACNAS – T*he National Diversity in STEM Virtual Conference.*
>
> You will receive an email next week with further instructions on how to register. In the meantime, if you have questions, please respond to this email.
>
> We look forward to your participation at the 2020 SACNAS conference!
>
> **Tim Smith**
> **Coordinator, Infrastructure & Knowledge**
>
>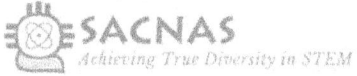
>
> tim@sacnas.org • (831) 459-0170 x223

Post-interview update letter:

Dear Yale Admissions Committee,

Happy 2021! I am writing to convey my continued enthusiastic interest in attending medical school at Yale as well as to provide several application updates that are located below. As the interview season is coming to a close, Yale has remained a stand-out in the collaborative, supportive culture that students foster and enjoy. From what I have gathered speaking to current students and faculty, I believe that the Yale System of Medical Education makes much of this vibrant culture possible. As someone who has very much enjoyed structuring and executing my gap year plans, I am confident that I would thrive as a student within the Yale System. Encouraging and cheering on my fellow classmates in achieving their goals would be one of my favorite roles within the YSM Family – a family I would love to join.

Thank you for considering my candidacy. Yale remains my top choice for medical school, and it would be a privilege to join the Class of 2025. Sending my best wishes to your team for a successful start to the New Year!

Yours sincerely,

Caroline Echeandia-Francis

Update 1: Article published in Oregon Faith Report about my volunteer work making masks for older adults during COVID-19 outbreak

In response to the onset of COVID-19 and the shortage of PPE, I had the opportunity to make masks for older adults and caregivers in senior housing communities to protect them from coronavirus. I am humbled to have these efforts featured in an article published by Oregon Faith Report: https://oregonfaithreport.com/2020/08/pre-med-student-memory-care-volunteer-makes-hundreds-of-masks-for-residents/. The masks are made as a volunteer initiative for Touchmark Senior Living in Portland, OR. Before the coronavirus outbreak, I volunteered in the memory care unit at Touchmark. I engaged with residents through life enrichment and wellness activities (physical exercise, art projects, brain games, puzzles, self-care, and current events). While unable to visit residents for the past several months due to COVID-19 safety restrictions, I have very much enjoyed contributing to the safety efforts of the Touchmark community through mask-making. It was an honor to have my work featured in the Oregon Faith Report, and I look forward to returning to the residents at Touchmark when it is safe to do so!

Update 2: CaregiverZone featured in Cambia Grove Impactful Innovation Exchange

I am proud to share that the company I co-founded – CaregiverZone – has been featured in Cambia Grove's Impactful Innovation Exchange: https://www.cambiagrove.com/caregiverzone. From discussing how to prevent falls among older adults to preventing loneliness among our aging population, CaregiverZone's online services provide research-backed information to incite conversation among those looking to make clear, confident, and personalized eldercare choices (caregiverzone.com). I served as CaregiverZone's President and was inspired to start the company in response to a growing need to aid aging adults and their loved ones in making informed decisions surrounding eldercare. Cambia Grove's Impactful Innovation Exchange provides a "comprehensive platform where changemakers can search for emerging and/or proven innovations to solve health care problems" – particularly those affecting older adults (Cambia Grove: Impactful Innovation Exchange). Through our spotlight in Impactful Innovation Exchange, CaregiverZone has reached a wider audience who have been able to access our resources and thus find answers to their most pressing eldercare questions.

Update 3: Research findings to be published in Annals of Neurology

Litvinchuk, A., Huynh, T.P.V., Shi, Y., Jackson, R., Finn, M.B., Manis, M., **Francis, C.M.,** *Tran, A., Sullivan, P.M., Ulrich, J., Hyman, B.T., Cole, T., Holtzman, D.M. (2021). The effects of ApoE4 reduction using antisense oligonucleotides in a mouse model of tauopathy. Annals of Neurology (Date: TBD)*

I am excited to share with the YSM Admissions Committee that a research project that I contributed to as part of the Holtzman lab is being published in the Annals of Neurology! The Holtzman lab researches Alzheimer's disease (AD) and specifically concentrates on investigating the apolipoprotein E (APOE) gene – the gene identified as the greatest genetic risk factor of late-onset AD. Our project examines the effect of reducing APOE expression on tauopathy. Tauopathies are a classification of neurodegenerative disease (such as AD) where the protein tau becomes misfolded in the brain, leading to tau aggregation in the form of neurofibrillary tangles. These tau tangles are one of the foremost biological hallmarks of Alzheimer's disease and are understood to play a key role in the progression of neurodegenerative processes that occur among those with AD (e.g., memory loss, personality changes, disorientation, difficulty learning new tasks, etc.). Thus, my mentors and I were eager to study possible links between the APOE gene and tau.

By lowering APOE expression, we reduced tau protein levels and aggregation by ~50%, thus protecting against tau pathology. Furthermore, we measured significantly decreased neurodegeneration (~20-25%), reduced neuroinflammation (~50%), and preserved synaptic density (~69%). Our results show that we must consider reducing APOE expression as a potential therapy for preventing and treating Alzheimer's disease. Further research is needed to investigate APOE-targeted therapy as a treatment. However, I am thrilled by its promise to protect against tau pathology and preserve the health of synapses and neurons.

CHAPTER 16

PAYING FOR MEDICAL SCHOOL

SCHOLARSHIPS

Medical school is expensive. No duh! Because of this unfortunate fact, one of the best ways to invest your time is by applying for outside medical school scholarships, and by 'outside,' I mean those are offered by organizations other than your medical school. Most medical schools consider all accepted students for their own awards, but by all means, apply to your medical school's scholarships if they ask you to write additional essays. Saint Louis University (SLU) was the only medical school that had me submit an additional application for a particular scholarship after I was admitted.

Besides the SLU scholarship, all my scholarship explications were to external organizations. As I write this, I have applied to 17 outside scholarships and plan to apply to at least nine more in the coming months. These awards range from $500-$10,000 in funds. Every little bit helps! Yet, the larger awards would be incredible to receive. Although outside scholarships are quite competitive, so is getting into medical school. You are already clearing a tall hurdle, so why not try and clear a few more? Also, they have to award the scholarship to someone! Why can't it be you?

Before worrying about how long the applications will take you (I totally understand application fatigue), know that I have submitted primary and secondary essays with minimal modifications for many scholarships. You have a slew of well-written essays at your fingertips – might as well put them to work.

When looking for outside scholarships to apply for, many medical schools have a list of outside awards on their website. **One of the most comprehensive and regularly updated lists that I have seen is from Case Western** (Case Western Reserve University School of Medicine, Outside Scholarships Inventory). I recommend looking through the lists of outside scholarships on at least six medical schools' websites and running an internet search for medical school scholarships. Cappex is the most comprehensive scholarship search engine that I have used.

Once your research is completed, then create an Excel sheet to compile the lists of awards that you are interested in applying for. On the Excel sheet, include the name of the scholarship, dates when the application opens and closes, the award amount, any relevant notes (e.g., number of recommendation letters), and a track of your progress. Inserted below is a screenshot of a sample Excel spreadsheet.

Sample Scholarship Spreadsheet:

Scholarship Name	Opens	Closes	Amount	Status	Link	Notes
American Indian Graduate Center Fellowship	Jan 1	June 1	$500-$5000	Submitted	https://www.aigcs.org/scholarships-fellowships/graduate-students/	Member of American Indian tribe or Alaskan Native Group
American Medical Association	Dec 1	Feb 1	$10,000	In progress	https://amafoundation.org/programs/scholarships/	In fourth year of study
American Society of Hematology	Aug 15	Feb 15	$5,000	Not started	https://www.hematology.org/awards/medical-student/honors-award	Research stipend; not scholarship

One of the best ways to narrow down medical school scholarships is to consider the following factors: area of medical interest, desire to care for underserved communities, regional ties, gender, sexual orientation, religion, race, ethnicity, and national origin. Many of the scholarships that I applied to were specifically geared toward women, Christians, residents of Oregon, those attending medical school in Connecticut, Latinas, graduate students, etc. My personal demographics helped narrow down which awards I was eligible for and wanted to apply to. So far, I have heard back from six scholarship programs, and I am honored to have been selected for three of these six scholarships. These funds will significantly impact the cost of my medical education - it is definitely worth applying! Because most of these scholarships are awarded after the April 30th commitment deadline for medical schools, any award will likely not be able to influence your financial decision in where to attend medical school.

Due to the sheer number of scholarships available, I am not able to comprehensively list every award out there. Below is a list of medical school scholarships for incoming and current students based on Case Western's outside scholarship list (Case Western Reserve University School of Medicine, Outside Scholarships Inventory). However, there are definitely going to be missing opportunities, so be sure to do your own research. Pro-tip – to get ahead of the game, keep a list of scholarships for current medical students so you know what awards to apply to as you progress through M1, M2, M3, and M4 years.

List of Medical School Scholarships:

- American Association of University Women Educational Foundation (AAUW) - Selected Professions Fellowships
- The American Heart Association (AHA) - AHA Scientific Council Student Scholarships
- American Indian Graduate Center (AIGC) - AIGC Fellowships, Gerald Peet Fellowship
- American Medical Association (AMA) Foundation - AMA Foundation Physicians of Tomorrow Scholarships
- American Medical Women's Association (AMWA) - Medical Education Scholarships
- American Society of Hematology (ASH) - ASH HONORS (Hematology Opportunities for the Next Generation of Research Scientists) Award
- American Society of Hematology (ASH) - ASH MMSAP (Minority Medical Student Award Program)
- Association of American Medical Colleges (AAMC) - Herbert W. Nickens Medical Student Scholarships
- Chinese American Physicians' Society (CAPS) - CAPS Scholarship
- Daughters of the American Revolution (DAR) - DAR Medical Scholarships
- Department of Defense - U.S. Air Force - Health Professions Scholarship Program
- Department of Defense - U.S. Army - F. Edward Hebert Armed Forces Health Professions Scholarship Program for Medicine
- Department of Defense - U.S. Navy - Health Professions Scholarship Program
- Department of Health and Human Services - Indian Health Service Scholarship Program - Health Professions Scholarship

- Department of Health and Human Services - National Health Service Corps (NHSC) Scholarship Program
- The Gamma Mu Foundation - Gamma Mu Foundation Scholarship Program
- Hispanic Scholarship Fund - College Scholarship Program
- The Japanese Medical Society of America, Inc. - Japanese Medical Society Scholarship
- Kaiser Permanente - Oliver Goldsmith, M.D. Scholarship
- Korean American Scholarship Foundation - Midwest Regional Scholarship
- The Kosciuszko Foundation - Tuition Scholarship Program
- The Kosciuszko Foundation - Dr. Marie E. Zakrzewski Medical Scholarship
- Mortar Board National Office - Fellowship Program
- Mustard Seed Foundation - Harvey Fellows Program
- The National Italian American Foundation (NIAF) - General Scholarships
- National Medical Fellowships, Inc. - General Scholarships and Awards
- National Medical Fellowships, Inc. - NMF Primary Care Leadership Program
- National Medical Fellowships, Inc. - United Health Foundation/NMF Diverse Medical Scholars Program
- National Hispanic Health Foundation - The Hispanic Health Professional Student Scholarship
- Osmosis - Health Education Impact Scholarship
- P.E.O. Sisterhood - P.E.O. Scholar Awards
- Paul and Daisy Soros Fellowships for New Americans - Paul and Daisy Soros Fellowships for New Americans
- Pisacano Leadership Foundation - Pisacano Scholars Leadership Program
- Point Foundation - Point Scholarship
- Polish-American Medical Society - Polish-American Medical Society Scholarship

- The Recovery Village - The Recovery Village Health Care Scholarship
- Sigma Chi Foundation - Sigma Chi Medical Scholarship
- Tylenol® - Tylenol® Future Care Scholarship
- Women in Medicine (WIM) - Leadership Scholarships

FINANCIAL AID

Applying for financial aid is a snooze fest, but it's important. Similar to applying for outside scholarships, you will want to make an Excel spreadsheet of all schools where you will apply for financial aid, as well as their financial aid protocols, deadlines, and necessary documents (FAFSA, CSS Profile, tax returns, W2s, etc.). Some schools want your FAFSA but not your CSS. Some schools want parental data, while others do not. Some schools have all interviewees submit financial information, while other schools only allow accepted students to apply for financial aid. Take note of these nuances in order to keep yourself organized and efficient.

My rule for applying for financial aid was to pump out the materials as quickly as possible. Schools risk not letting you know about your aid package before the commitment deadline if you submit the financial aid application late. Therefore, if finances are an important part of your medical school decision, submitting your financial aid applications as early as possible (at least before the school's deadline) is critical.

During the 2020-2021 application cycle, a section explained how COVID may have impacted your family's earnings. I'm not sure if this section or a similar section will be available on future applications, but if it is present, I highly suggest that you fill it out in detail. After explaining the impact of COVID on my family in addition to a job change that my dad made, I was asked by financial aid offices to submit additional documentation to show financial impact (2020 W2s and taxes in addition to 2019 W2s and taxes, a written statement from my dad, etc.). Most offices took this information into account. Washington University School of Medicine in St. Louis ended up awarding me an additional $6,450 in yearly aid from the provided documentation. Overall, if there has been a change to your financial circumstances that is not documented in the previous year's financial papers, be sure to discuss it with financial aid offices so that you can get the most assistance possible.

CHAPTER 17

REAPPLYING

Before we dive into talking about application results (acceptances, waitlists, and rejections), let's discuss what needs to happen when you have to reapply to medical school. The interview season usually winds down in February. If you haven't received any interviews by then, it's a good indicator that you will likely have to reapply to medical school. It's a total bummer, but if this is your dream career, it's totally worth it. Another scenario is receiving interviews but having no acceptances by April. If you are on a large number of waitlists, there are tips for helping to turn those into acceptances in the Waitlists section. Only rejections will warrant another application cycle. The key to a successful reapplicant – no matter what the circumstances – is finding out what went wrong the first time and then fixing those weaknesses for the next tango.

Some people say to act like you will have to reapply from day one of submitting your primary application. This may be good advice if you think there is an obvious hole in your application, but then I would have suggested waiting a cycle before applying in the first place. However, if you are a bit light on volunteering or research or perhaps have a lower MCAT, taking care of those things as you apply will allow you to send meaningful update letters that can score you an interview or acceptance.

WHAT WENT WRONG?

Nailing down what went wrong with your application will require input from others: Advisors, mentors, current medical students, admissions committee members, friends, and family. They all can bring insight as to where your application could be improved. I would focus on a few select people to receive feedback from, as too many opinions can be overwhelming and confusing. If at all possible, email the admissions committees at each school where you applied (especially those where you had an interview) to see if they give feedback. Consider reaching out to a current medical student at these schools to see if they can give their perspectives after explaining your situation. Some admissions committees do give feedback, which can be super helpful for reapplying to that school during an upcoming cycle.

In addition to getting feedback from others, get feedback from yourself! I recommend printing out your entire AMCAS primary application and going through it with three colored pens. Pretend that you are an admissions committee member with thousands of potential applicants and ask yourself 1) how does this applicant stand out, and 2) why does this person want to become a physician? Use one color to mark areas of your application that are strong (green perhaps), another color to mark areas that are so-so (yellow), and a third color to mark areas that need improvement (red). Assess the attributes that help your application stand out and where you see passionate answers to the question "why you want to be a physician." This exercise is a great starting point for assessing how you can become a stronger applicant.

APPLICATION REHAB

Many potential factors could be improved in an application. Even people sliding into Harvard Medical School have aspects that could have been improved. Although I am no HMS matriculant, I definitely could have earned more clinical hours over a greater span of years (most of my clinical volunteering occurred right before I submitted my application). My GPA – particularly my sGPA – could have been higher. Even my gap year activities could have been less choppy (perhaps continuing research rather than switching to entrepreneurship with CaregiverZone). We all have application components that can be improved.

When looking to rehabilitate your application, the first factors to note are those that may have kept you from earning an interview. Were there any red flags that weren't elegantly explained (institutional action, criminal record, downward GPA trend)? Were there any big boxes left unchecked (shadowing, volunteering, clinical exposure)? Were essays poorly written? Did your application lack a compelling personal narrative?

If your application checks out overall, but you still have not received any interviews, you are in the company of many others. Most of these cases come down to needing improved essays and articulating a narrative that pulls in your reader. An applicant who received multiple interviews but no acceptances should revisit their interview preparation. Particularly for those with only post-interview rejections, your interview was likely what held you back. See the Interviews chapter for tips on how to improve your interview skills. Be sure to practice interviewing with mentors, advisors, and friends.

After assessing your application, make a list of what needs to be rehabilitated and your plan moving forward. A lower GPA may need to be bolstered by additional classes or a post-bac or master's program. A low MCAT may lead to a retake. A top-heavy or state school-heavy school list might need adjustments. Sloppy essays will need to be rewritten with your personal narrative at the center. Minimal clinical hours should be boosted. Understanding the improvements to be made will help you create a timeline and identify which cycle you should target for your reapplication. Whatever you do, do not rush to reapply. Take your time to craft a strong application so you don't waste time and money applying for a third time if the second application is premature.

To give an example of a reapplication timeline, let's visit our friend Nyra. Nyra graduated from Washington University in St. Louis with an impressive resume of extracurriculars. She danced for two competitive school teams, held executive board positions for several school organizations, and served as a hotline crisis counselor for one of WashU's most competitive student groups. Nyra also led and organized a massive cultural event that takes place each year on campus, worked in a research laboratory, and was a counselor for students during their first-year orientation. During the summer, she traveled to India for an internship where she taught young girls about reproductive health. Each of Nyra's activities was intentional. Her involvement was sincere. Nyra had a resume that would get her considered by most, if not all, medical schools in the country. So what went wrong? As we've touched on before with Nyra's case, her weak points were her GPA and MCAT, which hovered around a 3.5 cGPA, 3.3 sGPA, and 508 MCAT. On top of that, she rushed her application and did not put much work into her essays. Despite having an incredibly compelling narrative about her long-standing work with women's health as well as personal experiences with reproductive health that tied into her story, her application was not well-articulated and fell flat. Nyra, expecting that there would be trouble due to her scores, applied to only a handful of in-state schools during the 2019-2020 cycle. She received no interview invitations and knew that she would have to reapply.

Looking at her application, Nyra chose to rehab her GPA and MCAT. She enrolled in a master's program after consulting with an advisor who recommended a master's degree rather than a post-bac program to show GPA improvement. She restudied for the

MCAT and began scoring above 520 on practice exams. Apart from metrics, Nyra continued to bulk her resume. She began working in a research laboratory and is in line to publish at least one first-author paper. She also continued her narrative surrounding women's health by volunteering at a women's and children's shelter. Thick quads, poppin' triceps – that CV was getting SWOL!

Nyra plans to reapply to medical schools during the 2021-2022 cycle. With her new MCAT score, an even better resume, an additional recommendation letter from her lab's PI, and a master's degree, I truly believe that Nyra will be a contender for any medical school in the country. A critical piece of her much-improved performance is her taking the time needed to improve her application. Nyra did not rush her reapplication. It is too soon yet to tell, but I have a hunch that this hard work will pay off for her in big ways.

CHAPTER 18

RESULTS

ACCEPTANCES

I skipped ahead to write this chapter a few days after a glorious and unexpected week of acceptances. Earning an acceptance to medical school is truly a triumph. Years of tireless hard work and hoop jumping come to a close. Of course, this win only unlocks another four years of hoops and exhausting work – but you will be immersed in medicine, doing what you love! Yay!

Nonexistent is the premed who has not imagined the moment when she receives her first acceptance to medical school. Each of us has spent waking hours over the years imagining what it would be like to open an email or answer a ringing phone and be greeted with "Congratulations! I am delighted to inform you...". Thoughts of joyful tears, frantically calling your parents to share the news, and pure elation are what fill the daytime fantasies of premedical students.

With these expectations in mind, viewing Reddit's premed forum may be puzzling once acceptances begin to be released. Although I do not have a Reddit account, I often visited the site throughout the application cycle to listen in on the conversation. People like me are known as Reddit lurkers. A number of posts that I have seen address how people felt unexpectedly subdued after earning an acceptance to medical school. These posts, as well as my own varied and unexpected reactions to acceptances, have prompted me to comment on the emotional reality behind an admittance into medical school.

My first admittance to medical school came on October 15th. For those familiar with the application cycle, October 15th has historically been the first day that schools release acceptances. This has changed recently, but for the 2020-2021 cycle, most rolling schools stuck to this timing. On the evening of October 14th, I was invited to a last-minute Zoom call with Case Western that would be taking place the following morning. The message wasn't specific about what the call was addressing, but I had a hunch that it was an acceptance surprise. The following morning, I woke up early to hop on the Zoom call, and my mom anxiously waited outside the office door as I logged into the call. After welcoming us with straight faces, the serious veneer was soon broken. Party hats flew on, and the impromptu welcoming committee exclaimed congratulations. I was thrilled to be accepted in such a touching manner. My mom rushed into the room and listened to the kind words spoken by the

Admissions Dream Team (what Case Western's admissions team has named themselves – a name that I think is well-deserved). I was ecstatic to be admitted to a medical school that I loved, but more than anything, I was relieved. I knew that I would become a physician.

What surprised me about finally being admitted to medical school was that the relief soon outweighed the excitement, and emotional exhaustion followed. The exhaustion came from six years of directed, purposeful work toward "the acceptance moment" as well as the months of interviews that still lay before me. It's almost absurd that a phone call or an email (in my case, a Zoom call) is truly life-changing. Truly life-changing in the sense that your trajectory is suddenly altered. One moment, you're on one side of a wall that you've been unremittingly stretching to peek over, and the next moment, you've found yourself, at last, on the other side. It's such a tremendous change that I don't think that I have been able to completely comprehend it in the months since finding myself on the other side of the wall. I know I will be in medical school soon, but until I'm there, I don't think that I'll quite understand that my career is beginning.

Beyond the emotional exhaustion, I was soon awash with anxiety. I had always expected the nerves to melt away once I knew that my fate was near-sealed and that I would become a physician. In reality, although I knew that I would be in medical school come summer, I still didn't know what that would look like. There were over a dozen post-interview decisions that awaited me. I couldn't plan for my life because I still couldn't see my next four years. Would I be in Cleveland or another city? Would I be close to my family? What would my classmates be like, and who were they? None of these questions could yet be answered. This uncertainty and inability to plan kept me anxious.

I am ashamed to say that there was another large source of my discomfort. I had an unhealthy focus on the schools I had yet to hear from. Because of this, my emotions would oscillate between restless and subdued. On October 15th, although I was delighted to have my acceptance to Case Western and then one to Tufts that came a few hours later, I kept obsessing over whether I would hear from UCLA. I spent most of the afternoon waiting for a Los Angeles number to ring my phone or an email from their office to ping my inbox. Unknown to me, an email from UCLA wouldn't arrive until six months later. Why couldn't I have celebrated my victories and then rest satisfied? Why was I obsessed with the unknown?

My disposition hit a low point on November 30th. That day, I was admitted to Northwestern Feinberg – a huge deal considering that Feinberg was one of my top choices going into the admissions cycle. If anyone had told me months prior (before the admissions cycle vortex began swirling) that I would be admitted to Feinberg, I would have lost my marbles. When the acceptance email arrived in my inbox on the evening of the 30th, I was overwhelmed. Disbelief that I had been accepted combined with joy. Yet, again, everything felt muted. Nervous hand-wringing returned as my focus re-settled on programs that I had not heard from. I felt that I couldn't truly celebrate my acceptance to Feinberg because I didn't even know if I would matriculate there. What was the point of getting excited about a program that I might not attend? I wish that I could have been one of those people who could push aside my worries and relish in these accomplishments. Looking at Reddit's premed community, it seems that I wasn't alone in this struggle. Although these experiences are a bit of a bummer, I'm sharing my own acceptance moments to give you a heads-up on what your own acceptance moments may look like. I never expected medical school acceptances to be wrapped up in complex emotions, but they were.

Before getting too doomy and gloomy, there is some good news to share! I did, in fact, have the magical acceptance moment. Yale was my top choice for medical school going into the admissions cycle. After interviewing with YSM (Yale School of Medicine) and all other programs, I began feeling confident that I would be happiest as a student there. Yale had told us that they would be releasing their admissions decisions by March 15th, yet on February 24th, I found myself scrolling through SDN to see if there were updates from other applicants. I scrolled to the bottom of the page, and there it was: a user named Lawlify had just been accepted to YSM. I knew that this meant one thing – decisions were out for everyone.

Hastily, I clamored to open my email, knowing that my YSM decision would be sitting in my inbox. As my inbox loaded, I repeated a few words to myself, "It's okay. The decision will be a waitlist or a rejection. It will be okay." Clearly, I was preparing for disappointment. I took a deep breath as my emails appeared before me. "Yale School of Medicine MD Acceptance" stared back at me. Needless to say, I totally freaked.

I gaped at the email for a solid 60 seconds before rushing to the bathroom. I was at work at my mom's company, but she was on a call, so I couldn't rush into her office and tell her. Instead, I sprang into the women's restroom and jumped up and down after making sure the stalls were empty. I was incandescently, purely joyful. I rushed back into the office so I could call my dad while my mom got off her work call. Of course, this was the ONE DAY that I had forgotten my cell phone at home. So, I sat. I sat at my desk, silently losing my mind, until I heard the click of the phone in my mom's office. Sharing my YSM acceptance with my mom and, soon after, my dad are moments I will cherish for the rest of my life.

My family and I knew that once Yale's acceptance came in, I would likely attend medical school there. At last, I was at peace. I could finally see around the bend what my next four years would look like. My medical school journey had come to a close.

Now, in actuality, the decision to commit to Yale was a bit more complicated than running off into the sunset with an acceptance letter in hand on my way to New Haven. Once scholarship offers came into the mix, the choice of where to matriculate became murky. The Deciding Where To Matriculate chapter will go into the process of comparing offers from my top choices and how I ultimately decided to enroll at YSM.

For many people, a mix of emotions comes with earning acceptances to medical school. I hope that sharing my own experiences can help you prepare for what to expect and, most importantly, feel less alone with the negative emotions that accompany this tangled process.

Another factor that shocked me is that I believed that if I got into Yale, I would be riding on cloud nine forever. Forever as in months or years. While I did experience days of elation, I soon returned to normal Caroline. Of course, I was thrilled to be matriculating to YSM that summer, but the emotional high wore off, as it always does. The hedonic treadmill caught up with me. Soon enough, I was my regular self: A very content self but back to normal, nonetheless. I had always imagined riding on months of pure invigoration if I were to get into my dream medical school. It's funny how quickly people – myself included – adapt to new circumstances. This is just another heads-up for anyone wondering what the emotional reality is behind medical school acceptances!

| Caroline's Medical School Application Cycle – Final Results |||
Applications (34)	Interviews (19)	Results
Baylor College of Medicine	Yes!	Waitlisted
Case Western Reserve University School of Medicine	Yes!	**Accepted**
Columbia University Vagelos College of Physicians and Surgeons		
Duke University School of Medicine		
Geisel School of Medicine at Dartmouth		
George Washington University School of Medicine and Health Sciences		
Harvard Medical School		
Icahn School of Medicine at Mount Sinai	Yes!	Waitlisted
Johns Hopkins University School of Medicine		
Keck School of Medicine at the University of Southern California		
Loyola University Chicago Stritch School of Medicine	Yes!	**Accepted**
Mayo Clinic Alix School of Medicine	Yes!	Waitlisted
New York University Grossman School of Medicine	Yes!	Rejected
Northwestern University The Feinberg School of Medicine	Yes!	**Accepted**
Oregon Health & Science University School of Medicine	Yes!	Withdrawal
Perelman School of Medicine at the University of Pennsylvania		
Saint Louis University School of Medicine	Yes!	**Accepted**
Stanford University School of Medicine		
The Warren Alpert Medical School of Brown University	Yes!	Waitlisted
Tufts University School of Medicine	Yes!	**Accepted**
University of California, Los Angeles David Geffen School of Medicine	Yes!	Waitlisted
University of California, San Diego School of Medicine	Yes!	Waitlisted

University of California, San Francisco, School of Medicine		
University of Chicago Division of Biological Sciences The Pritzker School of Medicine	Yes!	Waitlisted
University of Cincinnati College of Medicine		
University of Michigan Medical School	Yes!	**Accepted**
University of North Carolina at Chapel Hill School of Medicine		
University of Pittsburgh School of Medicine		
University of Virginia School of Medicine	Yes!	**Accepted**
Vanderbilt University School of Medicine	Yes!	**Accepted**
Wake Forest School of Medicine of Wake Forest Baptist Medical Center		
Washington University in St. Louis School of Medicine	Yes!	**Accepted**
Weill Cornell Medicine		
Yale School of Medicine	Yes!	**Accepted**

WAITLISTS

Waitlists are tough to grapple with. On the one hand, you are happy to still have a chance at being accepted. On the other hand, the difficult application process is dragged out even further. The good news is that I think each year, nearly every medical school takes people from their waitlist into the incoming class. At many schools, including top schools like Yale and Mayo, over 25% of the incoming class comes from the waitlist.

From my experience, medical schools really like you if they offer you a waitlist spot. It's challenging for medical schools to choose who is admitted outright and who is placed on the alternate list. Although I withdrew from each of my seven waitlist positions before May 1st (typically, waitlists begin moving on May 1st because the commit to enroll deadline is April 30th), I have some tips to share on how to get a seat in the incoming class off of the waitlist. I never had the opportunity to test these methods myself, but I have seen them work for others.

First, once you are put on a waitlist, I recommend reaching out to the admissions team to thank them for continuing to consider your candidacy and express your enthusiasm about the possibility of joining the incoming class. I would also reach out to your interviewers if you have their contact information. To your interviewers, send an update that you are on the waitlist and share how your conversation has left you excited about the possibility of joining the incoming class. Also, ask your interviewers if they have any tips for earning an acceptance off of the waitlist. While your interviews may no longer have a say in your admission, they might relay your comments back to the admissions office and advocate for your acceptance.

Second, depending on when you are put on the waitlist, I would send a minimum of one and a maximum of three letters to the admissions committee. For example, if you are placed on a waitlist in December and want to attend the program, I would send one or two updates between January and the end of March and then send a letter of interest or intent in April. If you are placed on a waitlist in March, I would send a combined update letter and letter of interest or intent in April. Programs will evaluate their waitlists continuously but will seriously start looking at who should be offered acceptances in April. Send a letter of intent in April to your dream waitlist schools. Send very strong letters of interest to all other waitlist schools. Overall, staying engaged and connected to the admissions team will show them that you are serious about joining the incoming class. When evaluating the alternate list, a program has two goals: 1) to choose someone who will balance the current class makeup (e.g., if there are currently 30 women enrolled and 40 men enrolled, women on the waitlist will likely be favored over men), and 2) to select someone who will enthusiastically accept the offered seat. While you have no control over the first factor (the current enrollee makeup), you have ample control over the second factor. The admissions team wants to choose people who want to be a part of the class, so put your best foot forward and show yourself as an engaged prospective student. None of these tips can guarantee a spot off the alternate list, but I think following through on this plan can give you a dang good shot at earning an acceptance.

The toughest waitlist that I received during my application cycle was to Mayo. I absolutely loved my interviews with Mayo; the administration was very engaged throughout the application process. For months, Mayo was where I thought I would end up for medical school, and I even decided to send a post-interview letter of intent. To be honest, despite Mayo's low acceptance rate, I thought I had my spot in the bag! I felt sunk when the acceptance calls for Mayo came and went, and I found myself with an empty voicemail. The school that I believed I was such a perfect fit for didn't exactly share my sentiments. I was grateful when the alternate list offer came into my inbox, but the excitement that I once had for the school had somewhat dulled. Waitlists are emotionally exhausting. Being strung along even further down the bumpy path of medical school admissions is grueling. Fortunately, by the time my waitlist for Mayo came, I had begun thinking that Yale would be the best fit for me. It ended up being a blessing that I was waitlisted at Mayo and didn't get stuck choosing between them and Yale. I still love Mayo ardently and look forward to applying to their residency programs!

REJECTIONS

Post-interview rejections are the most bitter of pills to swallow. It's one thing to get rejected without an interview – maybe the admissions team ran out of time to read your file, or maybe your application got randomly sandwiched between those of two Rhodes Scholars. Who knows?! But post-interview rejects definitely feel more personal. The school was excited to interview you and hand-selected your file out of thousands of others, only to have a first date and then say, "Eh, no thanks!" WTF?!

My post-interview rejection to NYU was a particularly salty one. My interview cohort was told on interview day that a few students are accepted outright, a few are rejected outright, and the vast majority of people are placed on hold for reconsideration. Can you guess where I found myself? That's right. I was flat-out rejected not even two weeks after my interview. Literally, I was in the first rejection batch to be sent out. LOL! It was hard to be given the boot at the tuition-free, top-ranked medical school. Ouchy! While I certainly felt down in the dumps for a bit, in truth, NYU was not at all a good fit for me. My interview was less than ideal. In part, it was my first MMI interview – a lot of their questions took me by surprise, and I accidentally didn't stick with my answer method because I was too thrown off by their questions. By the time my UMich interview came around, I was ready to rumble with MMI questions. Also, my interviewer asked me a no-no question, as I documented in the *What To Do if an Interview Bombs* section, which really turned me off from the school. Overall, I believe that the NYU admissions team made the best decision for both of us, but it still hurt to receive a swift no.

Had Yale been the school to reject me post-interview, I would have wallowed in sadness for a long time. There's nothing wrong with taking time to grieve a love lost. Even if that love is a dream school. When I applied to colleges, I was waitlisted at Harvard (my dream school) and eventually told that I would not be getting off of the waitlist. It was super painful to reconcile the loss of the college that I had dreamed of attending. To be honest, I was in a funk for about two years. Only within the last couple of years have I totally gotten over my heartbreak from that admissions decision. Part of what helped me overcome my heartbreak was the incredible experience I had at WashU. I graduated from WashU virtually certain that I would not have had a better experience at Harvard. WashU was just what I needed. The classes pushed me to learn effective critical thinking. My mentors were incredibly supportive and generous. The opportunities I was granted were enriching and made me a competitive medical school applicant. WashU was the home that I needed.

Although dealing with post-interview rejections is incredibly difficult, be sure to find time to set those emotions aside – even temporarily – to look at your medical school options. Maybe that option is another acceptance. Perhaps it is a band of waitlists. And possibly the remaining option is a reapplication. Whatever your next move forward is, be sure to approach it with gusto. Take a look at the programs where you have an acceptance. Work vigorously to get off of a waitlist. Diligently examine your previous application to determine what can be improved for the next application cycle. Don't let the rejections get you down forever. But don't let anyone make you feel guilty for mourning your losses. Make the most of your circumstances like I did at WashU, and the sky will be your limit!

CHAPTER 19

DECIDING WHERE TO MATRICULATE

As I hinted earlier, I expected my admission to Yale to be the slam dunk, one-and-done matriculation decision. In reality, it wasn't that simple. I think in my heart of hearts, I knew that I would attend YSM in the end, but this didn't change the difficulty of choosing among my other options. In this chapter, we will discuss researching your school choices, scholarship negotiation, and second-look events – all of which help you decide where to enroll. Before we begin, I'll share the thought process that led me to commit to YSM.

Of the schools to which I was admitted, I was able to narrow down to these top five: Northwestern Feinberg, University of Michigan, Vanderbilt, Washington University, and Yale. You will likely notice that a common factor among these five schools is that they are highly-ranked medical schools. The reason why I favored these high-ranking programs was because of the success rate of these programs in placing students into dermatology residency programs. I knew that dermatology was the specialty that I planned to pursue post medical school. Given that dermatology is one of the most competitive specialties, I sought to maximize my chance of success; applying from a top-ranked medical school would be a strong asset. I didn't want to get all the way to medical school and then not match into my specialty of choice because I was at a school where very few students each year matched into dermatology.

For my readers, looking at the match lists of your admitted and waitlisted schools can guide you to where their students match. Observe what specialties students match into, how many students are matching into those specialties, and what the specific matches are (which hospital/program). Dermatology seemed highly achievable at my top five schools based on my looking into these three questions.

Furthermore, it may seem counterintuitive, but I have come to learn that "top" medical schools tend to be more relaxed (have less strenuous grading) compared to other programs. I'm not sure why "top" programs are more relaxed, but I wanted to choose a school where I could focus on research, which is critical for matching into dermatology, and not be totally washed away by the stress of grading. More to this point, WashU became difficult in this regard because they split their class into thirds in terms of academic performance. I knew that being ranked into thirds would eat at my sanity during medical school and make it difficult for me to concentrate on other activities, especially because dermatology is more likely than other specialties to consider class rank. This ranking system was the biggest drawback of WashU. Similarly, Northwestern had Alpha Omega Alpha Honor Medical Society (AOA) for top students. While Northwestern's students told me that AOA wasn't important, I feared how important it would be for dermatology matching, which historically has heavily weighed AOA membership. In fact, it is reported in the 2019 match statistics that 49% of dermatology matches are AOA members (How to (Actually) Match into Dermatology, The Vibrant Med), which is particularly notable considering how many medical schools no longer have AOA.

UMich offered me an incredibly generous scholarship, as did Northwestern, and eventually, WashU even threw a little cash my way. These scholarships were what really made my decision-making difficult at another level. The debt that medical students enter into is significant. Considering how $100,000 in loans versus $200,000 in loans will affect your stress levels and quality of life as a resident physician should be taken seriously and discussed with your family and mentors. Ultimately, I chose to attend Yale, the more expensive program compared to UMich and Northwestern, because I felt that the extra debt was worth the "Yale experience." What I mean by the "Yale experience" is not only their no grades and no competition model (which I was thrilled about!) but more so that attending Yale would expose me to opportunities that I do not believe I would get at other institutions. In my first few months at Yale, these rarified opportunities have been abundant. I met and spoke with several of my biggest heroes: writers, statisticians, and politicians whom I do not think I would have otherwise met without the Yale magnet that attracts them to the university. I don't mean to sound pompous, but meeting these people has been one of the most enriching aspects of attending Yale. To me, these once-in-a-lifetime experiences have been worth the extra tuition money. I have also been able to significantly reduce the cost of attending Yale by applying to and being awarded several outside scholarships since the medical school does not offer merit aid.

I am also in the process of hunting down a single, lonely neurosurgeon to make my husband so I can graduate debt-free. Joking! Totally joking, totally just a joke... not to be taken seriously... at all... hehe!

Vanderbilt was the program that spoke to my heart in the same way that Yale did. As I learned more about the school, I saw myself thriving at Vandy. I loved that they had adopted Yale's minimal grades/no competition curriculum. I loved that Vandy was in Tennessee. The students were kind and engaged. I was a sucker for Vandy from the beginning. When examining Vandy further, I hesitated because they had quizzes every week during the M1 year, while Yale had none. Also, Yale had more dermatology matches each year, and Yale's matches were to better residency programs. Lastly, while Vandy offers merit aid, they choose not to send even a poor man's penny my way. On the other hand, Yale had no merit aid because they got rid of it years ago. While Vandy and Yale cost nearly the same amount to attend, you could say I was bitter (a bit butt hurt) that Vandy refused to pay this hussy some hush money even after I showed them my fat scholarships from UMich and Northwestern. The least they could have done if they ran out of scholarship money is offer me a ripe, juicy neurosurgeon with a ripe, juicy wallet to pay my bills. Am I right? What must a girl do to live like a queen around here?! And for all of you making a fuss about the med student-attending relationship dynamic, I have one question for you: why play for the rookie league when you can go pro? Now gimme that fist bump, baby!

What made Yale a standout medical school compared to my other options was the Yale System of Education (YSM's curriculum that emphasizes collaboration and minimal grading). Coming from WashU, which was collaborative but also academically challenging and therefore stressful, I valued a medical school where I could learn for my career rather than learn to get top scores on exams. Learning for one's career and not for a score is one of YSM's educational mottos. Medical school is full of people who are smarter than me and who are better test takers. Trying to outscore my peers to achieve the highest quartile ranking or earn Alpha Omega Alpha (Honor Medical Society) membership was *not* how I wanted to invest my time as a student. Being in an environment that rewards the minutiae of scoring in the 85th versus the 90th percentile on difficult exams would inundate me with stress and not allow me to direct sufficient attention toward research, volunteering, mentoring, and other activities. Moreover, I didn't want the minutiae of academic performance to determine what specialty I could match into. The feeling of every quiz and every exam pushing the needle on whether I could match into dermatology would be unbearable. Having experienced significant testing anxiety during my senior year of college, this was not a feeling to be ushered back into my psyche during medical school.

During orientation at YSM, our curriculum directors stated that they consider our pre-clerkship exams (known as qualifiers) to be pass/pass. It takes a lot to derail a YSM student. When these rare occurrences have happened, the derailment is most often rooted in notable personal life challenges rather than an inability to perform academically. Derailed students are also tended to by the administration in order to get them back on track. Admissions directors select YSM students who are highly self-motivated because of the relaxed nature of the school. Even with minimal hard markers of performance, YSM students perform exceptionally well on the USMLE exams and become expert physicians. Non-mandatory classes plus a few graded assessments mean that students are able to tailor their studying toward the USMLE Step Exams. Since Step 1 and Step 2 are the graded assessments that matter most to residency programs (soon to be just Step 2 with Step1 becoming pass/fail), it is wise to invest study time toward acing these two exams rather than memorizing a professor's long-winded tangents during a class lecture.

Clerkship grading is equally important as pre-clerkship grading. A MedBros video underscored the unique grading of YSM clerkships when Shaman, a YSM student, compared his educational experience to that of his sister, Puneet - a Mayo student. In the video, Puneet shared that she has felt more stress during Mayo clerkships than during her time at UC Berkeley because cutoffs to earn clerkship honors are incredibly high. Shaman added that he initially didn't believe the cutoffs that Mayo students needed to meet to earn honors, noting huge gaps between Mayo's cutoffs and those of other medical schools. Part of why clerkship grading at most medical schools is stress-inducing for students is because much of the grade depends on shelf exam performance. Shelf exams are taken during each of the core clerkships and test subject-based knowledge with officially licensed **NBME (National Board of National Examiners)** exams (Wolters Kluwer). These exams are difficult and require significant preparation time to score well, thus scoring within a range that earns clerkship honors. Balancing shelf exam studying with clerkship duties is a long-standing challenge for medical students, worsened by high honors cutoffs. While nearly all U.S. medical students deal with this challenge, YSM students do to less of an extent. YSM's shelf exams do not count toward clerkship grades. This means students do not need to pour over surgery material after coming home from a 12-hour surgery shift. Additionally, the cutoffs for honors at YSM are generous. These differences in clerkship grading between YSM and

Mayo were a large push for me to feel a stronger fit with YSM, and ultimately, I chose not to work the Mayo waitlist. Since competitive residencies heavily weight clerkship grades, those aspiring to become interventional radiologists, ophthalmologists, plastic surgeons, or, in my case, dermatologists are under more pressure. Medical school is taxing as is. The more that our environment can reduce stress, the better.

Whether researching medical schools by watching YouTube videos, speaking with current students and faculty, or pouring over match statistics, conducting a thorough inquisition is critical to choosing a school where you will thrive. Another consideration pushing me toward YSM over Mayo again came from Shaman and Puneet's conversation. Quick note - I promise that I am not trying to bash the Mayo Clinic through YSM comparison. I adore the Mayo Clinic and would have loved being a medical student there. In some ways, it may be more stressful than YSM, but it is an outstanding program. The people whom I met at Mayo were my favorite from interview season, and I am still in touch with both of my interviewers and a Mayo faculty member, even though I was waitlisted and chose to attend YSM. In Shaman and Puneet's conversation, Puneet remarked that YSM had an edge over Mayo because of the number of other graduate and undergraduate students that Yale medical students can interact with. Medical schools associated with larger universities allow students to befriend undergraduates as well as law, business, and Ph.D. students. This creates a much larger pool of people to interact with and exposes medical students to those outside the medical field. If someone is looking to find a spouse, being able to choose from a larger and more academically diverse pool is beneficial. At Mayo and other medical schools that are either removed from associated campuses (e.g., the medical school is miles away from the law and business schools) or do not have other associated programs (e.g., the medical school is a stand-alone program that is not affiliated with a larger university), there is a smaller group of people to befriend and date. Among this smaller group, it is likely that most people work in healthcare and, by nature, are less diverse in terms of academics and career choice.

While having access to affiliated programs and schools was not an obvious factor as I compared medical schools, I would now say that it is something important to consider. As a Yale medical student, I have recently joined a club for Yale law students and have already enjoyed get-togethers with club members. I love healthcare people but am extremely excited to build friendships with law students. Moreover, a new classmate and I are planning to study in the Law Library to find our husbands! Yay! Our mothers met before the White Coat Ceremony and devised their own plot to track how many hours we spend in the Law Library - they have to ensure that we are invested in Mission Hubby Hunting.

Mission Hubby Hunting is not the only way I will spend my free time. As someone looking to match into dermatology without taking a dedicated research year, I will be investing my non-studying hours into dermatology research, volunteering at the local free clinic, and mentoring local high school and college students who are interested in healthcare careers. The Yale System curriculum makes maximizing the hours spent on these activities (especially research) possible. Minimal assessments, a few mandatory activities, and pass/pass grading were designed to allow YSM students to spend their pre-clerkship months outside of the classroom. Yale wants to develop physicians who did not just train as medical students but who trained as medical students, researchers, global health specialists, local community leaders, and health policy experts. For those looking to match into a competitive specialty, having control over your time as a medical student is critical to allowing you to focus on both classes and meaningful research. When choosing a medical school, control over one's time is absolutely something to look into.

All prospective students need to consider a program's match list before deciding where to matriculate. Match lists show where graduating students have been matched for residency. Yet, not all match lists are created equal. The most competitive specialties, such as otolaryngology, plastic surgery, dermatology, and ophthalmology, will decorate the match lists of top medical schools and be completely absent from other medical schools' match lists. Typically, students from all U.S. M.D. programs have a shot at any competitive specialty. D.O. students, IMG students (international medical graduates), and Caribbean M.D. students have a much harder time matching into the most sought-after specialties. Although possible, D.O.s, IMGs, and Caribbean M.D.s usually need exceptionally high Step 1 and Step 2 scores in addition to remarkable research achievement to match into plastic surgery, radiation oncology, and the other top residencies. Furthermore, top medical schools will also send more of their graduates to top residency programs for all specialties. Is your dream to complete a residency at Massachusetts General Hospital or the Mayo Clinic? You will have a much easier time doing so if you attend a top medical school. Again, those not attending top medical schools can also match into top residency programs - it just can be more difficult to do so. Match lists are often region-specific. Medical schools in the Midwest can have a Midwest-centric match list. East Coast medical schools likely send a large portion of their graduates to East Coast residencies. The same goes for the West Coast. If you are set on living in a certain geographic region for residency, then the location of your medical school and how it impacts the match list is something to consider. The last word about location - residency programs associated with a medical school will often like taking their own students. For example, current Mayo medical students are probably in the best position to match to a Mayo residency - even in a better position than Harvard medical students wanting to match at Mayo. Connections to your home program are a huge advantage for residency matching.

The final five factors I considered before committing to YSM were the following:

> *One - I loved WashU as an undergraduate but wanted to try out a new university for medical school.* Many an undergraduate day was spent bouncing around Washington University School of Medicine (WUSM), so I was quite comfortable with the school and St. Louis as a city. I also knew many current WUSM students, so I felt socially comfortable. Comfort is a great thing, but I wanted to be pushed outside of my comfort zone for medical school, thus giving YSM an advantage over WUSM.

> *Two — Haters don't come for me, but the Yale name did come into play during decision-making.* Fellow WashU students share my pain in knowing what it is like for no one to know where you attended college. "Oh, you mean the University of Washington? I didn't know Washington State had a remote campus in Missouri?" These are the common responses to telling people that you attend WashU. Yale students do not have this same issue. To be clear, Yale's name recognition was not at all a massive factor in deciding where to attend medical school. But it certainly was a bonus to know that I wouldn't have to explain to people where I attend medical school. For everyone about to come after me - I chose WashU for college over Cornell and Notre Dame (two

schools with much broader name recognition). Name recognition means much less to me than a strong fit with a program.

Three - Access to world-class researchers and the Ivy League network. During my research on YSM, I discovered fantastic faculty and researchers with whom I could learn and work. Beyond Yale, I was introduced to the Ivy League network as a platform for connecting across the universities. While I believe this network is more useful to those in law or business, the medical school Ivy League network comes into play during research year and residency matching. Students at Ivy League medical schools will often match to Ivy League residency programs. The network was not largely influential when choosing YSM, but it was something to consider.

Four - Finances were the biggest negative of YSM. I had large scholarships to UMich as well as Northwestern (Feinberg). Although attending Yale costs significantly more than attending UMich and Northwestern (Feinberg), the value of low stress through the Yale System and the value of attending my dream medical school outweighed the financial downside. The lack of competition with my peers would give me the best chance to match into dermatology. Ultimately, I want to become a dermatologist, and I want to be happy in medical school - these factors meant more to me than taking out fewer student loans. Lastly, the outside scholarships that I have been awarded this year already exceed the scholarship that I was offered at Northwestern (Feinberg). Outside scholarships are not a guarantee, but they are an example of finding alternate ways to finance your medical education that can lead to taking out fewer loans.

Five - My gut told me to choose YSM. Before submitting my primary application, I had a feeling that Yale would be the right medical school for me. I set these feelings aside, never believing that I would be offered so much as an interview with the program. Following the interview and acceptance, I knew that if I didn't attend YSM, I would likely regret the decision forevermore. With only one chance to attend medical school, I wanted to choose the dream school that I never thought I would have the opportunity to join. And so I did.

GETTING TO KNOW YOUR MEDICAL SCHOOL OPTIONS

Even as the medical school acceptances and waitlists begin rolling in, the work isn't over. It's time for research, baby! You should aim to answer specific questions about your medical school options before the April 30th commitment deadline.

<u>What is the total cost of each program?</u> Living costs are much higher in New York, but you likely don't need a car. Apartments are cheaper in St. Louis, but a car might be needed. What is the curriculum and grading like? UCLA and UMich have one year of pre-clinicals, while Mayo has two years of pre-clinicals. Vanderbilt has weekly quizzes during pre-clinical courses, while Yale's quizzes are anonymous and optional. Nearly every student at Yale earns honors during clinical rotations, while at Mayo, you have to work your booty off to earn honors. For me, I loved the idea of minimal grades and more collaboration, but my friend at Perelman was terrified of the lack of grading at Yale. We each will have preferences for different curricula.

<u>What are the research opportunities?</u> Yale has an abundant offering of research programs for medical school students with stipends offered, including the START program (Summer to Advance Research Training) for incoming students. Other schools may leave it up to you to find research funding and summer research programs. When can you begin clinical involvement? Many schools have begun giving students significant clinical exposure starting in the first month of the M1 year. Others may have you wait until year three before interacting with patients.

<u>What is mentorship like for students?</u> The best mentors value time with students, while other mentors are unengaged and see mentorship as more of a requirement than a joy. Testing how strong a school is with mentorship can be difficult before you get there, but here are some strategies that I used. Email a few faculty members whose research excites you or who are practicing in a specialty that you are interested in. Introduce yourself as a prospective student who is accepted or waitlisted and ask about the possibility of joining them in the clinic or on their projects. See how they respond. At Yale, every faculty member I contacted enthusiastically responded and offered me an opportunity to join their work. This spoke volumes to me regarding these individuals' passion for working with medical school students. Additionally, reach out to one or two first-year residents who just graduated from the medical school. See what

they have to say about their mentorship experiences. I did this with a first-year dermatology resident at Yale New Haven Hospital who has attended Yale for medical school. He gave me the most helpful advice for matching into dermatology that I have ever received – he told me about the best mentors that he had worked with and prompted me to reach out to them. Because of his guidance, I hope to make one of these recommended physicians my primary mentor and will shadow him in the next few months. New residents will likely be more candid than current medical school students focused on hyping their school. I highly recommend finding a resident or two (who matched well) to reach out to. Don't worry if, among a number of communications, you find someone who is unresponsive. That's to be expected. Only start worrying if unresponsiveness or lack of engagement seems to be a common theme in the program.

Do you have a strong inkling of which specialty you would like to match into? Do you have specialties narrowed down to a top three? It would be worthwhile to assess the strength of a school's specialties. Some programs are leaders in neurology but weaker in OB/GYN. If you're a neurology fiend, then this may be the school for you, but if you love OB/GYN, another school might be a better fit. Faculty in your specialty of interest will likely be writing recommendation letters on your behalf for residency. For example, the letters from faculty at a particularly strong psychiatry program may hold more weight than those written by people at lesser-known psychiatry programs. While this can definitely be frustrating, connections to influential faculty can go a long way. Yet, it is important to note that an exceptional letter from a weaker program is much better than a mediocre letter from a top program. Similarly, if your potential schools have residency programs in your specialty(s) of interest, assess these programs. Schools like their own candidates. This means that you probably have a good chance of matching back to your medical school for residency. If you love the emergency medicine residency program at one school, it may be a good idea to attend medical school there in order to give you the best chance of staying with that school for residency. I did a lot of research on Yale's dermatology residency program and determined that I would love to stay at Yale for residency. From talking to the first-year dermatology resident whom I mentioned above to seeing that the dermatology residency program went out of its way to create a mentorship program for current Yale medical students, I felt that I would be thrilled to stay at Yale for residency.

Not to obsess about metrics, but assessing the USMLE Step One and Step Two scores (soon to be only Step 2 scores) earned by medical school students at your potential schools is important. These averages are easy to find with a quick online search. High Step scores indicate a strong curriculum and a hardworking student body. Lower Step scores may be something to discuss with current medical school students. While USMLE scores are not the be-all and end-all, they are important if you want to match into a competitive specialty. I personally believe that with outside resources, you can achieve a top Step score wherever you attend medical school, but it is still important to check out a school's strengths and weaknesses with regard to USMLE. Tied to USMLE scores is the strength of a medical school's match list. Take a look at both the specialties that people are matching into as well as the location and strength of the residency programs. Top medical schools match a lot of people into the most competitive specialties: radiology, ophthalmology, dermatology, plastic surgery, etc. Students at medical schools that are not top programs can certainly still match into these specialties, but they will likely have to work harder for these spots because there is such a wealth of opportunities at top medical schools. Unfortunately, Caribbean students typically have a harder time matching into the most competitive specialties, but I'm sure that there are still success stories (Kevin Jubbal, M.D., Caribbean Doctor Speaks the Truth on Caribbean Medical Schools). Reach out to those people and learn from the steps that they took! Also, if you want to match into California for residency, see if a medical school is matching students into California programs. It is typical for medical schools to have regionally strong match lists. For example, West Coast medical schools likely match a lot of their students into West Coast residencies. Programs in the Midwest, such as WashU, usually have strong ties to Northwestern, UChicago, Vanderbilt, and other Midwest programs. Yale and the other Ivies have their network. If your family is in Georgia and you want to be close to them for residency, a medical school within the region might be your best bet. But please note that if you make a strong case to match into Georgia and go to medical school in Oregon, you absolutely can still successfully complete residency in Georgia. These are all just factors to consider.

Lastly – it's a bit mushy – but be sure to see how happy the medical students are. Medical students will definitely be stressed, but stress is not the same thing as unhappiness. At WashU, I was super stressed but also very content. To assess happiness, I would look to

M4s who have lived through the toughest parts of the program. They will likely have the clearest perspectives on their happiness over the four years of medical school. Happy students are successful students. And you want to be both happy and successful.

NEGOTIATING SCHOLARSHIPS

Show me the money! Has anyone ever seen Jerry Maguire? If you are a lucky ducky who was awarded a medical school's merit scholarship, you may have more good things coming! Those puppies can multiply. Each year, many students successfully negotiate merit awards with medical schools when they were not initially given. To use myself as an example, I earned two outright merit awards, both worth $10,000 per year, from Northwestern Feinberg and Saint Louis University. I was incredibly grateful for these awards, as I did not at all expect to earn any merit scholarships with my 3.19 second semester freshman GPA.

Negotiating merit awards is like negotiating job offers. While negotiating makes me uncomfortable, it is still important to play the game. Once I received my merit awards, I emailed the admissions offices at the University of Michigan, Vanderbilt, Yale, and WashU to see if they could match the offer. **Pro tip: a lot of medical schools will say that they don't match scholarship offers but will actually work with you** if you approach them. While Vanderbilt and Yale could not match the scholarships, WashU said they would try to match if additional scholarship funds became available closer to April 30th. This was not a guarantee, but I appreciated their effort. UMich, to my delight and wonder, returned a week after my initial inquiry with an offer of $35,000 yearly! I was incredibly touched by UMich's offer, and this is why my decision of where to attend medical school came down to UMich and Yale. Ultimately, I did choose to attend Yale for medical school, but this was a very difficult choice because I also loved UMich. I know some people will think that I am crazy for not taking the scholarship offer and running to Ann Arbor, but I made the decision that was best for me. Just to be transparent, the flexible, low-stress, and collaborative environment created by the Yale System is what I wanted out of my medical school education. Although it will certainly take me longer to pay off my loans from Yale, I am only going to attend medical school once, and I want to go to the school where I will be happiest.

For those wondering how to write an email to negotiate scholarships, here is what I sent to UMich, Vanderbilt, WashU, and Yale. Also, be sure to be truthful about the amount that your scholarship is worth because schools will ask for documentation of your award. I sent Feinberg's offer to UMich at the request of their admissions office.

Scholarship negotiation email:

Dear University of Michigan Medical School Admissions Team,

I hope you are enjoying the start of Spring! I am greatly enjoying UMich's Second Look events and am thrilled to have the opportunity to join the incoming class.

Last week, I received a merit scholarship from The Feinberg School of Medicine, and I am wondering if there is an opportunity for a merit scholarship with UMich. While I am likely not eligible for need-based aid due to my family's 2019 income, our income has been reduced due to a job change last March, making finances an important part of my medical school decision. I am honored to have a spot in UMich's Medical School Class of 2025, and a scholarship would help tremendously in weighing my medical school options. Please let me know if you would like me to send documentation of my offer from Feinberg - I would be happy to do so. I greatly appreciate your consideration of my request.

With gratitude,

Caroline Echeandia-Francis

SECOND LOOK

Second Look events are a great way to feel out the medical schools that you are choosing among. Most likely, you have not been able to take a hard look at a medical school since you interviewed with them. Second Look, usually a day-long or multi-day-long event for admitted applicants, will reintroduce you to the curriculum, research and clinical opportunities, distinguished faculty, current students, other prospective students, and even alumni. I encourage anyone who is stuck between their choices to attend the Second Look events for each program and ask themselves, "Can I see myself thriving here as a medical student?" Because all of the program information (curriculum, research, volunteering, mentorship, etc.) is often similar and can become muddled, I recommend taking diligent notes at each Second Look event. When reviewing my acceptances to medical school, I even looked back at the notes that I took on interview day to see what my thoughts were in the months prior.

From attending Second Look events, connecting with faculty and current students, evaluating scholarship offers, and thoroughly researching each program, you should have a strong foundation of information to guide your matriculation decision. Don't forget to listen to your gut in the process. Gut feelings count, too. During my application cycle, my gut mostly oscillated between Mayo and Yale. Having committed to enroll at Yale hours before writing this, I can say with glee that my gut has had no regrets.

SELECTING YOUR SCHOOL AND WITHDRAWALS

Before closing out this guidebook, I want to take a moment to acknowledge how painful it was to withdraw my acceptances and waitlist positions. No one told me how hard withdrawing would be. Each medical school where I interviewed was important to me, and those where I was accepted or waitlisted were that much more important. Throughout the application cycle, I saw how excited faculty, staff, and students were to welcome us to their program and how eager they were to recruit us as incoming students. Like many other applicants, I built relationships with and formed attachments to these people. We bonded over our love of medicine and the possibility of shared time at their program. I could have seen myself as a student at each medical school where I applied. Saying goodbye to a possible life with a unique group of friends in a particular city wasn't easy. My hardest goodbyes were to Case Western (my first acceptance), Northwestern and UMich (who had both been very connected to prospective students and had given generous scholarships), Vanderbilt (where I thought I would matriculate before my Yale acceptance), and WashU (my lovely alma mater that had continued to support my journey toward becoming a physician). I ended up writing emails to each of the schools where I withdrew my application. It was important for me to let them know how much their program meant to me and how difficult the choice not to attend was to make. For me (and I hope for them, too), this was an important piece of closure to an emotional, exhausting, and completely rewarding application cycle. Once I was at peace with each program where I withdrew my application, I was able — with an open heart — to commit to enrolling at Yale School of Medicine.

To perk yourself up from withdrawals, share news of your final medical school selection with your recommenders. I sent them a pic of me in a Yale t-shirt, and you should do your own mini photoshoot! This is the type of follow-up that builds lifelong relationships with our mentors. After writing one of your letters, recommenders will be thrilled to have played an important role in helping you get into medical school. **Rejoice in the shared victory with letter writers and loved ones. You're going to be a doctor! You did it!**

ACKNOWLEDGEMENTS

To everyone who has read this guidebook, thank you. I hope my words have helped you along your path to becoming a physician. The road to a career in medicine is long and tiresome, but in the end, I believe that the expedition will be entirely worth it. At Yale's Second Look for admitted students, I remember Dean Nancy Brown speaking to what she wished she had known as a medical school student. Dean Brown shared, "I wish I had known how good it would be." She expanded, saying that medical school was hard, and she remembered times when she wanted to quit. Looking back on her career decades later, Dean Brown shared that she was happy with her choice to become a physician. She closed by remarking, "What a wonderful way to spend one's life by serving others through medicine." I hope that one day, each of us will share Dean Brown's sentiments when we look back on our careers. I have a hunch that we will.

I also want to acknowledge those who helped me become a medical student and, soon, a physician. While it is impossible to fit everyone on this list, these are some of the most influential people who have supported and encouraged me on my path to Yale School of Medicine. One thing is clear from these acknowledgments: it takes a village to achieve one's dreams. My victories are due to many others. Nothing of consequence was realized in isolation.

Mom and Dad
Who never stopped loving and supporting me and whose daughter I am proud to be

Claire
Who has always shared her joy and humor to make life feel lighter

Grandpa
Who makes me proud of where I come from and who I am

Patti Moir
Who has shown me the meaning of true friendship

Dr. Phat Huynh
Who pushed me to reach my potential and is a life-long mentor

Dr. David Holtzman
Who set the foundation for my love of research

Dr. Craig Smith, Dr. Mary Lambo, Dr. Kyle McCommis, Abigail Green
Who selflessly and repeatedly gave of themselves to help me achieve my dreams

Laura Back and the Mulberries
Who generously and unrelentingly encouraged my ambitions and who cheered me on throughout the application cycle

APPENDICES

Appendix A
2014-2018 Aggregate Medical School Matriculant Statistics for WashU Undergraduates

Aggregate Medical School Matriculant Statistics for WashU Undergraduates (2014-2018)

SCHOOL	GPA Middle 50%	GPA Mean	MCAT Middle 50%	MCAT Mean
Albert Einstein College of Medicine	3.64-3.83	3.72	94-97	94.81
Baylor College of Medicine	3.66-8.87	3.75	95-98	95.39
Boston University School of Medicine	3.62-3.88	3.75	95-98	95.33
Case Western Reserve University School of Medicine	3.58-3.83	3.68	95-98	95
Columbia University College of P & S	3.77-3.95	3.81	97-99	97.71
David Geffen School of Medicine at UCLA	3.80-3.92	3.85	94.5-99	94
Drexel University College of Medicine	3.38-3.64	3.51	84.5-91.5	87.25
Duke University School of Medicine	N/A	3.75	N/A	91
Emory University School of Medicine	3.43-3.79	3.57	87.75-97	91.56
FIU Herbert Wertheim College of Medicine	3.32-3.59	3.47	77.5-X	83.82
George Washington University Sch of Med & Hlth Sci	N/A	3.59	N/A	88.29
Georgetown University School of Medicine	3.24-3.83	3.56	87-92.5	87.80
Harvard Medical School	3.90-4.00	3.91	97-100	96.27
Hofstra Northwell School of Medicine at Hofstra University	N/A	3.47	N/A	90
Indiana University School of Medicine	3.20-3.70	3.49	79-94	82.64
Johns Hopkins University School of Medicine	3.87-4.00	3.93	96-100	97.46
Keck Sch. of Med. University of Southern California	N/A	3.52	N/A	90
Lewis Katz School of Medicine at Temple University	3.40-3.73	3.57	86.5-92.5	87.27
Loyola University Chicago Stritch School of Medicine	3.29-3.68	3.49	79.5-90.5	83.11
LSU School of Medicine in New Orleans	N/A	3.23	N/A	83.29
Medical College of Wisconsin	3.44-3.68	3.54	79-94	83.96

New York Medical College	3.23-3.52	3.37	80.75-93	85.67
New York University	3.70-3.96	3.82	97-99	97.50
Northwestern University Feinberg School of Medicine	3.88-3.98	3.90	96-98	97.30
Oregon Health and Science University	N/A	3.43	N/A	80.2
Perelman School of Medicine at the University of Pennsylvania	3.75-3.99	3.85	96-99.25	96.08
Rosalind Franklin University of Medicine and Science	3.32-3.62	3.47	80.5-91	86.27
Rush Medical College	3.36-3.58	3.48	81.25-92.5	85.5
Rutgers New Jersey Medical School	N/A	3.51	N/A	94.67
Rutgers Robert Wood Johnson Medical School	N/A	3.44	N/A	90.78
Saint Louis University School of Medicine	3.63-3.83	3.71	87-96	89.4
Sidney Kimmel Medical College at Thomas Jefferson University	3.50-3.63	3.54	82.25-94.25	88.19
Southern Illinois School of Medicine	N/A	3.26	N/A	82.83
Stanford University School of Medicine	N/A	3.84	N/A	95.14
State University of New York Downstate Medical Center	N/A	3.36	N/A	89.89
Stony Brook University School of Medicine	N/A	3.81	N/A	88.43
Texas A&M Uni. System HSC Col. of Medicine	N/A	3.38	N/A	86.14
Texas Tech Univ. Hlth. Sci. Ctr. Sch. of Medicine	N/A	3.33	N/A	93.5
The Ohio State Univ. Coll. of Med.	3.42-3.85	3.64	95-98	95
The University of Miami School of Medicine	3.25-3.65	3.39	83-94	88.6
The University of Oklahoma	N/A	3.49	N/A	86.13
The University of Vermont College of Medicine	N/A	3.67	N/A	88
Tufts University School of Medicine	3.54-3.79	3.64	83-96.25	89.58
Tulane University School of Medicine	3.23-3.50	3.34	82.25-90.5	84.05
University of Arizona College of Medicine-Tucson	N/A	3.57	N/A	87.4

University of Arkansas College of Medicine	3.19-3.46	3.40	64-85.5	74.45
University of California San Diego	N/A	3.68	N/A	93.86
University of Chicago - Pritzker	3.67-3.97	3.74	91-99	93.52
University of Cincinnati College of Medicine	3.40-3.76	3.57	83-95	89.73
University of Colorado School of Medicine	3.47-3.73	3.57	89.5-94	91.71
University of Florida	N/A	3.75	N/A	95.2
University of Hawaii John A. Burns Sch. of Med.	N/A	3.54	N/A	87.8
University of Illinois at Chicago-College of Medicine	3.30-3.77	3.52	83-95	87.72
University of Iowa, Carver College of Medicine	3.43-3.74	3.54	88.25-96.75	90.61
University of Kentucky College of Medicine	N/A	3.49	N/A	91
University of Louisville School of Medicine	N/A	3.48	N/A	86.8
University of Maryland School of Medicine	3.51-3.77	3.63	89.5-95.25	91.95
University of Massachusetts Medical School	3.47-3.80	3.62	83.75-94.75	88.6
University of Michigan Medical School	3.67-3.82	3.68	91-99	92.46
University of Minnesota Medical School-Minneapolis/Duluth	3.53-3.91	3.64	88-94.75	89.67
University of Missouri-Columbia School of Medicine	3.35-3.65	3.48	79.5-95	85.96
University of Nebraska College of Medicine	N/A	3.45	N/A	87.38
University of Pittsburgh School of Medicine	N/A	3.70	N/A	96.44
University of Texas Medical School at Houston	N/A	3.50	N/A	90.4
University of Texas Medical School at San Antonio	N/A	3.45	N/A	87.44
University of TN Health Science Cntr Coll. of Med.	N/A	3.48	N/A	86.17
University of Virginia School of Medicine	3.81-3.93	3.78	94-99	95

University of Washington School of Medicine	N/A	3.53	N/A	92.63
University of Wisconsin	3.53-3.93	3.75	87-97.5	92.36
USF Health Morsani College of Medicine	3.13-3.66	3.42	85.25-98	91.33
UT Southwestern (TMDSAS)	3.53-3.85	3.66	89.5-96.5	91.33
UT Southwestern (AMCAS, MD/PhD)	N/A	3.74	N/A	97.67
Vanderbilt University School of Medicine	3.89-3.98	3.91	97-99	97.53
Virginia Commonwealth University School of Medicine	N/A	3.46	N/A	85.17
Warren Alpert Medical School of Brown University	3.61-3.80	3.68	85.5-93.5	90.2
Washington University School of Medicine	3.67-3.98	3.80	97-100	97.56
Weill Medical College of Cornell University	3.68-3.95	3.79	92.25-98.75	94.93
Yale School of Medicine	N/A	3.68	N/A	92

Appendix B
List of Academic Term and Post-Baccalaureate Research and Clinical Fellowships

- American Red Cross - Fall/Winter/Spring Internships
- Banner Health - Academic Year Intern/Volunteer
- Cleveland Clinic Lerner Research Institute - Undergraduate Research Opportunities at Lerner
- Eunice Kennedy Shriver National Institute of Child Health and Human Development – Post-baccalaureate Intramural Research Training Award
- F. Hoffmann-LaRoche - numerous academic term internships available
- GlaxoSmithKline - numerous academic term internships available
- Johnson & Johnson - numerous academic term internships available
- National Institutes of Health – Post-baccalaureate Intramural Research Training Award (Postbac IRTA/CRTA)
- Regeneron Pharmaceuticals, Inc. - numerous academic term internships available
- Sanofi - numerous academic term internships available
- Tufts University Graduate School of Biomedical Sciences - Tufts Post-Baccalaureate Research Program
- University of California San Francisco - Breast Care Center Internship Program
- University of Cincinnati College of Medicine - The Post-baccalaureate Research Education Program at the University of Cincinnati College of Medicine

Appendix C
List of Summer Research and Clinical Fellowships

- Albert Einstein College of Medicine - Summer Undergraduate Research Program
- Alliance for Health Policy - Fellowship Host Site
- Alpha Genesis Incorporated - AGI Pre-Baccalaureate Program
- American Cancer Society - Alvan T. and Viola D. Fuller Research Fellowships
- American Heart Association - Undergraduate Student Summer Fellowship Program
- American Physiological Society - Summer Undergraduate Research Fellowships
- American Public Health Association - Public Health Policy Internship
- American Red Cross - Summer Internships
- American Society for Microbiology - Microbiology Fellowship for Undergraduate Students
- American Society for Pharmacology and Experimental Therapeutics - Summer Undergraduate Research Fellow Awards
- Amgen Scholars Program
- Arkansas IDeA Network of Biomedical Research Excellence - Summer Research Fellowships for Undergraduate Students
- Arthritis Foundation - Summer Science Internship Program
- Association of American Medical Colleges - Summer Health Professions Education Program (numerous university sites)
- Augusta University - Summer STAR Program
- Baylor College of Medicine Graduate School of Biomedical Sciences - Summer Undergraduate Research Training Program
- Baylor College of Medicine Human Genome Sequencing Center - Summer Undergraduate Research Program
- Baylor College of Medicine, Department of Surgery - DeBakey Summer Surgery Program
- Bingham and Women's Hospital - Summer Training in Academic Research and Scholarship
- Binghamton University - Research Experience for Undergraduates Summer Program

- Boston Children's Hospital Division of Newborn Medicine - Summer Student Research Program
- Boston College - Research Experience for Undergraduates
- Boston University - Summer Undergraduate Research Fellowship Program
- Boston University School of Medicine Graduate Medical Sciences - Summer Training as Research Scholars Program
- Boston University School of Public Health - Summer Institute for Research Education in Biostatistics
- Brandeis University - Research Experiences for Undergraduates Program
- Broad Institute - Broad Summer Research Program
- Brooklyn College - Psychology and Neuroscience Research Experiences and Undergraduates
- Brown University - Minority Health and Health Disparities International Research Training Program
- Burke University Institute - Summer Science Research Program
- California Institute of Technology - Summer Undergraduate Research Fellowships
- California Institute of Technology - WAVES Fellows Program
- California State University, Department of Biological Science - Minority Health and Health Disparities Research Training Program
- Carle Illinois College of Medicine - REACH Program
- Carle Illinois College of Medicine - Research and Education for the Advancement of Compassionate Healthcare Program
- Case Western Reserve University - Academic Careers in Engineering and Science Summer Undergraduate Research Program
- Case Western Reserve University Case Comprehensive Cancer Center - Cancer-Focused Summer Undergraduate Research Program
- Case Western Reserve University School of Medicine - Heart, Lung, and Blood Summer Research Program
- Case Western Reserve University School of Medicine, Department of Pharmacology - Summer Undergraduate Research Program
- Center for Engineering MechanoBiology - Undergraduate Summer Research Experience Program
- Center for the Environmental Implications for Nanotechnology - Research Experience for Undergraduates Program

- Center for the Neural Basis of Cognition - Summer Undergraduate Research Program in Computational Neuroscience
- Centers for Disease Control and Prevention - Collegiate Leaders in Environmental Health
- Centers for Disease Control and Prevention - Summer ORISE Fellowship Opportunity
- Charles B. Wang Community Health Center - Project Asian Health Education and Development
- Charles R. Drew University of Medicine and Science Division of Cancer Research and Training - Undergraduate Cancer Research Training Program
- Children's Hospital Colorado - Child Health Research Internship
- Children's Hospital Oakland Research Institute - Summer Student Research Program at CHORI
- Children's Hospital of Philadelphia - Injury Science Research Experiences for Undergraduates
- Children's Hospital of Philadelphia Research Institute - The CHOP Research Institute Summer Scholars Program
- Children's Hospital of Pittsburgh - Summer Research Training Program
- Christian Brothers University - Minority Health and Health Disparities International Research Training Program
- Cincinnati Children's Hospital Medical Center - Biomedical Research Internship for Minority Students
- Cincinnati Children's Hospital Medical Center - Summer Undergraduate Research Fellowship
- City of Hope Cancer Center - Eugene and Ruth Roberts Summer Student Academy
- City University of New York - Summer Undergraduate Research Program
- Clemson University - Biophysics Summer Research Experience for Undergraduates
- Cleveland Clinic Lerner Research Institute - Undergraduate Research Opportunities at Lerner
- Cleveland Clinic Lerner Research Institute Department of Biomedical Engineering - BME Undergraduate Student Position
- Cold Spring Harbor Lab - Undergraduate Research Program

- Colorado School of Public Health, Department of Biostatistics and Informatics - Colorado Summer Institute in Biostatistics
- Colorado State University, Department of Biochemistry and Molecular Biology - Summer Research Experience for Undergraduates in Molecular Biosciences
- Columbia University Medical Center - Summer Program for Under-Represented Students - A Biomedical Research Program
- Columbia University Vagelos College of Physicians and Surgeons - Summer Public Health Scholars Program
- Columbia University's Mailman School of Public Health - Biostatistics Epidemiology Summer Training Diversity Program
- Coriell Institute for Medical Research - Summer Experience Program
- Creighton University - Undergraduate Biomedical Research Program
- Crohn's & Colitis Foundation - Student Research Fellowship Awards
- Cystic Fibrosis Foundation - Student Traineeship Award
- Dana-Farber/Harvard Cancer Center - Continuing Umbrella of Research Experiences Program
- Dartmouth College - Academic Summer Undergraduate Research Experience
- DePaul University - Medical Informatics Experiences in Undergraduate Research
- Dialysis Clinic, Inc. - Collegiate Medical Summer Internship Program
- Diné College - Summer Research Enhancement Program
- Drexel University College of Medicine - Summer Undergraduate Research Fellowship
- Duke The Graduate School - Duke Summer Research Opportunity Program
- Duke University - Research Experience for Undergraduates
- Duke University School of Medicine, Department of Pharmacology & Cancer Biology - Summer Undergraduate Research in Pharmacology and Cancer Biology Fellowship Program
- Duquesne University - Biology CIRCLE Program
- Duquesne University - Chronic Pain Research Consortium Undergraduate Research Experience
- Duquesne University - Neurodegenerative Undergraduate Research Experience

- East Carolina University Brody School of Medicine - Summer Program for Future Doctors
- Eastern Virginia Medical School - Summer Scholars Program
- Ecole Polytechnique Fédérale de Lausanne School of Life Sciences - EPFL School of Life Sciences Summer Research Program
- Emory University School of Medicine, Department of Medicine - Summer Undergraduate Program in Renal Research
- Endocrine Society - Summer Research Fellowships
- Eunice Kennedy Shriver National Institute of Child Health and Human Development - Summer Internship Program in Biomedical Research
- F. Hoffmann-LaRoche - numerous summer internships available
- Feinstein Institutes for Medical Research - Feinstein Summer Research Internship Program
- Florida Agricultural and Mechanical University - Undergraduate Research Experience in Genomics, Proteomics and Bioinformatics
- Florida Atlantic University Harbor Branch Oceanographic Institution - Marine Science and Engineering Summer Internships
- Fox Chase Cancer Center - Undergraduate Summer Research Fellowship
- Fred Hutchinson Cancer Research Center - Pathways Undergraduate Researchers
- Fred Hutchinson Cancer Research Center - Summer Undergraduate Research Program
- Geisel School of Medicine - MD-Ph.D. Undergraduate Student Fellowship
- George Mason University - Aspiring Scientists Summer Internship Program
- Gerstner Sloan Kettering Graduate School of Biomedical Sciences - Summer Undergraduate Research Program
- Gilead Sciences, Inc. - numerous summer internships available
- Gillette Children's Specialty Healthcare - Summer Research Internship Program
- GlaxoSmithKline - numerous summer internships available
- The Graduate School of the Stowers Institute - Stowers Summer Scholars
- Hackensack University Medical Center - Summer Clinical Research Volunteer Program

- Hampton University - Minority Health International Research Training Program
- Hartford Hospital - Summer Student Pre-Med and Research Programs
- Harvard Medical School - Harvard Summer Research Program in Kidney Medicine
- Harvard Medical School and Brigham and Women's Hospital - Four Directions Summer Research Program
- Harvard Medical School Blavatnik Institute Biomedical Informatics - Summer Institute for Biomedical Informatics
- Harvard Medical School Blavatnik Institute Cell Biology - Cell Biology Research Scholars Program
- Harvard Stem Cell Institute - HSCI Internship Program
- Harvard T.H. Chan School of Public Health - Summer Internships in Biological Sciences in Public Health
- Harvard T.H. Chan School of Public Health, Department of Biostatistics - Summer Program in Biostatistics and Computational Biology
- Harvard T.H. Chan School of Public Health, Department of Epidemiology - Harvard Multidisciplinary International Research Training Program
- Harvard University - Immunology Undergraduate Summer Program
- Harvard University - Molecules, Cells, and Organisms Summer Research Opportunities at Harvard Internship Program
- Harvard University - Summer Honors Undergraduate Research Program
- Harvard-MIT Health Sciences and Technology - HST-Wellman Summer Institute for Biomedical Optics
- Harvard-MIT Health Sciences and Technology - HST-Wellman Summer Institute for Biomedical Optics
- Hauptman-Woodward Medical Research Institute - numerous summer internships available
- Health Career Connection - Summer HCC Internship Program
- Hepatitis B Foundation - College Internship Program
- The Hormel Institute - Summer Undergraduate Research Experience Internship
- Hospital for Special Surgery - Summer Internship
- Houston Methodist - Summer Undergraduate Research Internship
- Howard Hughes Medical Institute - Undergraduate Scholars Program

- Hunter College, Department of Biological Sciences - Summer Program for Undergraduate Research
- Huntington's Disease Society of America - The Donald A. King Summer Research Fellowship
- Icahn School of Medicine at Mount Sinai - Global Health Disparities Research Training Program
- Icahn School of Medicine at Mount Sinai - Summer Undergraduate Research Program
- Icahn School of Medicine at Mount Sinai, Ma'ayan Laboratory, Computational Systems Biology - Summer Research Program in Biomedical Big Data Science
- Indian Health Service Extern Program
- Indiana University Melvin and Bren Simon Comprehensive Cancer Center - Summer Research Program
- Indiana University School of Medicine - Summer Undergraduate Research Experience in the Biomedical Sciences
- Indiana University School of Medicine - Undergraduate Research for Future Physician Scientists
- Indiana University School of Medicine Stark Neurosciences Research Institute - Medical Neuroscience Undergraduate Summer Research Program
- Indiana University School of Medicine Wells Center for Pediatric Research - Pediatric Research Summer Student Internship Program
- Ionis Pharmaceuticals - numerous research internships available
- Irene & Eric Simon Brain Research Foundation - IES Brain Research Foundation Student Summer Fellowships in Neuroscience
- J. Craig Venter Institute - Internship Program
- The Jackson Laboratory - Summer Student Program
- John Innes Centre - International Undergraduate Summer School
- Johns Hopkins Bloomberg School of Public Health - Diversity Summer Internship Program for Undergraduates
- Johns Hopkins Institute for Nanobiotechnology - Nanotechnology for Biology and Bioengineering Research Experience for Undergraduates Program
- Johns Hopkins Whiting School of Engineering - Research Experience for Undergraduates in Computational Sensing and Medical Robotics
- Johnson & Johnson - numerous summer internships available

- Joslin Diabetes Center - Summer Student Research Internship
- Juvenile Diabetes Research Foundation - JDFR's College Internship Program
- Kansas State University - Summer Undergraduate Research Opportunity Program
- Keck Graduate Institute - Summer Undergraduate Research Experience
- Kennedy Krieger Institute - Maternal Child Health Careers/Research Initiatives for Student Enhancement Undergraduate Program
- The Leadership Alliance - Summer Research Early Identification Program
- Lehigh Valley Health Network - Research Scholar Program
- Loma Linda University School of Medicine, Center for Health Disparities and Molecular Medicine - Undergraduate Training Program
- Louis de la Parte Florida Mental Health Institute - Summer Research Institute
- Louisiana Biomedical Research Network - LBRN Summer Research Program
- Louisiana State University Health Sciences Center, Department of Pharmacology, Toxicology and Neuroscience - Summer Undergraduate Pharmacology Experience in Research
- Louisiana State University School of Medicine, Department of Genetics - Research Experiences for Undergraduates in the Basic Sciences, Genomics, and Biochemistry
- Loyola University Chicago Stritch School of Medicine, Department of Molecular Pharmacology and Neuroscience - Discover Pharmacology Summer Undergraduate Research Fellowship
- Loyola University Medical Center, Department of Microbiology and Immunology - Undergraduate Summer Research Program
- Lupus Foundation of America - Gina M. Finzi Student Fellowship
- Magee-Women's Research Institute and Foundation - College Summer Internship Program
- Maine Medical Center Research Institute - Summer Student Research Program
- Marquette University College of Health Sciences, Department of Biomedical Sciences - Marquette Biomedical Sciences Summer Undergraduate Research Program

- Marquette University, Department of Biological Sciences - Undergraduate Summer Research Program
- Marshfield Clinic Research Institute - Summer Research Internship Program
- Masonic Medical Research Institute - Summer Fellowship Program
- Massachusetts General Hospital - Summer Research Trainee Program
- Massachusetts Institute of Technology - Bernard S. and Sophie G. Gould MIT Summer Research Program in Biology
- Mayo Clinic Biomedical Ethics Research Program - Summer Undergraduate Program in Biomedical Ethics
- Mayo Clinic College of Medicine and Science - Summer Undergraduate Research Fellowship
- McLaughlin Research Institute for Biomedical Sciences - numerous summer internships available
- Medical College of Wisconsin - Diversity Summer Health-Related Research Education Program
- Medical College of Wisconsin Graduate School - Summer Program for Undergraduate Research
- Medical University of South Carolina College of Graduate Studies - Summer Undergraduate Research Program
- Medical University of South Carolina College of Medicine - Drug Abuse Research Training Summer Research Fellowship Program
- Meharry Medical College - Meharry Cancer Summer Undergraduate Research Program
- MetroHealth - The Chester Summer Scholars Program
- Michigan State University College of Veterinary Medicine - Biomedical Research for University Students in Health Sciences Summer Research Program
- Michigan State University, Department of Pharmacology and Toxicology - The ASPET Summer Undergraduate Research Fellowship
- Minneapolis Heart Institute Foundation - Clinical Research Internship
- Moffitt Cancer Center - Summer Undergraduate Program to Advance Research Knowledge
- Monell Center - The Monell Science Apprenticeship Program
- Monmouth University School of Science - Summer Research Program
- Morehouse College Public Health Sciences Institute - Project IMHOTEP

- Morehouse College Public Health Sciences Institute - Public Health Leader Fellowship Program
- Mount Desert Island Biological Laboratory - IDeA Networks of Biomedical Research Excellence Program
- Mount Desert Island Biological Laboratory - National Science Foundation Research Experiences for Undergraduates Program
- Mount Desert Island Biological Laboratory - Science Education Partnership Award College of the Atlantic Undergraduate Fellowships
- Mount Desert Island Biological Laboratory - Undergraduate Student Summer Fellowships
- National Cancer Institute - Cancer Research Interns Program
- National Cancer Institute - Center for Cancer Research Summer Internships
- National Cancer Institute - Division of Cancer Epidemiology and Genetics Summer Program
- National Cancer Institute - Introduction to Cancer Research Careers
- National Cancer Institute - NCI Frederick Summer Programs
- National Cancer Institute - NIH Summer Internship Program
- National Cancer Institute - Summer Curriculum in Cancer Prevention
- National Center for Toxicological Research - NCTR Summer Student Research Participation Program
- National Eye Institute - NEI Summer Intern Program
- National Heart, Lung, and Blood Institute - Summer Institute in Biostatistics
- National Heart, Lung, and Blood Institute - Summer Internship in Biomedical Research
- National Human Genome Research Institute - Summer Internship Program in Biomedical Research
- National Institute for Mathematical and Biological Systems - Summer Research Experiences
- National Institute of Arthritis and Musculoskeletal and Skin Diseases - Scientific Summer Student Program
- National Institute of Biomedical Imaging and Bioengineering - Biomedical Engineering Summer Internship Program
- National Institute of Diabetes and Digestive and Kidney Diseases - NIDDK Diversity Summer Research Training Program for Undergraduate Students

- National Institute of Diabetes and Digestive and Kidney Diseases - Short-Term Research Experience for Underrepresented Persons
- National Institute of Environmental Health Sciences - NIH Summer Internship Program in Biomedical Research
- National Institute of Health - Summer Internship Program in Biomedical Research
- National Institute of Neurological Disorders and Stroke - Summer Program in the Neurological Sciences
- National Institute on Drug Abuse - NIDA Summer Research Internship Program
- National Institute on Drug Abuse Center for GWAS in Outbred Rats - Research Experiences for High School and Undergraduate Students
- National Science Foundation Engineering Research Center for Revolutionizing Metallic Biomaterials - Research Experiences for Undergraduates
- Nemours Children's Health System - Nemours Summer Undergraduate Research Program
- New York Blood Center, Lindsley F. Kimball Research Institute - Summer Internship for Undergraduates
- New York City Health Department - HRTP: A Public Health Internship Program
- New York University Center for Neural Science - Summer Undergraduate Research Program
- New York University Grossman School of Medicine Division of General Internal Medicine and Clinical Innovation - Program for Medical Education Innovations and Research Summer Scholars
- New York University Grossman School of Medicine Musculoskeletal Research Center - Interdisciplinary Orthopedic Research Opportunities
- New York University Grossman School of Medicine Vilcek Institute of Graduate Biomedical Sciences - Summer Undergraduate Research Program
- New York University Grossman School of Medicine, Ronald O. Perelman Department of Emergency Medicine - Emergency Medicine Project Healthcare Summer Volunteer Program
- New York University Grossman School of Medicine, Ronald O. Perelman Department of Emergency Medicine - Emergency Medicine Research Associate Internship

- North Carolina State University - Biotechnology Sequencing-Based Undergraduate Research Experience
- Northeastern University College of Science, Department of Biology - Summer Research Experiences for Undergraduates Program at Northeastern
- Northern Illinois University Institute for the Study of Environment, Sustainability and Energy - Research Experience for Undergraduates
- Northwestern University Feinberg School of Medicine Robert H. Lurie Comprehensive Cancer Center of Northwestern University - Cancer Undergraduate Research and Education
- Novartis Institutes for Biomedical Research - NIBR Summer Internship
- Office of Naval Research - Naval Research Enterprise Internship Program
- Ohio State University College of Pharmacy - Summer Undergraduate Research Fellowships
- Ohio University Heritage College of Osteopathic Medicine - National Science Foundation Research Experience for Undergraduates
- Ohio University Heritage College of Osteopathic Medicine - Summer Undergraduate Research Fellowship
- Ohio University Heritage College of Osteopathic Medicine - Summer Scholars
- Oregon Health and Science University Center for Diversity and Inclusion - Equity Research Program
- Oregon Health and Science University Oregon Institute for Occupational Health Sciences - Occupational Health Sciences Summer Internship
- Oregon Health and Science University Oregon National Primate Research Center - Summer Fellowship Program
- Oregon Health and Science University Oregon National Primate Research Center - Provost Scholar Program
- Oregon Health and Science University School of Medicine Neuroscience Graduate Program - Vollum/NGP Undergraduate Summer Research Program
- Oregon Health and Science University School of Medicine, Department of Medical Informatics and Clinical Epidemiology - Undergraduate Data Science Internship
- Parkinson's Foundation - Summer Fellowships

- Penn State College of Medicine - American Heart Association Undergraduate Student Fellowship Program
- Penn State College of Medicine - Short-Term Educational Program for Underrepresented Persons
- Penn State College of Medicine - Summer Undergraduate Research Internship Program
- Pepperdine University - Pepperdine University Seaver College Summer Undergraduate Research Program in Biology
- Plum Island Animal Disease Center - Research Participation Program
- Princeton Neuroscience Institute - PNI Summer Internship Program
- Purdue University College of Pharmacy - Summer Research Fellowships
- Purdue University, Department of Biochemistry - Research Experience for Undergraduates Molecular and Biochemical Analysis of Proteins
- Regeneron Pharmaceuticals, Inc. - numerous summer internships available
- Rhode Island IDeA Network of Biomedical Research Excellence - Summer Undergraduate Research Fellowships
- Rhodes College - Minority Health and Health Disparities International Research Training Program
- Rockefeller University - Chemers Neustein Summer Undergraduate Research Fellowship Program
- Roswell Park Comprehensive Cancer Center - Summer Programs College Research Experience
- Rowan University Graduate School of Biomedical Sciences - Summer Undergraduate Research Experience
- Rowan University Henry M. Rowan College of Engineering - National Science Foundation Research Experience for Undergraduates Site in Biomedical Materials, Devices, Therapeutics, and Emerging Frontiers
- Rutgers Center for Advanced Biotechnology and Medicine - CABM Summer Undergraduate Research Experience
- Rutgers Center for Computational and Integrative Biology - Research Experience for Undergraduates
- Rutgers Ernest Mario School of Pharmacy - Summer Undergraduate Research Fellowship
- Rutgers Institute for Health, Health Care Policy, and Aging Research - Project L/EARN Undergraduate Research Training

- Rutgers Robert Wood Johnson Medical School, Department of Neuroscience and Cell Biology - Summer Undergraduate Research Program in Neuroscience
- Rutgers School of Graduate Studies - Research in Science and Engineering
- Rutgers School of Graduate Studies - Summer Undergraduate Research Program
- San Diego State University - Minority Health and Health Disparities International Research Training Program
- San Jose State University - Research by Undergraduates using Molecular Biology Applications
- Sanford Research - Sanford Program for Undergraduate Research
- Sanford Research - Summer Undergraduate Research Experience Social-Behavioral Research Training in American Indian Community-Based Projects
- Sanofi - numerous summer internships available
- Sansum Diabetes Research Institute - numerous summer internships available
- Scripps Research - Summer Undergraduate Research Fellows
- SENS Research Foundation - SRF Summer Research Program
- Siemens Foundation - Siemens Foundation PATH Fellowships
- Society of Toxicology - numerous summer internships available
- The Spanish National Cancer Research Centre - Summer Training Programme
- St. Jude Children's Research Hospital - Pediatric Oncology Education Program
- Stanford School of Medicine - Canary Cancer Research Education Summer Training Program
- State University of New York at Albany - University at Albany Summer Research Program
- State University of New York at Buffalo - Collaborative Learning and Integrated Mentoring in the Biosciences Undergraduate Program for Summer Research
- State University of New York at Buffalo Jacobs School of Medicine and Biomedical Sciences - Summer Undergraduate Research Experience

- State University of New York at Buffalo The Institute for Strategic Enhancement of Educational Diversity - The iSEED Summer Research Experience Program
- State University of New York Downstate Health Sciences University - Exploring Health Careers
- State University of New York Downstate Health Sciences University - Early Medical Education Program
- State University of New York Downstate Health Sciences University - Summer Program in Translational Disparities and Community Engaged Research
- State University of New York Downstate Health Sciences University The School of Graduate Studies - Downstate Summer Research Program
- State University of New York Upstate Medical University - Mercy Works SYNERGY Summer Internship Program at Upstate
- State University of New York Upstate Medical University - Presidential Scholars Summer Internship Program
- State University of New York Upstate Medical University - Summer Undergraduate Research Fellowship Physician Scientist Program
- State University of New York Upstate Medical University College of Graduate Studies - Summer Undergraduate Research Fellowship Program
- Stony Brook University Renaissance School of Medicine - American Association for Pharmacology and Experimental Therapeutics Summer Undergraduate Research Fellowship
- Texas A&M University College of Medicine - Summer Research Program
- Texas Biomedical Research Institute Southwest National Primate Research Center - SNPRC Summer Internship Program
- Texas Commission on Environmental Quality - Mickey Leland Environmental Internship Program
- Texas Tech University Health Sciences Center Graduate School of Biomedical Sciences - Amarillo Biomedical Research Internship
- Texas Tech University Health Sciences Center Graduate School of Biomedical Sciences - Summer Accelerated Biomedical Research
- Thomas Jefferson University College of Life Sciences - Summer Undergraduate Research Programs
- Translational Genomics Research Institute - Helios Scholars at TGen

- Tufts University Graduate School of Biomedical Sciences - Building Diversity in Biomedical Sciences for Undergraduates
- Tulane University National Primate Research Center - Summer Research Program
- Tulane University School of Science and Engineering - Summer MAterials Research @ Tulane Research Experience for Undergraduates
- U.S. Food and Drug Administration - Medical Device Fellowship Internship Program
- U.S. Food and Drug Administration - National Center for Toxicological Research Summer Student Research Participation Program
- U.S. Food and Drug Administration The Center for Drug Evaluation and Research Summer Research Participation Program
- University of Alabama at Birmingham School of Medicine - Preparing for Graduate and Medical Education Summer Program
- University of Alabama at Birmingham School of Medicine - Summer in Biomedical Science Undergraduate Research Program
- University of Alabama at Birmingham School of Medicine, Department of Neurobiology - Summer Program in Neuroscience
- University of Alabama at Birmingham Sparkman Center for Global Health - Summer Global Health Internships
- University of Arizona Biosphere 2 - Research Experiences for Undergraduates Summer Program
- University of Arizona College of Engineering - Research Experiences for Undergraduates
- University of Arizona Graduate College - Minimizing Health Disparities
- University of Arizona Graduate College - Summer Research Institute
- University of Arkansas for Medical Sciences - Summer Undergraduate Research Program to Increase Diversity in Research
- University of Arkansas for Medical Sciences College of Medicine, Department of Biochemistry and Molecular Biology - Summer Undergraduate Research Fellowship Program
- University of Arkansas for Medical Sciences, Department of Pharmacology and Toxicology - Summer Undergraduate Research Fellowship Program
- University of California Davis Health, Department of Pathology and Laboratory Medicine - Hugh Edmondson Research Internship
- University of California Irvine Outreach, Research Training and Minority Science Programs - Bridges to Baccalaureate

- University of California Irvine Outreach, Research Training and Minority Science Programs - Minority Health and Health Disparities International Research Training Program
- University of California Los Angeles Brain Research Institute - Brain Research Institute Summer Undergraduate Research Experience
- University of California Los Angeles David Geffen School of Medicine - UCLA Pre-Medical Enrichment Program
- University of California Los Angeles Fielding School of Public Health - UCLA Public Health Scholars Training Program
- University of California Los Angeles Graduate Programs in Bioscience - Summer Program for Undergraduate Research Life and Biomedical Sciences
- University of California Los Angeles Institute for Quantitative and Computational Biosciences - Bruins-In-Genomics Summer Undergraduate Research Program
- University of California Los Angeles School of Nursing - Summer Research Program
- University of California San Diego - American Heart Association Undergraduate Student Research Fellowships
- University of California San Diego Graduate Division - Summer Training Academy for Research Success
- University of California San Diego School of Medicine - Medical Scientist Training Program Summer Undergraduate Research Fellowship Program
- University of California San Diego School of Medicine, Department of Pharmacology - Summer Undergraduate Research Fellowships Program
- University of California San Francisco Graduate Division - Summer Research Training Program
- University of California San Francisco, Department of Epidemiology and Biostatistics - Pre-Health Undergraduate Program
- University of Central Florida Nanoscience Technology Center - Research Experiences for Undergraduates
- University of Chicago Center for Global Health - Summer Research Fellowship
- University of Chicago Pritzker School of Medicine - Chicago Academic Medicine Program I

- University of Chicago Pritzker School of Medicine - Chicago Academic Medicine Program II
- University of Chicago Pritzker School of Medicine - Pritzker School of Medicine Experience in Research
- University of Chicago, Marine Biological Laboratory - Biological Discovery in Woods Hole Summer Opportunity for Undergraduate Research
- University of Cincinnati College of Medicine - American Society of Pharmacology and Experimental Therapeutics Summer Undergraduate Research Fellowship Program at the University of Cincinnati
- University of Cincinnati College of Medicine - Summer Undergraduate Research Fellowships
- University of Cincinnati College of Medicine - Summer Undergraduate Research Fellowship in Neuroscience
- University of Cincinnati College of Medicine Neuroscience Graduate Program - Research Innovation in Neuroscience Education for Underserved Populations
- University of Cincinnati College of Medicine, Department of Biomedical Informatics - Summer Undergraduate Research Fellowship in Biomedical Informatics
- University of Colorado Anschutz Medical Campus - Graduate Experience for Multicultural Students
- University of Colorado Boulder - Summer Multicultural Access to Research Training
- University of Colorado Boulder, Department of Chemical and Biological Engineering - Young Scholars Summer Research Program
- University of Colorado Cancer Center - Cancer Research Experience for Undergraduates
- University of Colorado Gates Center for Regenerative Medicine - Gates Summer Internship Program
- University of Connecticut Richard D. Berlin Center for Cell Analysis and Modeling - Summer Undergraduate Research Internships in Cell Analysis and Modeling
- University of Connecticut School of Medicine and School of Dental Medicine - Health Disparities Clinical Summer Research Fellowship Program
- University of Connecticut School of Medicine and School of Dental Medicine - Summer Research Fellowship Program Aetna Health Professions Partnership Initiative

- University of Connecticut The Graduate School - Undergraduate Summer Research Internship Program in Biological and Biomedical Sciences
- University of Connecticut, Department of Physiology and Neurobiology - Research Experience for Undergraduates Program
- University of Florida - Summer Undergraduate Research at Florida
- University of Florida College of Medicine, Department of Neuroscience - Summer Neuroscience Internship Program
- University of Florida College of Medicine, Department of Pharmacology and Therapeutics - Summer Undergraduate Research Fellowship Program
- University of Florida Whitney Laboratory for Marine Biosciences - The Whitney Laboratory Research Experience for Undergraduate Program
- University of Georgia - Nanotechnology and Biomedicine REU Site @ UGA
- University of Georgia - Population Biology of Infectious Diseases REU Site @ UGA
- University of Georgia - Summer Undergraduate Research Experience in Neuroscience
- University of Hawai'i Cancer Center - Cancer Research Education, Advancement, Training and Empowerment Program For Undergraduate Sophomores and Juniors
- University of Illinois Chicago College of Pharmacy - Summer Undergraduate Research Fellowship Program
- University of Illinois Urbana-Champaign The Grainger College of Engineering, Department of Bioengineering - Research Experiences for Undergraduates Program
- University of Iowa Carver College of Medicine - Summer Undergraduate MSTP Research Program
- University of Iowa Carver College of Medicine, Department of Biochemistry and Molecular Biology - Biochemistry Summer Undergraduate Research Fellowship
- University of Iowa Carver College of Medicine, Department of Microbiology and Immunology - Summer Research Experience for Undergraduates in Microbiology
- University of Iowa College of Public Health, Department of Biostatistics - Iowa Summer Institute in Biostatistics

- University of Iowa College of Public Health, Department of Global Public Health - Minority Health and Health Disparities International Research Training Program
- University of Iowa Graduate College - Biomedical Scholars Summer Undergraduate Research Program
- University of Iowa Graduate College - Summer Research Opportunities Program
- University of Iowa The Nanoscience and Nanotechnology Institute - Nano Research Experience for Undergraduates Program
- University of Kansas Medical Center, Department of Pharmacology, Toxicology and Therapeutics - Summer Undergraduate Research Fellowship Program
- University of Kansas School of Pharmacy, Department of Pharmaceutical Chemistry - Summer Undergraduate Research Program
- University of Kansas, Department of Molecular Biosciences - Research Experiences for Undergraduates Program
- University of Kentucky College of Engineering - Summer Research Experiences for Undergraduates
- University of Kentucky College of Medicine, Department of Molecular and Cellular Biochemistry - Summer Program in Biochemical Sciences
- University of Kentucky College of Medicine, Department of Pharmacology and Nutritional Sciences - Summer Undergraduate Research Fellowship
- University of Lausanne School of Life Sciences - Summer Research Program for Undergraduate Life Science Students
- University of Louisville School of Medicine, Department of Physiology - Undergraduate Summer Program in Cardiovascular Research for those from Under-Represented or Under-Served Populations
- University of Louisville, Kentucky Biomedical Research Infrastructure Network - Undergraduate Summer Biomedical Research Program
- University of Maine College of Natural Sciences, Forestry, and Agriculture - Research Experience for Undergraduates Accelerating New Environmental Workskills
- University of Maryland Marlene and Stewart Greenebaum Comprehensive Cancer Center - Nathan Schnaper Intern Program in Translational Cancer Research
- University of Massachusetts Medical School Graduate School of Biomedical Sciences - Summer Undergraduate Research Program

- University of Miami Miller School of Medicine - Summer Undergraduate Research Fellowship Program
- University of Michigan - Michigan Health Sciences Undergraduate Research Academy
- University of Michigan - Summer Undergraduate Research Experience in Physics at the University of Michigan
- University of Michigan - Undergraduate Research Opportunity Program
- University of Michigan College of Literature, Science, and the Arts - Summer Undergraduate Research Experience in Biophysics at the University of Michigan
- University of Michigan College of Literature, Science, and the Arts - Chemistry Research Experiences for Undergraduates Program
- University of Michigan College of Pharmacy - Research Experiences for Undergraduates Program in the Structure and Function of Proteins
- University of Michigan Frankel Cardiovascular Center - The Frankel CVC Summer Undergraduate Research Fellowship Program
- University of Michigan Life Sciences Institute - Perrigo Undergraduate Summer Fellowship
- University of Michigan Medical School - UM-SMART Undergrad Summer Program
- University of Michigan Medical School Neuroscience Graduate Program - Neuroscience Undergraduate Research Opportunity Program
- University of Michigan Medical School Neuroscience Graduate Program - Summer Intensive Research Experiences in Neuroscience
- University of Michigan Medical School, Department of Cancer Biology - Cancer Research Summer Internship Program
- University of Michigan Medical School, Department of Molecular and Integrative Physiology - Summer Undergraduate Research Fellowship Program
- University of Michigan Medical School, Department of Molecular and Integrative Physiology - Short Term Educational Program toward Digestive and Metabolic Physiology
- University of Michigan Medical School, Department of Molecular and Integrative Physiology - Summer Undergraduate Research in Physiology Summer Fellowship Program
- University of Michigan Medical School, Department of Pharmacology - Department of Pharmacology Summer Research Programs

- University of Michigan Medical School, Department of Pharmacology - ASPET Institutional Summer Undergraduate Research Fellowship
- University of Michigan Medical School, Department of Pharmacology - Charles Ross Summer Fellowship for Underrepresented Students
- University of Michigan Medical School, Kresge Hearing Research Institute - Summer Program for the Deaf and Hard-of-Hearing
- University of Michigan Rackham Graduate School - Summer Research Opportunity Program
- University of Michigan School of Public Health - Big Data Summer Institute
- University of Michigan School of Public Health - Future Public Health Leaders Program
- University of Michigan School of Public Health - Summer Enrichment Program
- University of Minnesota Lillehei Heart Institute - Summer Research Scholars Program
- University of Minnesota Medical School - Life Sciences Summer Undergraduate Research Program
- University of Minnesota School of Public Health - Summer Institute in Biostatistics
- University of Mississippi Medical Center School of Graduate Studies in Health Sciences - Summer Undergraduate Research Experience
- University of Mississippi The Center of Research Excellence in Natural Products Neuroscience - Summer Undergraduate Research Program
- University of Missouri College of Engineering - Summer Research Experiences for Undergraduates in Neuroscience
- University of Missouri School of Medicine - Summer Research Internship in Medical Sciences
- University of Missouri, Department of Psychological Sciences - MU Alcohol Research Training Summer School and Internship Program
- University of Montana The College of Health Professions and Biomedical Sciences, Department of Biomedical and Pharmaceutical Sciences - Center for Environmental Health Sciences Summer Undergraduate Research Program
- University of Montana, Department of Chemistry and Biochemistry - REU Summer Research Program
- University of Nebraska College of Medicine - MD-Ph.D. Summer Undergraduate Research Program

- University of Nebraska College of Medicine, Department of Pathology and Microbiology - Summer Undergraduate Research Program
- University of Nebraska Lincoln - Minority Health Disparities Initiative Research Experience for Undergraduates
- University of Nebraska Lincoln - REU Redox Biology
- University of Nebraska Lincoln - Undergraduate Research Opportunities in Biomedical Engineering Devices
- University of Nebraska Medical Center - Summer Undergraduate Research Program
- University of Nebraska Medical Center Eppley Institute for Research in Cancer and Allied Diseases - Summer Undergraduate Research Program
- University of Nebraska Medical Center Eppley Institute for Research in Cancer and Allied Diseases - Paid Internship Opportunities for Native American Undergraduates
- University of New Mexico School of Medicine - Undergraduate Pipeline Network Summer Research Program
- University of North Carolina at Chapel Hill - Science Enrichment Preparation Program
- University of North Carolina at Chapel Hill School of Medicine - Summer of Learning and Research
- University of North Carolina at Chapel Hill School of Medicine - Summer Research Experience for Undergraduates in Biological Mechanisms at UNC-Chapel Hill
- University of North Carolina at Chapel Hill School of Medicine - Medical Education Development Program
- University of North Carolina at Chapel Hill School of Medicine, Department of Pharmacology - Carolina Summer Fellowship Program
- University of Notre Dame, Department of Biological Sciences - Research Experiences for Undergraduates
- University of Notre Dame, Department of Chemistry and Biochemistry - International Research Experiences for Students
- University of Oklahoma Health Sciences Center Graduate College - Summer Undergraduate Research Experience
- University of Oklahoma Stephenson Cancer Center - Cancer Undergraduate Research Experience
- University of Oregon - UO R25 Summer Research Program

- University of Oregon - UO Research Experiences for Undergraduates Summer Program in Molecular Biosciences
- University of Pennsylvania Biomedical Graduate Sciences - Summer Undergraduate Internship Program
- University of Pennsylvania Perelman School of Medicine - Summer Undergraduate Research Program for Educating Radiation Scientists
- University of Pennsylvania Perelman School of Medicine - Undergraduate Clinical Scholars Program
- University of Pennsylvania Perelman School of Medicine Center for Molecular Studies in Digestive and Liver Diseases, Department of Medicine - Undergraduate Student Scholars Program
- University of Pittsburgh Center for Neuroscience - Summer Undergraduate Research Program
- University of Pittsburgh Human Engineering Research Laboratories - American Student Placements in Rehabilitation Engineering Research Experience for Undergraduates
- University of Pittsburgh School of Medicine - Summer Premedical Academic Enrichment Program
- University of Pittsburgh School of Medicine Graduate Studies - Summer Undergraduate Research Program
- University of Pittsburgh Vascular Medicine Institute - Pittsburgh Undergraduate Research Diversity Program
- University of Pittsburgh, Department of Computational and Systems Biology - Training and Experimentation in Computational Biology REU
- University of Puerto Rico-Río Piedras - Puerto Rico-Chemical Learning Integrated in Materials and Biomolecular Applications
- University of Rochester Center for Visual Science - Summer Fellowship Program
- University of Rochester Medical Center Golisano Children's Hospital, Department of Pediatrics - Strong Children's Research Center Summer Program
- University of Rochester Medical Center Schmitt Program on Integrative Neuroscience - Undergraduate Summer Research Fellowships
- University of Rochester Medical Center The Center for Advocacy, Community Health, Education and Diversity - Summer Undergraduate Research Fellowship
- University of Rochester School of Medicine and Dentistry - Summer Scholars Program

- University of Rochester School of Medicine and Dentistry - Summer Undergraduate Research Fellowship
- University of South Carolina Center for Colon Cancer Research - Summer Undergraduate Minority Research Program
- University of South Florida, Department of Molecular Pharmacology and Physiology - Summer Undergraduate Research Program
- University of Southern California Dana and David Dornsife College of Letters, Arts and Sciences - Latino Mental Health Research Training Program
- University of Tennessee Health Science Center - Tennessee Institute for Pre-Professionals Pre-Health Internship Program
- University of Tennessee Health Science Center - Tennessee Institute for Pre-Professionals Pre-Health Internship Program PLUS
- University of Texas at Austin Cockrell School of Engineering - Biomedical Engineering CUReS Cancer Scholars
- University of Texas at Austin Dell Medical School - Summer Undergraduate Research Fellowship
- University of Texas at Del Paso - Summer Mentoring and Research Training: Methods in Neuroscience of Drug-abuse Program
- University of Texas Health Science Center at Houston McGovern Medical School - GradSURP
- University of Texas Health Science Center at Houston McGovern Medical School - Micro-SURP
- University of Texas Health Science Center at San Antonio Long School of Medicine, Department of Pharmacology - Summer Undergraduate Research Fellowship
- University of Texas Health Science Center at San Antonio Long School of Medicine, Department of Cellular and Integrative Physiology - Summer Physiology Undergraduate Researcher Program
- University of Texas Medical Branch Graduate School of Biomedical Sciences - Neuroscience Summer Undergraduate Research Program
- University of Texas Southwestern Graduate School of Biomedical Sciences - Quantitative and Physical Sciences Summer Undergraduate Research Fellowship
- University of Texas Southwestern Graduate School of Biomedical Sciences - Summer Undergraduate Research Fellowship Stem Cell
- University of Texas Southwestern Graduate School of Biomedical Sciences - Summer Undergraduate Research Fellowship

- University of Texas Southwestern Graduate School of Biomedical Sciences - Summer Undergraduate Research Institute for the Study of Kidney Disease
- University of Texas, MD Anderson Cancer Center - Cancer Prevention Research Training Program Summer Research Experience
- University of Texas, MD Anderson Cancer Center - CPRIT-CURE Summer Undergraduate Program
- University of Texas, MD Anderson Cancer Center - Summer Imaging Research Program
- University of Texas, MD Anderson Cancer Center - Summer Undergraduate Research Program
- University of Texas, MD Anderson Cancer Center - U54 Partnership for Excellence in Cancer Research Summer Training Program
- University of Texas, MD Anderson Cancer Center - University Outreach Summer Program
- University of Texas, MD Anderson Cancer Center, Department of Translational Molecular Pathology - Interdisciplinary Translational Education and Research Training Undergraduate Summer Research Training
- University of Utah - Huntsman Cancer Institute Pathmaker Summer Research Program
- University of Utah - Summer Program for Undergraduate Research
- University of Utah School of Medicine, Department of Pediatrics - Genomics Summer Research for Minorities Internship
- University of Utah School of Medicine, Department of Pediatrics - Native American Summer Research Internship
- University of Virginia Center for Global Health Equity - Minority Health International Research Training Orientation
- University of Virginia School of Medicine - Summer Research Internship Program
- University of Virginia School of Medicine, Department of Surgery - Summer Diabetes Research Internship
- University of Washington - Center for Neurotechnology Research Experience for Undergraduates
- University of Washington Center for Neurotechnology - Research Experience for Undergraduates
- University of Washington Environmental and Occupational Health Sciences - Supporting Undergraduate Research Experiences in Environmental Health

- University of Washington Harborview Injury Prevention and Research Center - Pediatric Injury Prevention Student Internship Training Program
- University of Washington Medicine, Department of Neurological Surgery - Neurological Surgery Summer Student Program
- University of Washington School of Pharmacy, Department of Medicinal Chemistry - Pharmacology Science Summer Diversity Program
- University of Washington, Department of Genome Sciences - UW Genome Sciences Summer REU
- University of Wisconsin Madison - REU: Integrated Biological Sciences Summer Research Program
- University of Wisconsin Madison Biostatistics and Medical Informatics - Undergraduate Summer Program in Biomedical Data Science
- University of Wisconsin Madison Graduate School - Summer Research Program Opportunity
- University of Wisconsin Madison Neurosciences Training Program - Integrated Biological Sciences Summer Research Program
- University of Wisconsin Madison, Department of Molecular and Environmental Toxicology - Summer Research Opportunities Program
- University of Wisconsin Madison, Department of Psychology - REU: Psychology Research Experience Program
- Van Andel Institute Graduate School - Summer Internship Program
- Vanderbilt School of Medicine, Vanderbilt Summer Science Academy - The BP-ENDURE Program
- Vanderbilt School of Medicine, Vanderbilt Summer Science Academy - MSTP Summer Research Program
- Vanderbilt School of Medicine, Vanderbilt Summer Science Academy - Summer Enrichment Research Program in Education and Neuroscience Training
- Vanderbilt School of Medicine, Vanderbilt Summer Science Academy - Undergraduate Clinical Research Internship Program
- Vanderbilt School of Medicine, Vanderbilt Summer Science Academy - Aspirnaut Undergraduate Discovery Science Experience in Renal Biology and Disease
- Vanderbilt School of Medicine, Vanderbilt Summer Science Academy - The Molecular and Cellular Biology Summer Program
- Vanderbilt School of Medicine, Vanderbilt Summer Science Academy - Vanderbilt Summer Diabetes Research Program

- Vanderbilt School of Medicine, Vanderbilt Summer Science Academy - Vanderbilt Minority Summer Research Program
- Vanderbilt School of Medicine, Vanderbilt Summer Science Academy - Department of Biomedical Informatics Summer Research Internship Program
- Vanderbilt School of Medicine, Vanderbilt Summer Science Academy - Vascular Biology-Short Term Training Program for Minority Students
- Vanderbilt School of Medicine, Vanderbilt Summer Science Academy - Vanderbilt-Ingram Cancer Center: Discover Cancer Research Program
- Vanderbilt School of Medicine, Vanderbilt Summer Science Academy - VI4 Germs, Defenses, & Diseases Undergraduate Research Program
- Vanderbilt School of Medicine, Vanderbilt Summer Science Academy - Vanderbilt Vaccine Center
- Vanderbilt University College of Arts and Sciences - Research Experience for Undergraduates in Chemical Biology
- Virginia Commonwealth University Division for Health Sciences Diversity - Summer Academic Enrichment Program
- Virginia Commonwealth University Philips Institute for Oral Health Research - Summer Research Program
- Wadsworth Center, Department of Health - Research Experience for Undergraduates
- Wake Forest School of Medicine Institute for Regenerative Medicine - WFIRM Summer Scholars Program in Regenerative Medicine
- Wake Forest School of Medicine, Department of Biomedical Engineering - Biomedical Engineering Summer Research Program
- Wake Forest School of Medicine, Department of Internal Medicine - Excellence in Cardiovascular Sciences Summer Research Program
- Washington State University Cahnrs Department of Horticulture - Research Experience for Undergraduates in Plan Genomics and Biotechnology
- Washington State University College of Veterinary Medicine - Summer Undergraduate Research Experience
- Washington State University The College of Pharmacy and Pharmaceutical Sciences - Summer Research Fellowship
- Washington State University The Gene and Linda Voiland School of Chemical Engineering and Bioengineering - REU Program
- Washington University in St. Louis - WUSTL ENDURE

- Washington University in St. Louis Institute for Public Health - Summer Research Program: Aging and Neurological Diseases Track
- Washington University in St. Louis Institute for Public Health - Summer Research Program: Public and Global Health Track
- Washington University in St. Louis Siteman Cancer Center - Leah Menshouse Springer Summer Opportunities Program
- Washington University in St. Louis Siteman Cancer Center - Siteman Cancer Center Diversity in Cancer Research Summer Program
- Washington University in St. Louis The Division of Biology and Biomedical Sciences - Biomedical Research Apprenticeship Program
- Washington University School of Medicine in St. Louis Institute of Clinical and Translational Sciences - Advanced Summer Program for Investigation and Research Education
- Washington University School of Medicine in St. Louis Mallinckrodt Institute of Radiology - Summer Research Program at the Mallinckrodt Institute of Radiology
- Washington University School of Medicine in St. Louis McDonnell Genome Institute - Opportunities in Genomics Research Undergraduate Scholars Program
- Wayne State University School of Medicine Cancer Biology Graduate Program - Undergraduate Summer Research Fellowships
- Wayne State University School of Medicine Center for Molecular Medicine and Genetics - Summer Undergraduate Research Program
- Wayne State University School of Medicine Office of Biomedical Graduate Programs - Summer Undergraduate Research Experience
- Wayne State University School of Medicine, Department of Physiology - Summer Undergraduate Research Fellowship
- Weill Cornell Medicine Graduate School of Medical Sciences - Advancing Cornell Career Experiences for Science Students Summer Internship Program
- Weill Cornell Medicine Graduate School of Medical Sciences - Advancing Cornell Career Experiences for Science Students
- Weill Cornell Medicine Medical College - Travelers Summer Research Fellowship Program
- Weill Cornell Medicine Tri-Institutional MD-Ph.D. Program - Gateways to the Laboratory Summer Program
- West Virginia University Cancer Institute - Summer Undergraduate Cancer Research Program

- West Virginia University School of Medicine, Department of Neuroscience - Summer Undergraduate Research Internships
- Yale School of Medicine, Department of Internal Medicine - Yale Summer Undergraduate Medical Research
- Yale University - Program in Physics, Engineering, and Biology

Appendix D
Out-of-State Applicant vs. In-State Applicant Friendliness Table (*Accepted, 2022*)

School	State	Overall Acceptance Rate	In-State Acceptance Rate	Out-of-State Acceptance Rate	Ratio of In-State vs. Out-of-State Acceptance Rate	**In-State Advantage**
Albert Einstein College of Medicine	NY	3.3%	7.2%	2.3%	3.13	Material
Augusta University	GA	10.9%	23.2%	0.9%	27.19	**Huge**
Baylor College of Medicine	TX	4.3%	11.0%	1.5%	7.52	**Huge**
Boston University	MA	4.5%	5.5%	4.4%	1.25	Negligible
Brown University (Alpert)	RI	2.6%	16.7%	2.4%	6.87	**Huge**
California University of Science and Medicine	CA	3.8%	6.1%	0.2%	37.31	**Huge**
Case Western Reserve University	OH	5.9%	8.8%	5.6%	1.58	Modest
Columbia University	NY	3.6%	3.7%	3.6%	1.01	None
Cooper Medical School of Rowan University	NJ	3.9%	10.3%	1.9%	5.45	**Huge**
Cornell University (Weill)	NY	3.4%	3.6%	3.3%	1.1	None
Dartmouth College (Geisel)	NH	2.4%	9.7%	2.3%	4.14	**Huge**
Drexel University	PA	6.1%	21.2%	4.8%	4.44	**Huge**
Duke University	NC	2.9%	4.8%	2.7%	1.77	Modest

East Tennessee State U. (Quillen)	TN	4.7%	14.5%	1.3%	10.81	**Huge**
Eastern Virginia Medical School	VA	3.4%	11.0%	2.2%	5.11	**Huge**
Edward Via College of Osteopathic Medicine	VA	13.2%	29.9%	10.8%	2.78	Material
Emory University	GA	2.9%	6.3%	2.6%	2.38	Material
Florida Atlantic University (Schmidt)	FL	2.5%	3.9%	1.3%	2.94	Material
Florida International University (Wertheim)	FL	4.3%	7.6%	2.0%	3.8	Material
Florida State University	FL	4.0%	6.9%	0.2%	30.02	**Huge**
Georgetown University	DC	2.4%	8.8%	2.4%	3.69	Material
Hackensack Meridian School of Medicine	NJ	5.8%	14.0%	3.6%	3.89	Material
Harvard University	MA	2.8%	3.2%	2.7%	1.18	None
Hofstra University	NY	6.5%	10.0%	5.0%	1.98	Modest
Howard University	DC	2.9%	18.0%	2.8%	6.46	**Huge**
Icahn School of Medicine at Mount Sinai	NY	3.4%	4.6%	3.1%	1.47	Negligible
Indiana University – Indianapolis	IN	8.0%	44.4%	2.9%	15.08	**Huge**
Johns Hopkins University	MD	5.1%	5.3%	5.1%	1.03	None
Kaiser Permanente	CA	1.1%	1.2%	1.0%	1.16	None
Lake Erie College of Osteopathic University	PA	5.2%	11.7%	4.2%	2.74	Material

Lincoln Memorial University (DeBusk)	TN	17.6%	62.2%	14.3%	4.36	**Huge**
Marian U. College of Osteopathic Medicine	IN	5.5%	28.6%	3.6%	7.88	**Huge**
Marshall University (Edwards)	WV	5.5%	51.8%	1.2%	43.97	**Huge**
Mayo Clinic School of Medicine (Alix)	MN	4.0%	3.9%	4.0%	1	None
Medical University of South Carolina	SC	14.3%	33.7%	2.6%	12.93	**Huge**
Michigan State U. College of Osteopathic Medicine	MI	7.0%	25.9%	3.6%	7.22	**Huge**
New York Medical College	NY	3.5%	9.6%	2.2%	4.26	**Huge**
New York University (Grossman)	NY	2.1%	1.8%	2.2%	0.83	None
New York University – Long Island	NY	1.5%	3.0%	0.9%	3.28	Material
Northeast Ohio Medical University	OH	6.6%	16.9%	3.4%	5.01	**Huge**
Northwestern University (Feinberg)	IL	5.6%	5.1%	5.6%	0.9	None
Nova SE U. Patel College of Osteopathic Medicine	FL	13.1%	17.7%	11.6%	1.53	Modest
Nova Southeastern University	FL	4.9%	6.7%	3.7%	1.8	Modest
Ohio State University	OH	5.2%	14.2%	3.3%	4.31	**Huge**
Ohio University	OH	6.9%	35.1%	0.8%	44.77	**Huge**
Oklahoma State University	OK	5.5%	43.6%	0.8%	53.73	**Huge**

Oregon Health and Science University	OR	3.1%	20.4%	1.1%	19.09	**Huge**
Quinnipiac University	CT	3.1%	11.9%	2.7%	4.48	**Huge**
Rowan University College of Osteopathic Medicine	NJ	6.2%	21.4%	3.5%	6.08	**Huge**
Rush University	IL	3.8%	6.0%	3.4%	1.74	Modest
Rutgers New Jersey Medical School – Newark	NJ	5.4%	14.4%	2.0%	7.28	**Huge**
Rutgers Robert Wood Johnson Med School – N. Brunswick	NJ	4.8%	13.2%	1.8%	7.32	**Huge**
SUNY Upstate Medical University	NY	7.7%	12.9%	3.6%	3.57	Material
Saint Louis University	MO	6.1%	10.0%	5.8%	1.72	Modest
Stanford University	CA	1.4%	1.3%	1.4%	0.92	None
Stony Brook University – SUNY	NY	7.5%	11.9%	4.6%	2.59	Material
Temple University (Katz)	PA	4.5%	13.4%	3.4%	3.87	Material
Texas A&M University	TX	7.1%	7.5%	5.5%	1.35	Negligible
Texas Christian University	TX	1.4%	2.0%	1.3%	1.59	Modest
Texas Tech U. Health Sciences Center	TX	5.1%	5.5%	3.0%	1.83	Modest
Thomas Jefferson University (Kimmel)	PA	3.5%	8.2%	2.9%	2.78	Material
Touro University California	CA	6.7%	11.2%	3.5%	3.18	Material
Tufts University	MA	4.0%	7.9%	3.6%	2.18	Material

U. of Texas Health Science Center – Houston (McGovern)	TX	5.8%	7.1%	1.0%	7.42	**Huge**
U. of Texas Health Science Center – San Antonio	TX	6.4%	6.7%	4.9%	1.37	Negligible
U. of Texas Southwestern Medical Center	TX	6.0%	6.9%	3.2%	2.15	Material
University at Buffalo (SUNY) – Jacobs	NY	5.2%	10.0%	1.5%	6.71	**Huge**
University of Alabama – Birmingham	AL	5.0%	30.3%	1.9%	15.6	**Huge**
University of Arizona – Tucson	AZ	2.3%	15.0%	0.9%	17.39	**Huge**
University of Arkansas for Medical Sciences	AR	13.2%	50.8%	1.7%	29.71	**Huge**
University of California – Davis	CA	2.2%	3.5%	0.2%	15.92	**Huge**
University of California – Irvine	CA	3.0%	3.4%	2.0%	1.71	Modest
University of California – Los Angeles (Geffen)	CA	2.2%	2.6%	1.9%	1.35	Negligible
University of California – Riverside	CA	2.1%	2.7%	0.1%	42.73	**Huge**
University of California – San Diego	CA	3.0%	4.0%	1.7%	2.36	Material
University of California – San Francisco	CA	2.6%	3.7%	1.8%	2.08	Material
University of Central Florida	FL	5.4%	7.6%	3.6%	2.12	Material

University of Chicago (Pritzker) Medical	IL	3.2%	4.1%	3.1%	1.31	Negligible
University of Cincinnati	OH	6.2%	11.3%	4.8%	2.36	Material
University of Colorado	CO	3.6%	20.2%	2.5%	7.97	**Huge**
University of Connecticut	CT	4.8%	23.7%	2.0%	12.04	**Huge**
University of Florida	FL	4.3%	6.6%	1.6%	4.09	**Huge**
University of Hawaii – Manoa (Burns)	HI	5.5%	26.1%	1.5%	17.28	**Huge**
University of Illinois	IL	8.4%	18.8%	4.6%	4.05	**Huge**
University of Iowa (Carver)	IA	7.0%	36.0%	4.4%	8.23	**Huge**
University of Kansas Medical Center	KS	7.8%	36.2%	2.0%	17.79	**Huge**
University of Kentucky	KY	7.5%	35.4%	2.4%	14.77	**Huge**
University of Louisville	KY	5.9%	37.7%	2.4%	15.92	**Huge**
University of Maryland	MD	4.1%	15.5%	1.6%	10	**Huge**
University of Massachusetts – Worcester	MA	7.2%	17.1%	4.4%	3.93	Material
University of Miami (Miller)	FL	3.2%	5.8%	2.4%	2.43	Material
University of Michigan – Ann Arbor	MI	3.5%	6.4%	3.0%	2.1	Material
University of Minnesota	MN	5.1%	18.8%	2.1%	8.8	**Huge**
University of Missouri	MO	6.0%	21.3%	1.5%	14.02	**Huge**
University of Missouri – Kansas City	MO	12.0%	32.9%	6.4%	5.17	**Huge**

University of Nebraska Medical Center	NE	9.2%	39.9%	3.5%	11.44	**Huge**
University of Nevada – Reno	NV	7.3%	26.0%	1.4%	18.96	**Huge**
University of New England	ME	8.2%	31.8%	7.8%	4.1	**Huge**
University of New Mexico	NM	7.2%	42.6%	1.4%	29.37	**Huge**
University of North Carolina – Chapel Hill	NC	4.1%	17.0%	1.1%	14.91	**Huge**
University of North Texas Health Science Center	TX	8.4%	9.3%	4.1%	2.29	Material
University of Oklahoma	OK	7.6%	40.5%	1.2%	33.97	**Huge**
University of Pennsylvania (Perelman)	PA	3.8%	4.1%	3.8%	1.07	None
University of Pittsburgh	PA	3.5%	9.4%	2.7%	3.51	Material
University of Rochester	NY	5.8%	7.1%	5.5%	1.29	Negligible
University of South Carolina	SC	7.0%	30.0%	1.9%	15.39	**Huge**
University of South Florida	FL	6.3%	5.2%	7.2%	0.72	None
University of Southern California (Keck)	CA	4.0%	5.7%	2.2%	2.56	Material
University of Tennessee Health Science Center	TN	8.7%	26.4%	1.6%	16.47	**Huge**
University of Utah	UT	4.6%	17.1%	2.1%	8.23	**Huge**
University of Vermont	VA	4.4%	45.9%	3.9%	11.76	**Huge**
University of Virginia	VT	8.5%	14.3%	7.5%	1.9	Modest

University of Washington	WA	3.7%	18.1%	0.6%	30.35	**Huge**
University of Pikeville	KY	11.6%	36.9%	10.4%	3.56	Material
University of Toledo	OH	4.3%	15.4%	1.6%	9.91	**Huge**
University of Wisconsin – Madison	WI	6.3%	24.6%	3.4%	7.28	**Huge**
Vanderbilt University	TN	4.7%	8.3%	4.5%	1.82	Modest
Virginia Commonwealth University	VA	4.9%	13.8%	3.3%	4.22	**Huge**
Virginia Tech Carilion School of Medicine	VA	1.8%	2.9%	1.6%	1.79	Modest
Wake Forest University	NC	2.4%	7.4%	1.9%	3.93	Material
Washington University in St. Louis	MO	7.5%	8.8%	7.4%	1.18	None
Wayne State University	MI	6.6%	15.3%	4.6%	3.3	Material
West Virginia School of Osteopathic Medicine	WV	11.0%	49.3%	10.0%	4.94	**Huge**
West Virginia University	WV	3.3%	37.3%	1.8%	21.03	**Huge**
William Carey U. College of Osteopathic Medicine	MS	13.1%	24.0%	12.8%	1.88	Modest
Wright State University (Boonshoft)	OH	3.1%	15.6%	1.0%	16.17	**Huge**
Yale University	CT	4.8%	5.4%	4.7%	1.15	None

ABOUT THE AUTHOR

Caroline Echeandia-Francis is a member of the Yale School of Medicine Class of 2026. She also served as a student member of YSM's Admissions Committee. Upon graduation, she plans to pursue a career in dermatology while continuing to advise those applying to medical school.

Caroline completed her undergraduate education at Washington University in St. Louis (WashU) and worked for two years before attending medical school. She spent significant time at WashU conducting research into Alzheimer's disease through which she was a contributing author on multiple publications. She also served as a teaching assistant for two science courses, mentored first year students, helped organize and run orientation for incoming students, and volunteered with older adults at local memory care facilities. These formative experiences shaped her approach to medical school admissions and inspired her to share her insights by authoring this book.

Outside of medicine, Caroline remains involved in her community and enjoys pickleball, golf, Colorado Buffaloes football, and time with family and friends. She continues to mentor aspiring medical students through her writing as well as her medical school advisory services. You can learn more and reach Caroline at www.PrepMDadvising.com.

www.ingramcontent.com/pod-product-compliance
Lightning Source LLC
Chambersburg PA
CBHW050547160426
43199CB00015B/2563